Decision Making in
VITREORETINAL SURGERIES

Decision Making in VITREORETINAL SURGERIES

Editor-in-Chief

Sushma Ratna Jayanna
MBBS DNB (Ophth) FICO (UK) FLVPEI
Vitreoretina Consultant
Department of Vitreoretina and Pediatric Retina
Narayana Nethralaya
Bengaluru, Karnataka, India

Foreword

Lingam Gopal

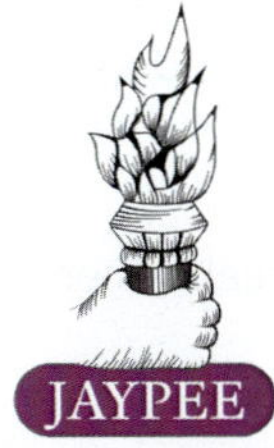

JAYPEE BROTHERS MEDICAL PUBLISHERS
The Health Sciences Publisher
New Delhi | London

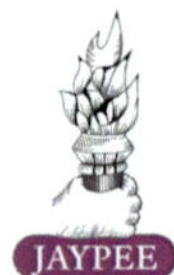

Jaypee Brothers Medical Publishers (P) Ltd

Headquarters
EMCA House, 23/23-B
Ansari Road, Daryaganj
New Delhi 110 002, India
Landline: +91-11-23272143, +91-11-23272703
+91-11-23282021, +91-11-23245672
e-mail: jaypee@jaypeebrothers.com

Corporate Office
4838/24, Ansari Road, Daryaganj
New Delhi 110 002, India
Phone: +91-11-43574357
Fax: +91-11-43574314
e-mail: jaypee@jaypeebrothers.com

Overseas Office
JP Medical Ltd.
83, Victoria Street, London
SW1H 0HW (UK)
Phone: +44-20 3170 8910
e-mail: info@jpmedpub.com

EU GPSR Authorised Representative
Logos Europe, 9 rue Nicolas Poussin
17000, La Rochelle, France
Phone: +33 (0) 6 67 93 73 78
e-mail: contact@logoseurope.eu

Website: www.jaypeebrothers.com
Website: www.jaypeedigital.com

Inquiries for bulk sales may be solicited at: jaypee@jaypeebrothers.com

Decision Making in Vitreoretinal Surgeries

First Edition: **2026**

ISBN: 978-93-7806-892-8

Printed at: Samrat Offset Pvt. Ltd.

प्रारूप आरजी - 2
Form RG - 2

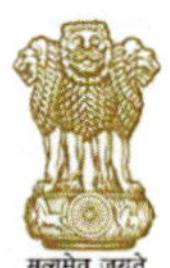

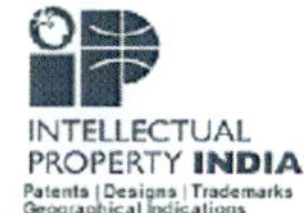

भारत सरकार
Government of India
व्यापार चिन्ह रजिस्ट्री
Trade Marks Registry

क्रमांक
No. 2442588

व्यापार चिन्ह अधिनियम, 1999

Trade Marks Act, 1999

व्यापार चिन्ह के रजिस्ट्रीकरण का प्रमाणपत्र, धारा 23 (2), नियम 56 (1)

Certificate of Registration of Trade Mark, Section 23 (2), Rule 56 (1)

व्यापार चिन्ह संख्या / **Trade Mark No.** 3436251 दिनांक /**Date** 19/12/2016 ज. संख्या /**J. No.** 1930

यह प्रमाणित किया जाता है कि जिस प्रकार चिन्ह की समाकृति इसके साथ संलग्न है, वह ....
के बारे में दिनांक ....नाम से रजिस्ट्रीकृत हो चुका है|
Certified that Trade Mark / a representation is annexed hereto, has been registered in the name(s) of :-
JAYPEE BROTHERS MEDICAL PUBLISHERS PRIVATE LIMITED, 4838/24, ANSARI ROAD, DARYAGANJ, NEW DELHI-110002, Body Incorporate, Service Provider, (Body Incorporate)

In Class 41 Under No. 3436251 as of the date 19 December 2016 in respect of

PUBLICATION SERVICES RELATING TO BOOKS, NOTE-BOOKS, MAGAZINES, BROCHURES, PAMPHLETS, MANULAS, PUBLICATION OF PRINTED MATTERS, ELECTRONIC PUBLICATON INCLUDED IN CLASS-41

JAYPEE BROTHERS MEDICAL PUBLISHERS

मेरे निर्देश पर आज .... के .... मास के .... वे दिन को इस पर मुद्रा लगायी गई

Sealed at my direction, this 07th day of August, 2020

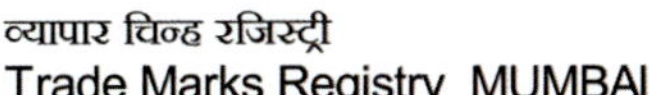
व्यापार चिन्ह रजिस्ट्री
Trade Marks Registry MUMBAI

व्यापार चिन्ह रजिस्ट्रार
Registrar of Trademarks

रजिस्ट्रीकरण आवेदन की तारीख से १० वर्ष के लिए है और तदोपरांत वह १० वर्ष की कालावधि के लिए और प्रत्येक १० वर्ष की कालावधि के अवसान पर भी नवीनीकृत किया जा सकेगा।

Registration is for 10 years from the date of application and may then be renewed for a period of 10 years and also at the expiration of each period of 10 years.

यह प्रमाणपत्र विधि कार्यवाहियों में प्रयोग के लिए या विदेश में रजिस्ट्रीकरण अभिप्राप्त करने के लिए नहीं है

This certificate is not for use in legal proceedings or for obtaining Registration abroad.

टिप्पणी - इस व्यापार चिन्ह के स्वामित्व में कोई परिवर्तन होने पर, या कारोवार के मुख्य स्थान के पते में या भारत में तामील के लिए पते में परिवर्तन होने पर परिवर्तन के लिए आवेदन तुरंत किया जाना चाहिए.

Note: Upon any change of ownership of this Trademark, or change in address, of the principal place of business or address for service in India a request should **AT ONCE** be made to register the change.

INTELLECTUAL PROPERTY **INDIA**
PATENTS | DESIGNS | TRADE MARKS
GEOGRAPHICAL INDICATIONS

सत्यमेव जयते

प्रारूप आरजी - 2
Form RG - 2
क्रमांक No. 3772319

व्यापार चिन्ह रजिस्ट्री, भारत सरकार Trade Marks Registry, Government Of India
व्यापार चिन्ह अधिनियम, 1999 Trade Marks Act, 1999
व्यापार चिन्ह के रजिस्ट्रीकरण का प्रमाणपत्र | Certificate of Registration of Trade Mark
(धारा 23 (2), नियम 56 (1)) | Section 23 (2), Rule 56 (1)

व्यापार चिन्ह संख्या / Trade Mark No. : 5191318
दिनांक / Date : 28-10-2021
ज. संख्या / J. No. : 2158

प्रमाणित किया जाता है कि व्यापार चिन्ह / जिसका प्रतिरूप इसके साथ संलग्न है, वह .... के नाम से .... वर्ग में .... संख्या के अधीन दिनांक .... को .... के संबंध में रजिस्ट्रीकृत किया गया है|

Certified that Trade Mark / a representation is annexed hereto, has been registered in the name(s) of :- JAYPEE BROTHERS MEDICAL PUBLISHERS PRIVATE LIMITED, 4838/24, ANSARI ROAD, DARYAGANJ, NEW DELHI-110002., Body Incorporate, (Body Incorporate)

In Class 41 Under No. 5191318 as of the date 28 October 2021 in respect of

Publication Services , Electronic Publication , Issue of Publications, Publication of Books and Textbooks, Publication of Booklets, Publication of Brochures, Publication of Journals, included Under Class-41.

Trade Mark as annexed

आज वर्ष 20........................ के .... माह के .... वें दिन को मेरे निर्देश पर मुद्रांकित किया गया

Sealed at my direction, this 19th day of October , 2024

उन्नत पी पंडित

व्यापार चिन्ह रजिस्ट्री मुंबई
Trade Marks Registry MUMBAI

व्यापार चिन्ह रजिस्ट्रार
Registrar of Trademarks

रजिस्ट्रीकरण आवेदन की तारीख से १० वर्ष के लिए है और तदोपरांत वह १० वर्ष की अवधि के लिए और प्रत्येक १० वर्ष की अवधि की समाप्ति पर भी नवीनीकृत किया जा सकेगा।
यह प्रमाणपत्र विधि कार्यवाहियों में प्रयोग के लिए या विदेश में रजिस्ट्रीकरण प्राप्त करने के लिए नहीं है
टिप्पणी : इस व्यापार चिन्ह के स्वामित्व में कोई परिवर्तन होने पर, या कारोबार के मुख्य स्थान के पते में या भारत में सेवा के लिए पते में परिवर्तन होने पर परिवर्तन को दर्ज करने के लिए एक बार अनुरोध किया जाना चाहिए.
Registration is for 10 years from the date of application and may then be renewed for a period of 10 years and also at the expiration of each period of 10 years.
This certificate is not for use in legal proceedings or for obtaining Registration abroad.
Note: Upon any change of ownership of this Trademark, or change in address, of the principal place of business or address for service in India a request should AT ONCE be made to register the change.

व्यापार चिन्ह के लिए अनुलग्नक / Annexure of Trade Mark Certificate

क्रमांक / No. **3772319**

व्यापार चिन्ह संख्या / Trade Mark No. **5191318**

दिनांक / Date **28-10-2021**

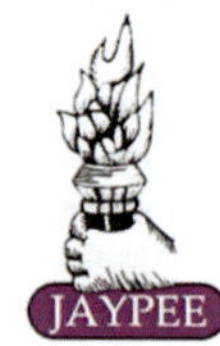

Dedicated to

The exceptional art and artists of
vitreoretinal surgeries across the globe.

Contributors

Amer F Alsouldi MD
Vitreoretina Fellow
Associated Retinal Consultants
Royal Oak, Michigan, USA

Antonio Capone Jr MD
Professor
Associated Retinal Consultants/
Oakland University William
Beaumont School of Medicine
Royal Oak, Michigan, USA

Arkaprava Pradhan DNB FICO MRCS (Ed)
Associate Consultant
Shri Bhagwan Mahavir
Department of Vitreoretinal
Services
Sankara Nethralaya
Chennai, Tamil Nadu, India

Atul Arora MS MCH
Consultant (Ophthalmology)
Department of Telemedicine
Postgraduate Institute of Medical
Education and Research
Chandigarh, India

Ayushi Mohapatra MBBS DNB FMRF
Assistant Consultant
Vitreoretina Services
Shri Bhagwan Mahavir
Department of Vitreoretinal
Services
Sankara Nethralaya
Chennai, Tamil Nadu, India

Chaitanya YVK MS
Senior Resident
Advanced Eye Centre
Department of Ophthalmology
Postgraduate Institute of Medical
Education and Research
Chandigarh, India

Chaitra Jaydev DOMS PhD
Senior Consultant
Department of Vitreoretinal Services
Narayana Nethralaya
Bengaluru, Karnataka, India

CK Nagesha MS FMRY
Consultant
Department of Vitreoretinal Services
Narayana Nethralaya
Bengaluru, Karnataka, India

Deeksha Katoch MS
Additional Professor
Advanced Eye Centre
Department of Ophthalmology
Postgraduate Institute of Medical
Education and Research
Chandigarh, India

Divya Balakrishnan FRCS FNB
Senior Consultant
Department of Vitreoretinal Diseases
Little Flower Hospital
Ernakulam, Kerala, India

Gaurav Malwe MS
Senior Vitreoretina Fellow
Department of Vitreoretina
Narayana Nethralaya
Bengaluru, Karnataka, India

Jay Chhablani MD
Professor
Department of Ophthalmology
UPMC Vision Institute
University of Pittsburgh
Pittsburgh, PA, USA

Lisa J Faia MD
Associate Professor
Associated Retinal Consultants/
Oakland University William
Beaumont School of Medicine
Royal Oak, Michigan, USA

Manoj Shettigar MS
Consultant
Department of Vitreoretinal Services
Anant Bajaj Retina Institute
LV Prasad Eye Institute
YSR Kadapa, Andhra Pradesh, India

Matthew GJ Trese DO MA
Assistant Professor
Associated Retinal Consultants/
Oakland University William Beaumont
School of Medicine
Royal Oak, Michigan, USA

Meenakshi Mahesh DNB FVRS FAICO
Consultant
Department of Vitreoretinal
Services and Ocular Oncology
Sankara Eye Hospital
Bengaluru, Karnataka, India

Muna Bhende MS FMRF
Senior Consultant and Director
Shri Bhagwan Mahavir
Department of Vitreoretinal
Services
Sankara Nethralaya
Chennai, Tamil Nadu, India

Naresh Kumar Yadav DOMS FRCS
Senior Consultant
Department of Vitreoretinal
Services
Narayana Nethralaya
Bengaluru, Karnataka, India

P Mahesh Shanmugam
DO FRCSED PhD
Head
Department of Vitreoretinal
Services and Ocular Oncology
Sankara Eye Hospital
Bengaluru, Karnataka, India

Padmaja Kumari Rani
MS FRCS FICO FNB
Senior Consultant and Network Associate Director
Department of Teleophthalmology
Anant Bajaj Retina Institute
LV Prasad Eye Institute
Hyderabad, Telangana, India

Pradeep Susvar FRCS
Senior Consultant and Professor
Shri Bhagwan Mahavir
Department of Vitreoretinal Services
Medical Research Foundation
Sankara Nethralaya
Chennai, Tamil Nadu, India

Pramod S Bhende MS
Senior Consultant
Shri Bhagwan Mahavir
Department of Vitreoretinal Services
Medical Research Foundation
Sankara Nethralaya
Chennai, Tamil Nadu, India

Priya BV MS
Head
Department of Vitreoretinal Services
Narayana Nethralaya
Bengaluru, Karnataka, India

Saloni Kapoor MD
Vitreoretina Fellow
Department of Ophthalmology and Visual Sciences
University of Iowa
Iowa City, IA, USA

Saumya Johri MS
Vitreoretina Fellow
Department of Vitreoretina
Narayana Nethralaya
Bengaluru, Karnataka, India

Shreeya Jain MS
Vitreoretinal Fellow
Department of Vitreoretina
Anant Bajaj Retina Institute
LV Prasad Eye Institute
Hyderabad, Telangana, India

Simakurthy Sriram MD
Consultant
Department of Vitreoretinal Services
Sankara Eye Hospital
Hyderabad, Telangana, India

Subhadra Jalali MS
Senior Consultant and Network Director (Quality)
Newborn Eye Health Alliance (NEHA)
Anant Bajaj Retina Institute
LV Prasad Eye Institute
Hyderabad, Telangana, India

Subhashchandra Doralli
DOMS DNB (Ophth)
Senior Consultant
Department of Vitreoretinal Services
Narayana Nethralaya
Bengaluru, Karnataka, India

Sushma Ratna Jayanna
MBBS DNB (Ophth) FICO (UK) FLVPEI
Vitreoretina Consultant
Department of Vitreoretina and Pediatric Retina
Narayana Nethralaya
Bengaluru, Karnataka, India

Taraprasad Das MS
Distinguished Ophthalmologist
Vice-Chair Emeritus
LV Prasad Eye Institute
Hyderabad, Telangana, India

Virangi Doshi DNB FVRS
Consultant
Department of Vitreoretinal Services
RJ Sankara Eye Hospital
Navi Mumbai, Maharashtra, India

Vishali Gupta MS
Professor
Department of Ophthalmology
Postgraduate Institute of Medical Education and Research
Chandigarh, India

Vivek Dave MS DNB FLVPEI
Senior Consultant and Network Head
Anant Bajaj Retina Institute
LV Prasad Eye Institute
Hyderabad, Telangana, India

Foreword

It is indeed my pleasant task to write this foreword to this excellent book on *Decision Making in Vitreoretinal Surgeries*.

In this era of information overload, there are several avenues to update oneself in the field of vitreoretinal (VR) surgery. Standard textbooks give us an overview of the subject while individual articles in journals focus on cases, techniques or complications. Most VR surgeons (especially the novice surgeons) would have felt many a time a difficulty in decision making—to operate or not; to reoperate or not; what is the best technique to adopt in a given situation, etc. Unfortunately, there is no one source of information that can serve as a quick reference to guide the surgeon. Sushma Ratna Jayanna and her colleagues have addressed this unmet need by way of publishing this book aptly titled *Decision Making in Vitreoretinal Surgeries*.

This multiauthor book covers the most common indications for vitreoretinal surgery. Some very experienced vitreoretinal surgeons were selected to do the difficult task of distilling all the information available and presenting it in an easy-to-understand format. The central piece of each chapter is the well-structured algorithm that reduces complex issues surrounding an indication for surgery into relatively nonoverlapping compartments. One understands that medicine is a gray area with considerable overlap in features. However, the first step in any decision-making process is to draw some artificial boundaries that enable us to decide whether to operate or not and what technique to adopt in a given case. In addition to the algorithm, the authors provide common clinical scenarios to illustrate the dilemmas one faces in clinical decision making and key points as take-home messages.

There is no pretense to do an in-depth review of literature nor was the book meant to address all variations in clinical presentation that one comes across.

Overall, the book provides a quick reference for the busy practitioner as well as novice surgeon in the surgical management of vitreoretinal disorders. The editor and the authors must be congratulated in bringing out this much needed ready reckoner for surgical vitreoretinal practice.

Lingam Gopal
MS DNBE MSc (Epidemiology)
Senior Consultant
Sankara Nethralaya
Medical Research Foundation
Chennai, Tamil Nadu, India

Preface

For a surgeon, knowing when to operate is as crucial as knowing how to operate. The technical skills of vitreoretinal surgery can be mastered within a few years, but the wisdom to decide when and when not to intervene is something we pursue throughout our professional lives. It is in this space between skill and judgment that the true art of surgery resides, where the mind, heart, and hand must work in an extraordinary synchrony, which no artificial intelligence can replicate.

When M/s Jaypee Brothers Medical Publishers (P) Ltd, New Delhi, India proposed the idea of a book on *Decision Making in Vitreoretinal Surgeries*, I immediately felt the connect and the importance of such project. The concept resonated deeply, as the ability to decide the right moment and the right approach often determines success more than the act of surgery itself. To me, this book was also an opportunity to bring together some of the most distinguished retinal surgeons across the world who have turned their collective wisdom of decision making into an exceptional form of art. This book elaborates not just on how the surgeries are performed, but why certain decisions shape their outcomes. Each chapter in this book begins with algorithms that outline the general approach followed by real-world case scenarios, where surgeon's thought process behind every crucial step is mirrored in the form of detailed flowcharts.

I hope this book serves as a valuable guide for retinal surgeons at every stage of their careers from those just beginning their journey to those with years of experience behind them. As this book holds not only the practical strategies but also the collected wisdom of countless hours in the operating room. May it inspire thoughtful judgment, precise execution, and above all, the confidence to make decisions that truly define excellence in vitreoretinal surgeries.

Sushma Ratna Jayanna

Contents

Video Contents

Scan QR code to access the above listed Videos. Instruction is there on the front of flap cover.

Abbreviations

ARN	:	Acute Retinal Necrosis
AMD	:	Age-related Macular Degeneration
AC Maintainer	:	Anterior Chamber Maintainer
BCVA	:	Best Corrected Visual Acuity
BE	:	Both Eyes
BIOM	:	Binocular Indirect Ophthalmomicroscope
BRVO	:	Branch Retinal Vein Occlusion
CRA	:	Chorioretinal Atrophy
CRD	:	Combined Retinal Detachment
CNVM	:	Choroidal Neovascularization Membrane
CSR	:	Central Serous Retinopathy
d/d	:	Differential Diagnosis
DR	:	Diabetic Retinopathy
EIMA	:	Endophthalmitis Infectivity Measurement Algorithm
ERM	:	Epiretinal Membrane
FA	:	Fluorescein Angiography
FEVR	:	Familial Exudative Vitreo Retinopathy
FTMH	:	Full Thickness Macular Hole
GRT	:	Giant Retinal Tear
HST	:	Horseshoe Tear
ILM	:	Internal Limiting Membrane
INQ	:	Inferonasal Quadrant
IOFB	:	Intraocular Foreign Body
IOL	:	Intraocular Lens
IOP	:	Intraocular Pressure
ITQ	:	Inferotemporal Quadrant
LE	:	Left Eye
LSV	:	Lens Sparing Vitrectomy
MLD	:	Minimum Linear Diameter
MVR Blades	:	Micro-vitreo-retinal Blades
OCT	:	Optical Coherence Tomography
PFCL	:	Perfluorocarbon Liquid
PFO	:	Perfluoro-octane
PFV	:	Persistent Fetal Vasculature
PPL	:	Pars Plana Lensectomy
PPV	:	Pars Plana Vitrectomy
PR	:	Pneumatic Retinopexy
PRP	:	Panretinal Photocoagulation
PVD	:	Posterior Vitreous Detachment
PVR	:	Proliferative Vitreoretinopathy
RD	:	Retinal Detachment
RE	:	Right Eye
ROP	:	Retinopathy of Prematurity
RPE	:	Retinal Pigment Epithelium
RRD	:	Rhegmatogenous Retinal Detachment
SB	:	Scleral Buckle
SNQ	:	Superonasal Quadrant
SOR	:	Silicone Oil Removal
SRF	:	Subretinal Fluid
STQ	:	Superotemporal Quadrant
TA	:	Triamcinolone Acetonide
TRD	:	Tractional Retinal Detachment
VEGF	:	Vascular Endothelial Growth Factor
VH	:	Vitreous Hemorrhage
VMT	:	Vitreomacular Traction

CHAPTER 1

General Principles in Retinal Surgeries

Sushma Ratna Jayanna, Subhashchandra Doralli, Naresh Kumar Yadav

PRINCIPLES OF RETINAL DETACHMENT

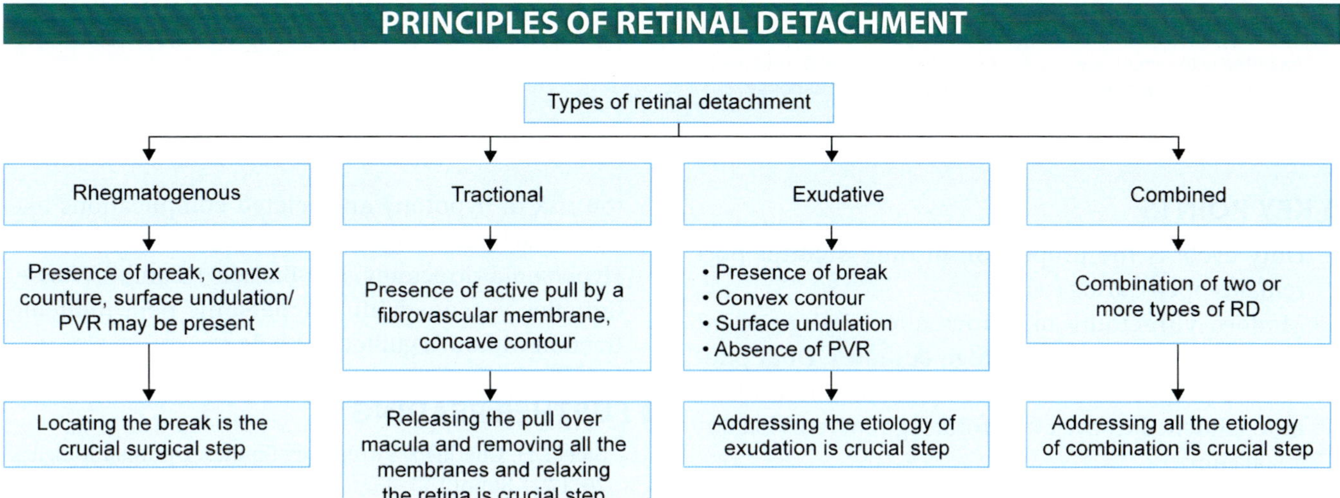

KEY POINTS

- Performing a detailed dynamic indirect ophthalmoscopic examination is vital step in management of retinal detachments.
- Recognizing the type of retinal detachment is crucial for selecting effective surgical approach.
- Simple imaging modalities such as ultrawide field color fundus photos such as OPTOS, ultrasound B-scans, and OCT are useful tools for distinguishing between the various forms of detachment.
- It is crucial to devote ample time to patient counseling so that patients can thoroughly grasp the details of their condition, the need for several surgeries, positioning guidelines, travel limitations, and possible complications—including cataracts, elevated intraocular pressure, infection, bleeding, and the risk of redetachment—prior to intervention.

FURTHER READING

1. Blair K, Czyz CN. Retinal Detachment. Treasure Island (FL): StatPearls Publishing; 2025.
2. Lin JB, Narayanan R, Philippakis E, Yonekawa Y, Apte RS. Retinal detachment. Nat Rev Dis Primers. 2024; 10(1):18.
3. Moisseiev E, Loewenstein A, Moshiri A, Yiu G. The Management of Retinal Detachment: Techniques and Perspectives 2018. J Ophthalmol. 2019;2019:8185619.

VITRECTOMY FLUIDICS

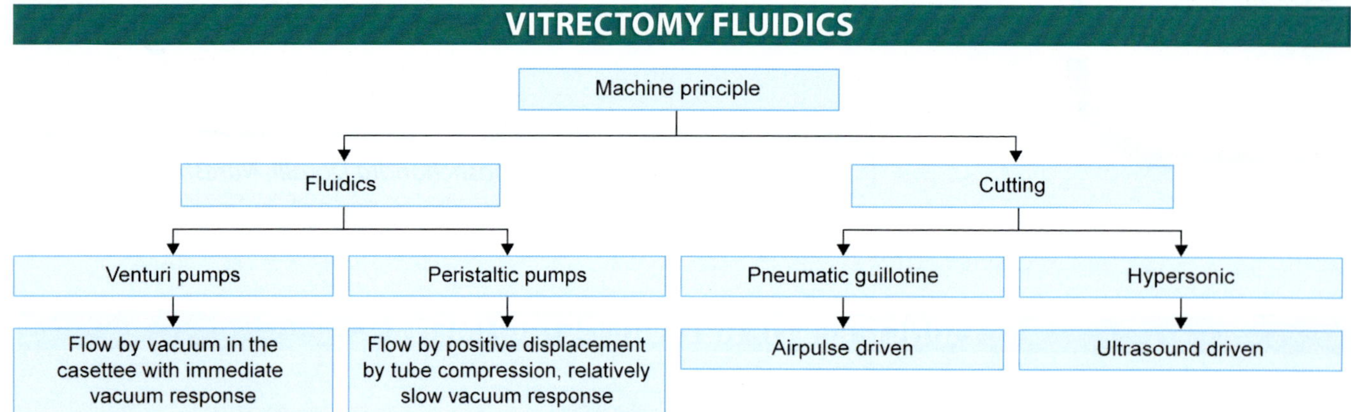

KEY POINTS

- Duty cycle is the proportion of time a cutter port remains open during a cut.
- Modern vitrectomy machines allow independent duty cycle control even at high cut rates. Dual pneumatic probes, such as Alcon Constellation, allow independent duty cycle control at high cut rates (5,000–7,500 cpm).
- Modern vitrectomy systems now achieve up to 30,000 cuts per minute and use real-time sensors to maintain stable intraocular pressure (IOP). This minimizes the risk of hypotony and related complications like choroidal hemorrhage.
- Hypersonic vitrectomy, like Bausch + Lomb's Vitesse, liquefies vitreous with a hypersonic pen, reducing traction without a guillotine blade.

FURTHER READING

1. Steel DH, Charles S. Vitrectomy fluidics. Ophthalmologica. 2011;226 Suppl 1:27-35.
2. Teixeira Pinto AG, Diniz B. Vitrectomy Principles and Systems. In: Ferreira MA (Ed). Diseases of the Retina and Vitreous. Cham: Springer; 2025.

SURGICAL INSTRUMENTS: PRINCIPLES AND USES

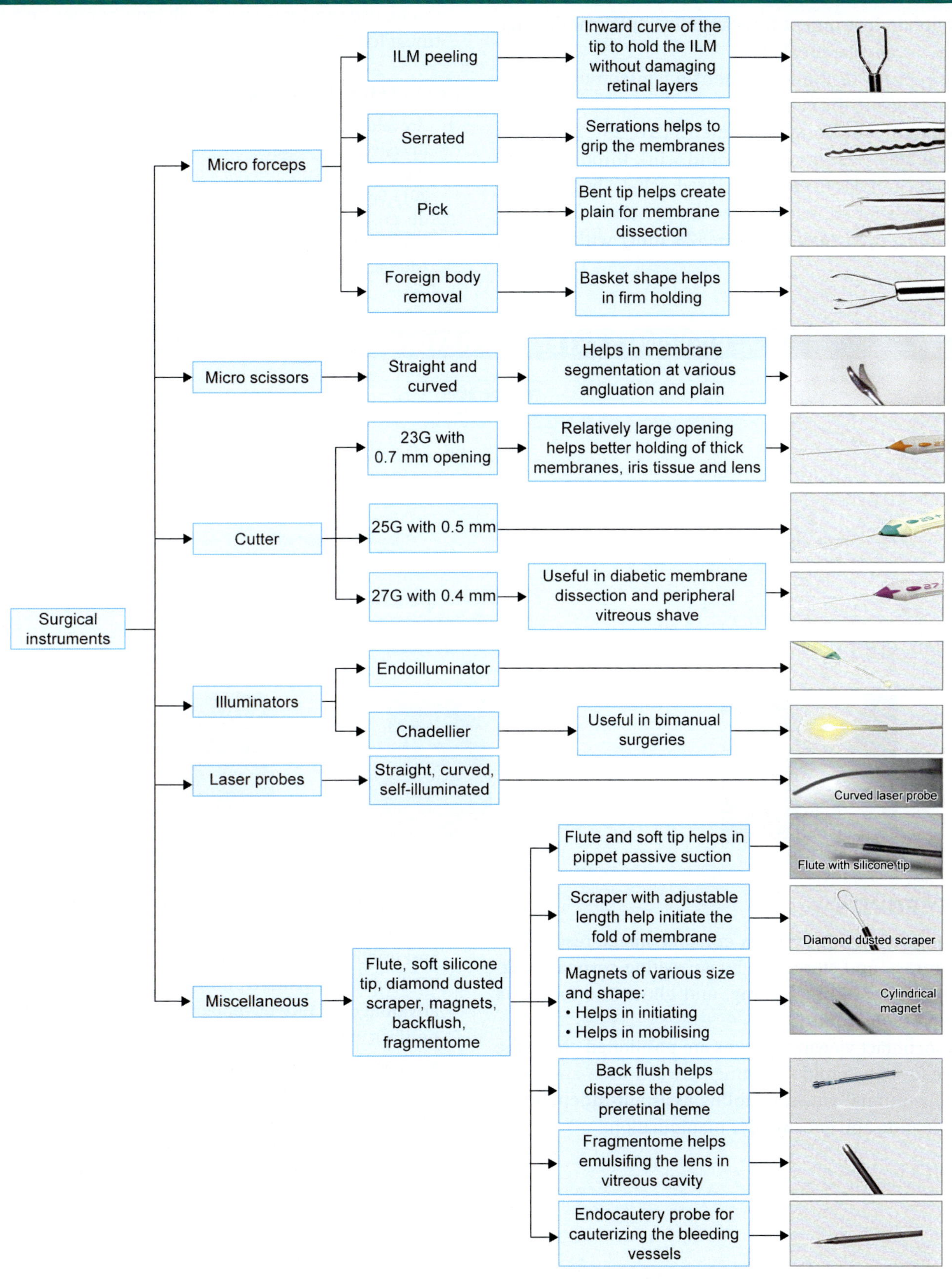

KEY POINTS

- Maintain instrument tips carefully to prevent damage and intraocular breakage.
- Inspect tip of the instrument for intactness before entering into the eye.
- Standard vitrectomy instruments (23-, 25-, 27-gauge) have 28.8–32.6 mm shafts and work through 4 mm microcannulas to ensure a closed, self-sealing system.
- Longer-shafted instruments are preferred for highly myopic eyes (axial length >28 mm) with 36-mm shafts.
- In pediatric eyes with short axial length and flexible sclera, use shorter trocars or silicone stoppers to adjust trocar length.

FURTHER READING

1. Arevalo JF, Berrocal MH, Arias JD, Banaee T. Minimally invasive vitreoretinal surgery: is sutureless vitrectomy the future of vitreoretinal surgery? J Ophthalmic Vis Res. 2011;6(2):136-44.
2. de Oliveira PR, Berger AR, Chow DR. Vitreoretinal instruments: vitrectomy cutters, endoillumination and wide-angle viewing systems. Int J Retina Vitreous. 2016;2:28.

VIEWING SYSTEMS IN RETINAL SURGERIES

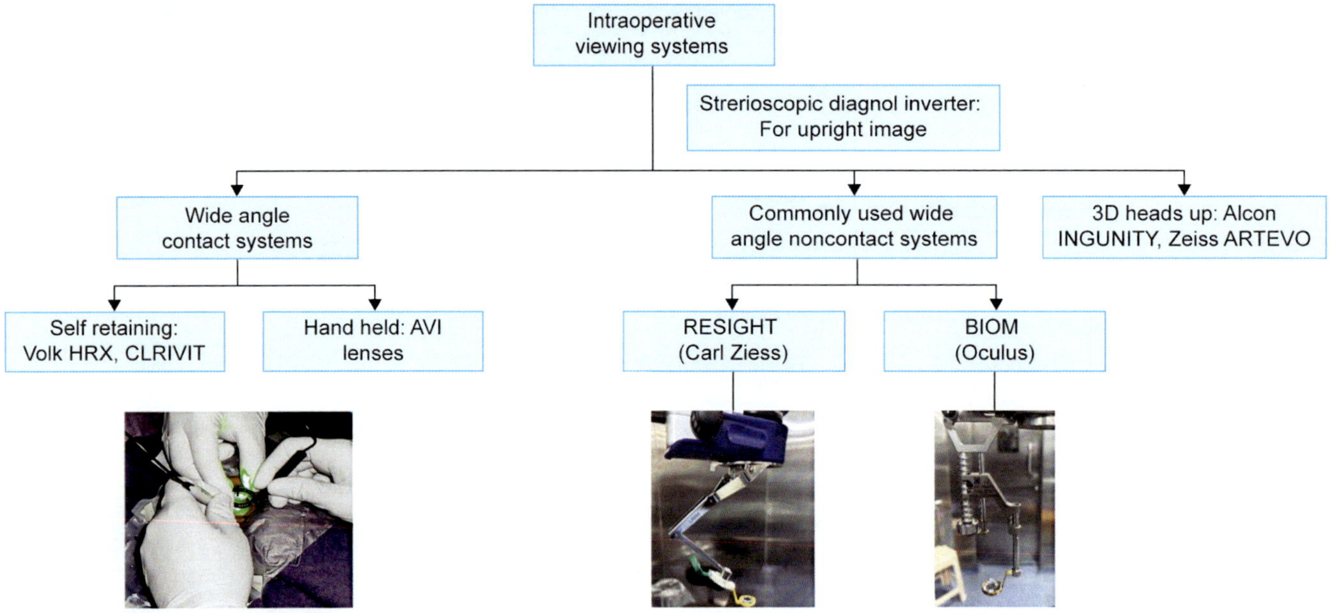

Intraoperative viewing systems

Strerioscopic diagnol inverter: For upright image

Wide angle contact systems

- Self retaining: Volk HRX, CLRIVIT
- Hand held: AVI lenses

Commonly used wide angle noncontact systems

- RESIGHT (Carl Ziess)
- BIOM (Oculus)

3D heads up: Alcon INGUNITY, Zeiss ARTEVO

KEY POINTS

- Contact viewing systems enhance image resolution, contrast, and stereopsis by correcting corneal irregularities, without fogging, and allow fine focus via microscope control.
- Noncontact viewing systems are positioned above the eye for easy, rapid switching between wide-angle and conventional views, enabling assistant-independent operation and effective eye manipulation.
- Chandelier illumination allows bimanual surgery in complex rhegmatogenous retinal detachment (RRD) and tractional retinal detachment (TRD).
- 3D heads-up visualization system offers significant advantages in PPV by replacing traditional microscope oculars with a high-definition screen, improving surgeon comfort, visualization, improved field of depth, and teaching capabilities.
- Endoscopic vitrectomy uses intraocular endoscope to visualize and treat retinal pathologies when the view is hampered by corneal opacity.

FURTHER READING

1. Agranat JS, Miller JB. 3D Surgical Viewing Systems in Vitreoretinal Surgery. Int Ophthalmol Clin. 2020;60(1):17-23.
2. Razavi P, Cakir B, Baldwin G, D'Amico DJ, Miller JB. Heads-Up Three-Dimensional Viewing Systems in Vitreoretinal Surgery: An Updated Perspective. Clin Ophthalmol. 2023;17:2539-52.
3. Tieger MG, Rodriguez M, Wang JC, Obeid A, Ryan C, Gao X, et al. Impact of contact versus non-contact wide-angle viewing systems on outcomes of primary retinal detachment repair (PRO study report number 5). Br J Ophthalmol. 2021;105(3):410-3.

INTRAOPERATIVE DYES: TYPES AND PRINCIPLES

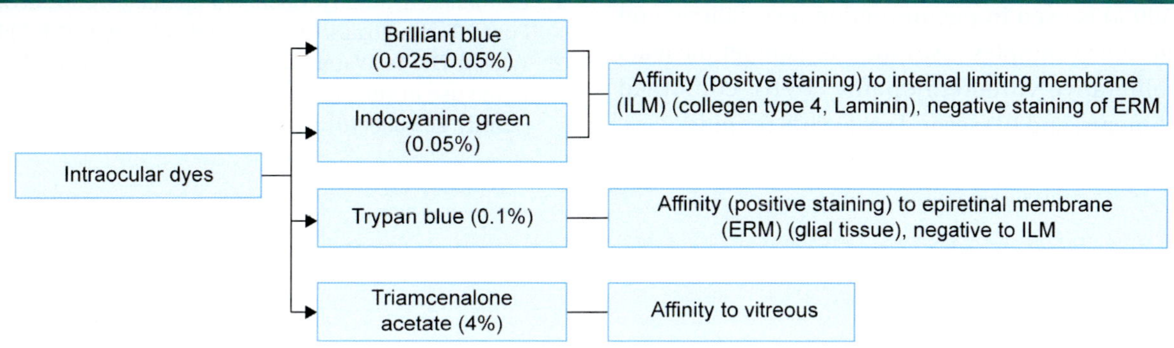

KEY POINTS

- Dyes can be injected using the "dry" technique (under air after fluid-air exchange for macular concentration but with higher exposure risk) or the "wet" technique (in a fluid-filled eye, often with "heavy" dyes that settle at the macula).
- Two dyes may be used sequentially or together (e.g., trypan blue for ERM, followed by Brilliant blue for ILM) to enable complete removal of multiple retinal layers (double staining).
- Certain dyes, like ICG, have absorption spectra that overlap with surgical light, increasing the risk of photochemical retinal damage.
- Prompt and thorough removal of dye after staining is essential to minimize retinal cell exposure and toxicity.

FURTHER READING

1. Bergamo VC, Caiado RR, Maia A, Magalhães O Jr, Moraes NSB, Rodrigues EB, et al. Role of Vital Dyes in Chromovitrectomy. Asia Pac J Ophthalmol (Phila). 2020;10(1):26-38.
2. Farah ME, Maia M, Rodrigues EB. Dyes in ocular surgery: principles for use in chromovitrectomy. Am J Ophthalmol. 2009;148(3):332-40.

INTRAOCULAR TAMPONADES: PROPERTIES AND USES

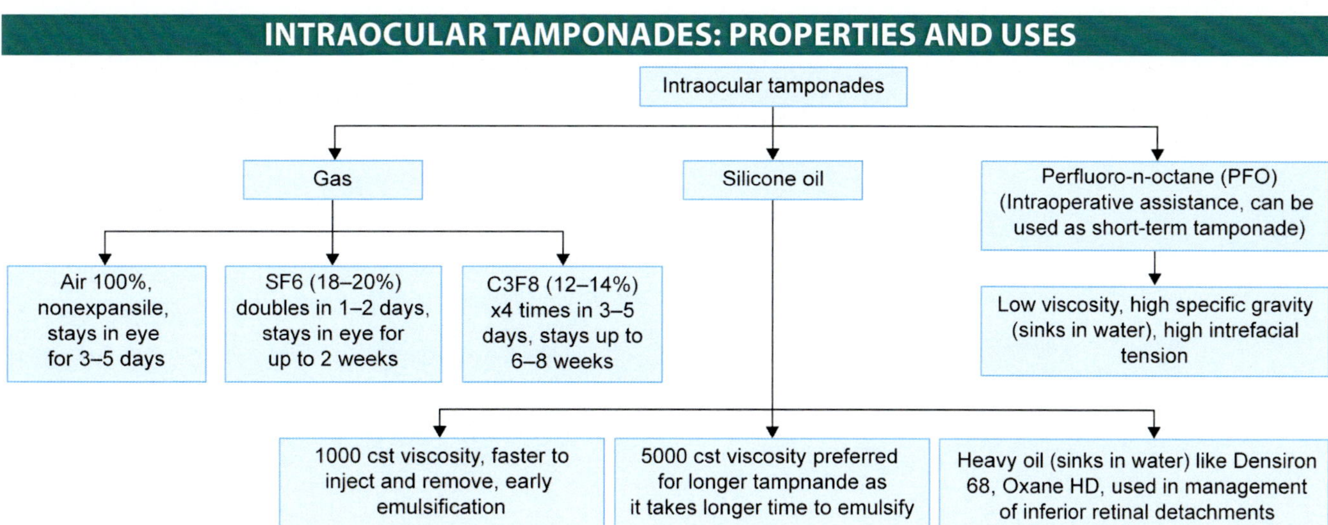

KEY POINTS

- Choice of tamponade depends on location of the retinal break. Gases (SF6 and C3F8) suit superior breaks due to buoyancy, while heavy silicone oil or strict positioning address inferior breaks.
- Nonexpansile gases are used for macular hole repair surgeries and simple retinal detachment (RD). Pure gas (100%) is used in pneumoretinopexy. Silicone oil is preferred in complex cases such as giant retinal tears or proliferative vitreoretinopathy (PVR), combined detachments, and RD secondary to viral retinitis.
- Complications include increased intraocular pressure (from gas expansion or oil overfill or oil emulsification) and cataract progression.
- Patients with intraocular gas must avoid air travel and nitrous oxide anesthesia due to the risk of rapid gas expansion.

FURTHER READING

1. Deobhakta A, Rosen R. Retinal Tamponades: Current Uses and Future Technologies. Curr Ophthalmol Rep. 2020;8(3):144-51.
2. Wilson DI, Te Water Naude AD, Snead MP. Refinements in the use of silicone oil as an intraocular tamponade. Eye (Lond). 2024;38(10):1810-5.

CHAPTER 2

Decision Making in Surgical Management of Rhegmatogenous Retinal Detachments

Ayushi Mohapatra, Muna Bhende

ALGORITHM FOR MANAGEMENT OF RHEGMATOGENOUS RETINAL DETACHMENT

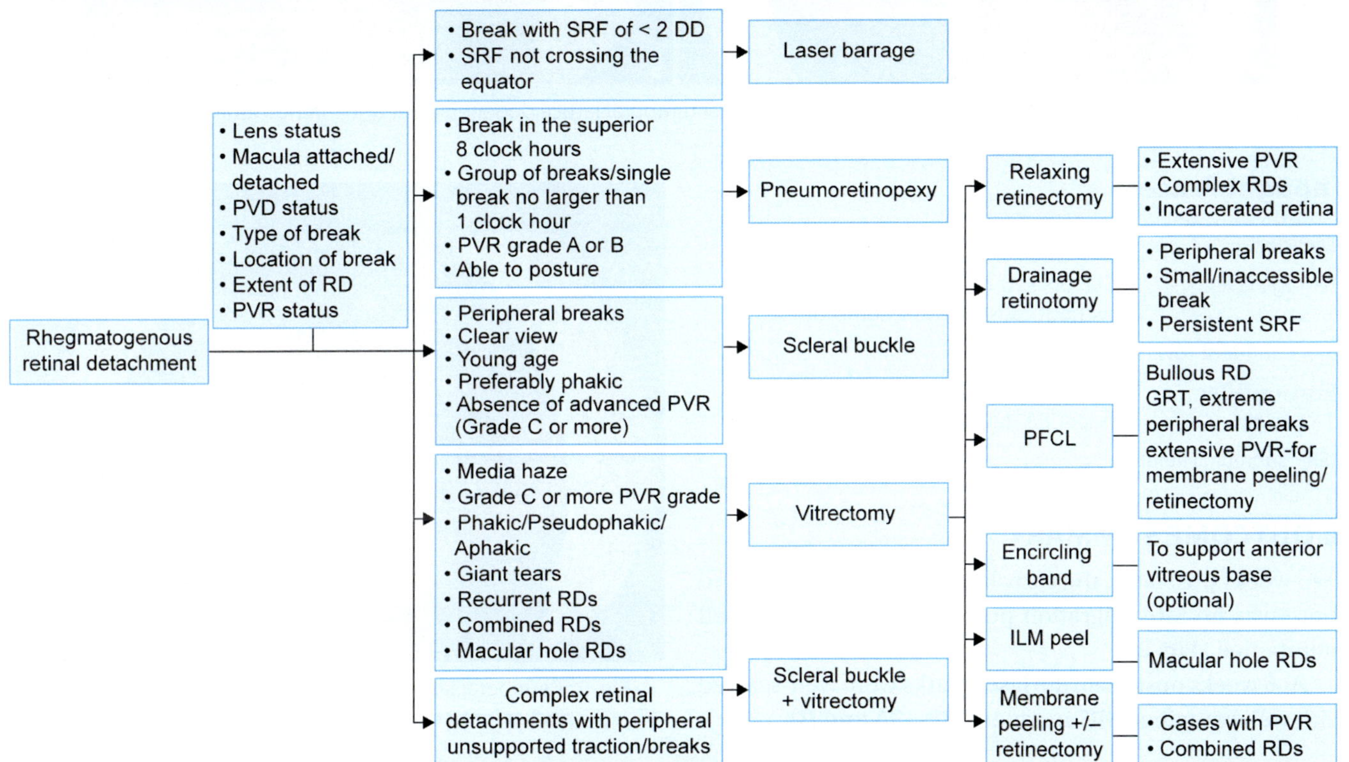

CASE SCENARIO 1: ROLE OF LASER BARRAGE IN MANAGEMENT OF RRD

Case Summary

A 21-year-old male with nil comorbidities presented with sudden drop in vision in the right eye for 2 months. On evaluation, the right eye was noted to have a rhegmatogenous retinal detachment involving macula and was planned for surgical intervention **(Figs. 1A and B)**.

His left eye, on evaluation, revealed a best-corrected visual acuity (BCVA) of 6/6 with 14 mm Hg of intraocular pressure with a two separate pockets of subretinal fluid (SRF) at the temporally and inferior periphery with multiple lattice degenerations within the pockets—with posterior edge of SRF anterior to the equator. Patient was phakic with -8 D of myopia bilaterally.

Treatment Plan

Barrage laser around the SRF pockets and the lattice degenerations

↓

Reassess after 1–2 weeks for any extension of SRF beyond the laser borders

(SRF: subretinal fluid)

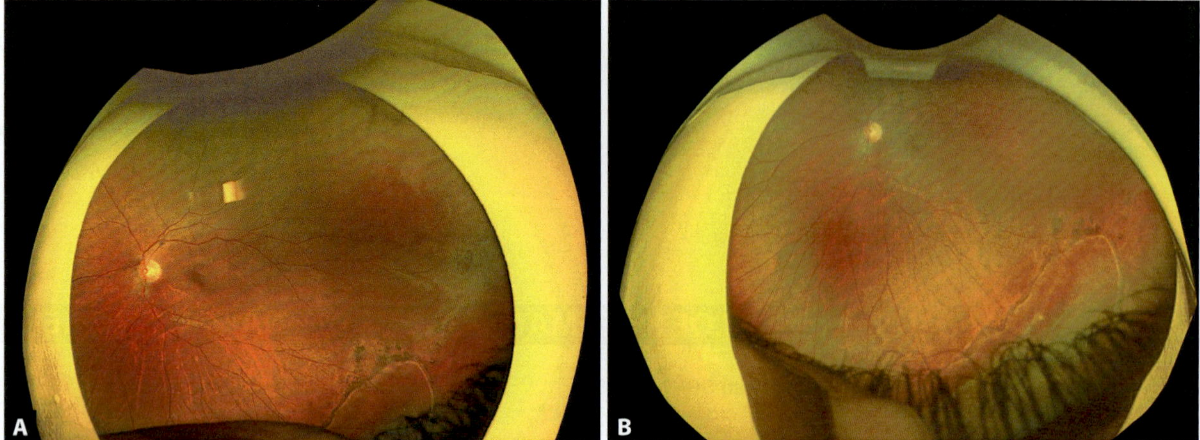

Figs. 1A and B: Ultra-widefield image of left eye with peripheral temporal lattice degenerations and inferior subretinal fluid. (Case 1)

Thought Process

Decision	*Rationale*
Barrage laser	SRF pockets can be limited by laser without causing visual compromise
3–4 confluent rows	Presence of SRF
Reassess after 1–2 weeks	To ensure no migration of SRF till the laser CRA develops

(SRF: subretinal fluid)

OUTCOME SUMMARY

Two weeks post laser, the early laser scars were noted and there was no SRF migration posteriorly. BCVA was well maintained **(Fig. 2)**.

At 6 weeks post laser, the laser marks were well-scarred with well contained SRF margins **(Figs. 3A and B)**.

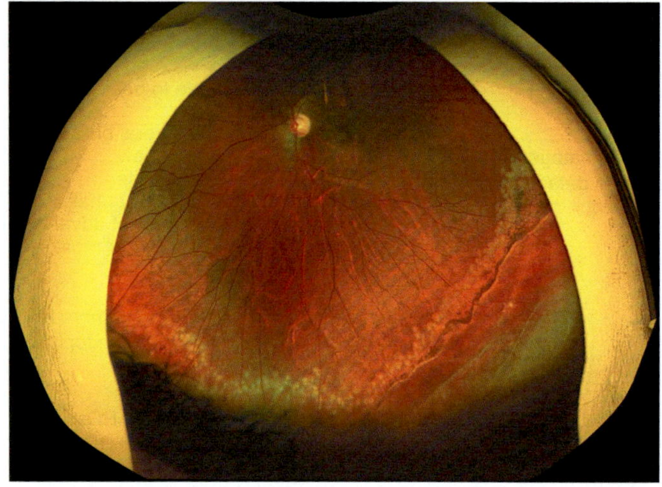

Fig. 2: Peripheral lattice degenerations and subretinal fluid pocket immediately post-barrage laser. (Case 1)

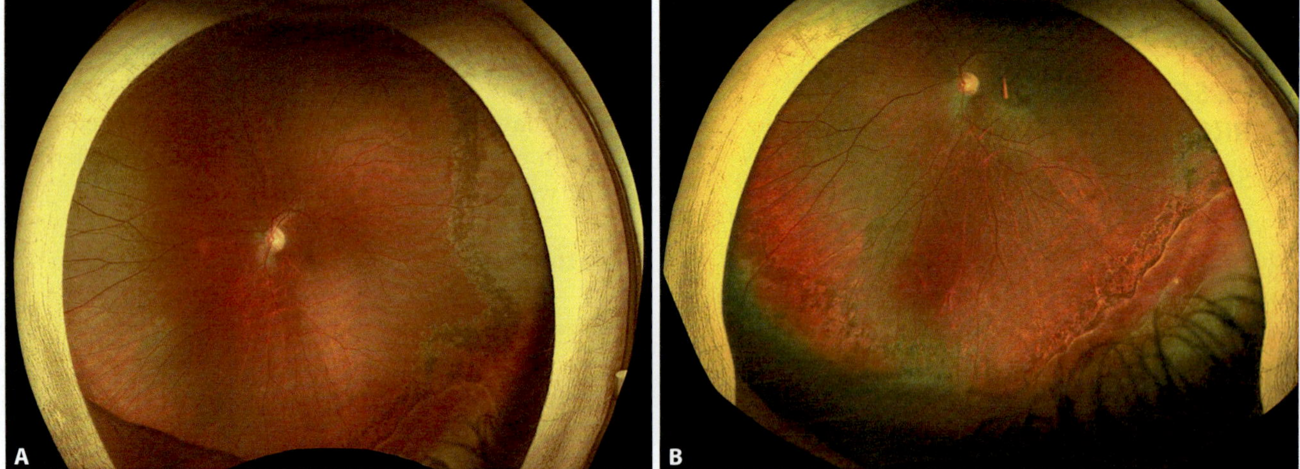

Figs. 3A and B: Peripheral lattice degenerations and subretinal fluid pocket 6 weeks post-barrage laser. (Case 1)

KEY POINTS

- Demarcation laser photocoagulation (DLP) is done to create confluent adhesions between retina and RPE around a break or detachment to create a barrier against further spread of subretinal fluid.
- The criteria for DLP published by Okun et al. include width of detachment not greater than five times the diameter of the largest break, and less than 2 clock hours in size with the posterior extent not extending beyond the equator.
- The progression of retinal detachment requiring surgical intervention can be seen in 20% of such cases and hence a close follow-up is necessary.

FURTHER READING

1. Okun EC, Cibis PA. Photocoagulation in "limited" retinal detachment and breaks without detachment. In: McPherson A (Ed). New and Controversial Aspects of Retinal Detachment. New York: Harper and Row; 1968. pp. 164-72.
2. Xu D, Levin HJ, Garrigan H, Wibbelsman TD, Obeid A, Pandit RR, et al. Outcomes and Complications of In-Office Laser Demarcation of Peripheral Rhegmatogenous Retinal Detachments. Ophthalmic Surg Lasers Imaging Retina. 2020;51(8):428-34.

CASE SCENARIO 2: MANAGEMENT OF FOCAL RRD WITH HST

Case Summary

A 61-year-old male with nil comorbidities presented with floaters in the right eye for 3 months. Patient was phakic, his BCVA was noted to be 6/7.5 in both eyes with 11 mm Hg intraocular pressure in right eye. On examination, he was noted to have a temporal retinal detachment with macula uninvolved and single HST **(Fig. 4)**.

Treatment Plan

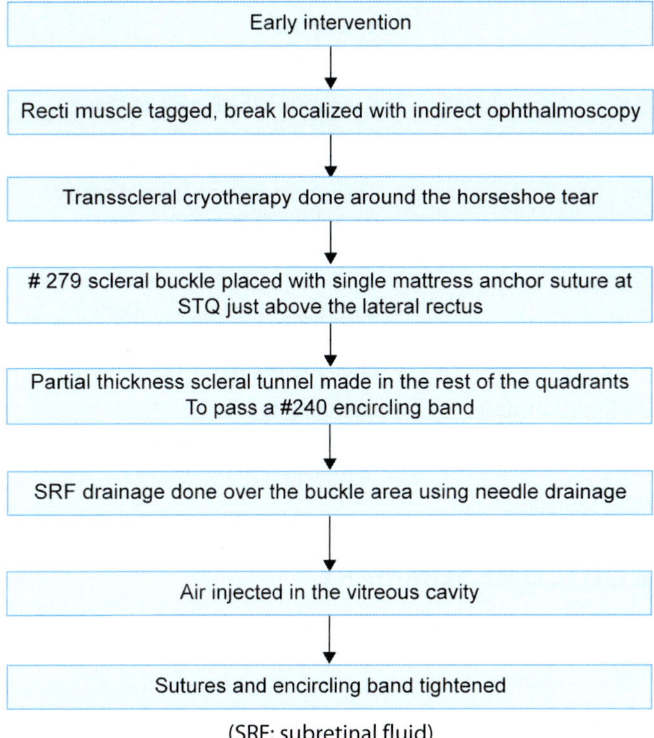

(SRF: subretinal fluid)

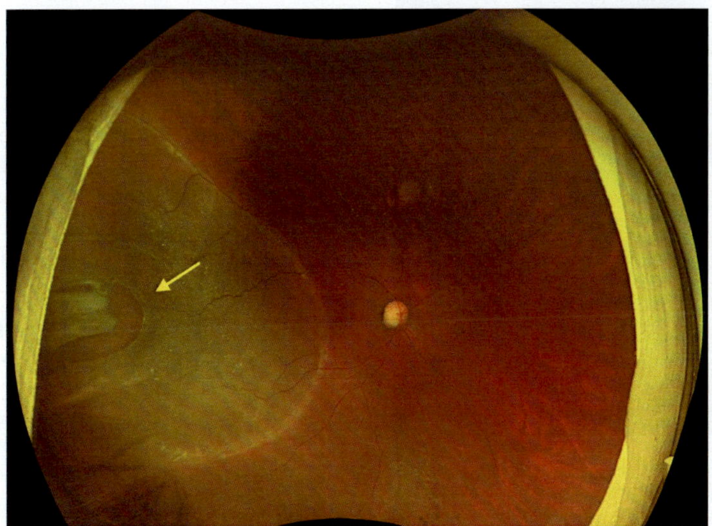

Fig. 4: Ultra-widefield image of right eye with temporal horseshoe tear (yellow arrow) and temporal retinal detachment with macula still attached. (Case 2)

Thought Process

Decision	*Rationale*
Immediate intervention	Macula sparing retinal detachment
SB	Clear view, single peripheral break
#279 buckle segment	Posterior edge of HST at 8 mm from muscle insertion
SRF drainage	To permit the apposition of the break to the buckle
Encircling band	To support vitreous base (optional)
SRF drainage within the buckle area	• Can tighten the buckle to stop egress of fluid from the opening once adequate drainage is done • To support drainage site in case of iatrogenic damage • In case of iatrogenic retinal damage, the break with shallow fluid will be covered by the buckle indent • *Caution:* Avoid draining through an open break-careful localization
Air injection after drainage	• Optional step • To build up IOP after drainage, to flatten out fish mouthing

(SRF: subretinal fluid)

OUTCOME SUMMARY

Immediate postoperative period—posterior pole was attached with minimal SRF temporally **(Fig. 5)**.

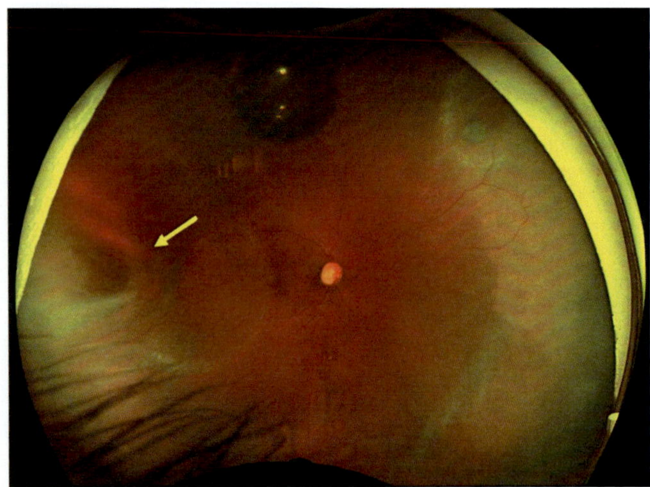

Fig. 5: Postoperative day 4 with temporal horseshoe tear supported by the buckle indent (yellow arrow) with surrounding cryo edema and shallow resolving subretinal fluid and a small air bubble in the superior vitreous cavity. Fresh laser marks are seen around a horseshoe tear in attached retina at 1 o'clock. (Case 2)

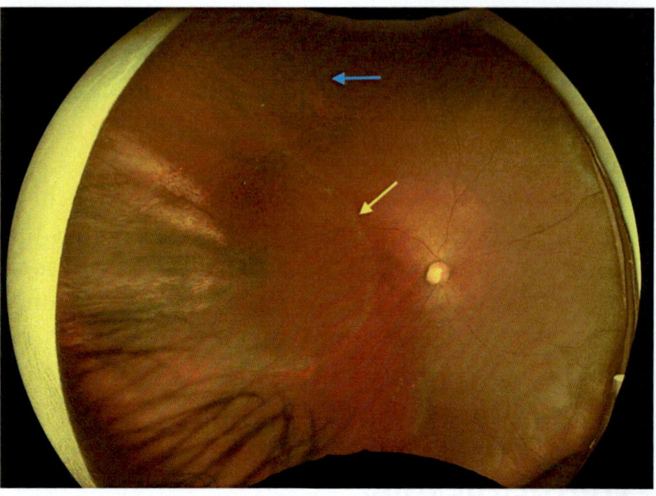

Fig. 6: 6 weeks postoperative fundus with cryo scars around the horseshoe tear temporally, well supported by the buckle indent with clinically attached retina and a demarcation line (yellow arrow). An area of pigment dropout noted at STQ periphery (blue arrow). (Case 2)

At 6 weeks postoperatively, BCVA was noted to be 6/9 with intraocular pressure of 16 mm Hg **(Fig. 6)**.

Other options: Segmental buckle and pneumatic retinopexy.

KEY POINTS

- Timely surgery in macula-sparing retinal detachment is essential to prevent foveal involvement and preserve vision.
- Scleral buckle can be regarded as one of the options in phakic eyes with single peripheral break.

FURTHER READING

1. Fallico M, Alosi P, Reibaldi M, Longo A, Bonfiglio V, Avitabile T, et al. Scleral Buckling: A Review of Clinical Aspects and Current Concepts. J Clin Med. 2022;11(2):314.
2. Mahmoudi S, Almony A. Macula-Sparing Rhegmatogenous Retinal Detachment: Is Emergent Surgery Necessary? J Ophthalmic Vis Res. 2016;11(1):100-7.

CASE SCENARIO 3: MANAGEMENT OF RRD WITH BREAKS IN MULTIPLE QUADRANT

Case Summary

A 22-year-old high myope (–13 Diopter) came with complaints of occasional floaters in both eyes. She had a 6/9 BCVA in the left eye with a clear lens, 12 mm Hg IOP and multiple peripheral pockets of SRF with multiple

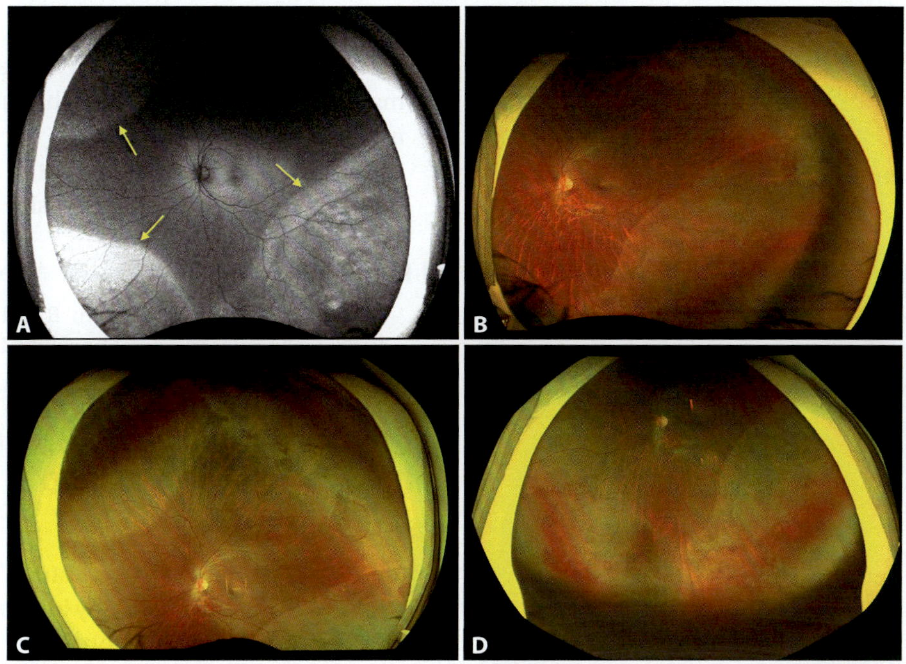

Figs. 7A to D: Ultra-widefield autofluorescence and fundus photo of left eye with multiple lattice degenerations and holes with 3 separate pockets of subretinal fluids (yellow arrows), the inferotemporal pocket extending beyond equator. (Case 3)

lattice degenerations and breaks within. The inferotemporal pocket extended beyond equator posteriorly **(Figs. 7A to D)**. The macula was attached. Her other eye had a similar picture.

Treatment Plan

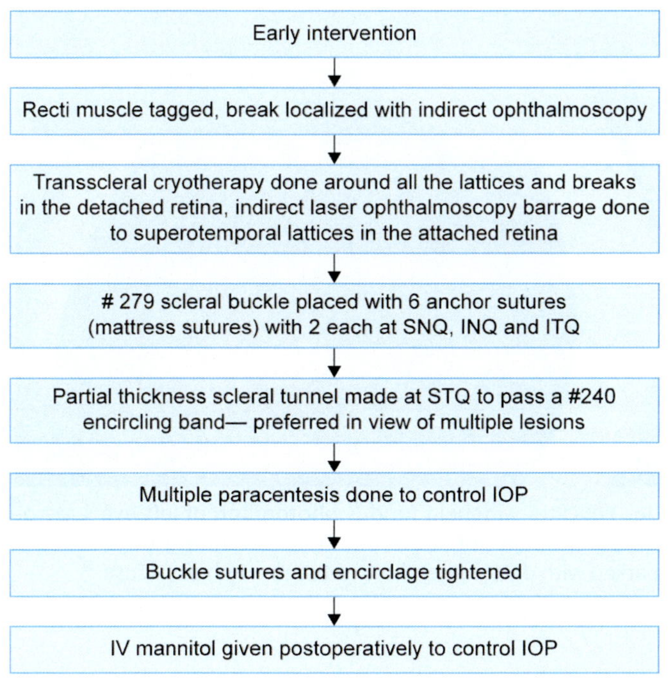

Thought Process

Decision	*Rationale*
Immediate intervention	Macula sparing retinal detachment
SB	Clear view, multiple peripheral breaks, depressible breaks
SRF drainage deferred	Very shallow SRF
LIO to lesions in attached retina	To avoid complications (additional inflammation and RPE pigment dispersion) of excess cryo
Multiple paracentesis	• Nondrainage 3 quadrant buckle • To control IOP intraoperatively and achieve buckle effect
IV mannitol—immediate postoperative	• Nondrainage 3 quadrant buckle • To prevent postoperative IOP spike

(RPE: retinal pigment epithelium; SRF: subretinal fluid)

OUTCOME SUMMARY

On postoperative day 1, the patient had a flat posterior pole with shallow SRF around the previous breaks with all breaks in previously detached retina well supported by the buckle indent. IOP was 14 mm Hg.

At 2 weeks postoperatively, the residual SRF had reduced **(Fig. 8)**. BCVA was maintained and IOP was 16 mm Hg. A similar clinical picture was noted postoperatively 6 weeks **(Fig. 9)**.

Other options: Segmental buckles or pars plana vitrectomy.

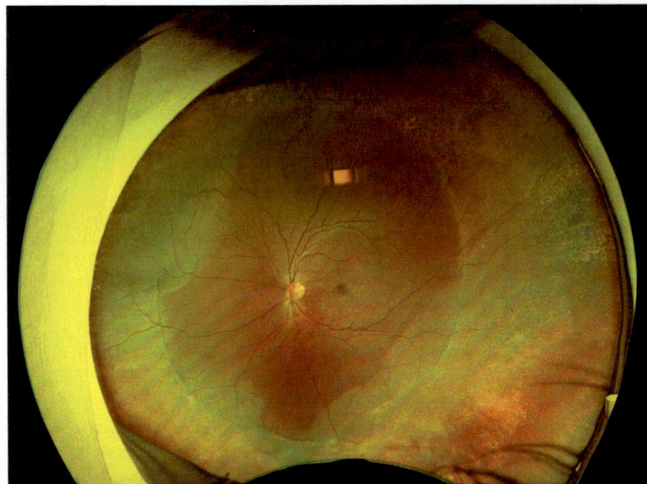

Fig. 8: 2 weeks postoperative ultra-widefield fundus photograph showing reduced subretinal fluid with early cryo scarring and all lesions flat over the buckle indent. Shallow fluid is seen posterior to the buckle, not communicating with the breaks. (Case 3)

KEY POINTS

- Scleral buckle is an effective treatment option for macula sparing retinal detachment associated with multiple peripheral breaks.
- Intra and postoperative IOP control is essential in non-drainage procedures with extensive buckles.

FURTHER READING

1. Shanmugam PM, Ramanjulu R, Mishra KCD, Sagar P. Novel techniques in scleral buckling. Indian J Ophthalmol. 2018;66(7):909-15.

CASE SCENARIO 4: PNEUMORETINOPEXY IN MANAGEMENT OF RRD

Case Summary

A 47-year-old high myope with Marfan's syndrome, status post-lensectomy, and vitrectomy bilaterally for subluxated lens presented with recent onset of floaters in the left eye. He was aphakic with 6/18 BCVA in the left eye with +14D aphakic correction, IOP was 12 mm Hg. There was a superotemporal retinal hole with pocket of SRF (>2 disk diameter) but anterior to equator with SRF tracking inferiorly in the temporal periphery. Macula was attached **(Fig. 10)**.

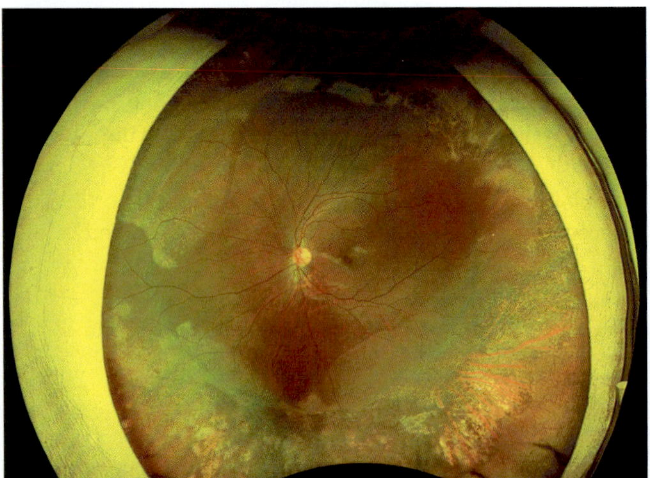

Fig. 9: 6 weeks postoperative ultra-widefield fundus photograph showing resolved subretinal fluid with scarring around the lesions and all peripheral lattice degenerations and break flat over the buckle indent. (Case 3)

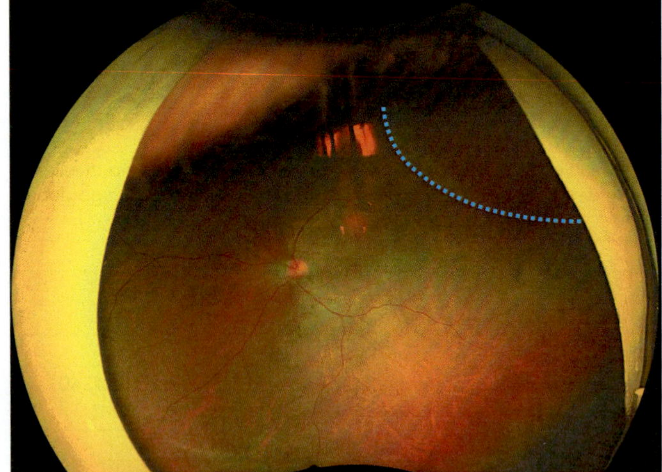

Fig. 10: Ultra-widefield fundus photograph of left eye superotemporal pocket of subretinal fluid extending till arcades—marked with dotted lines (hole not seen on photo). (Case 4)

Treatment Plan

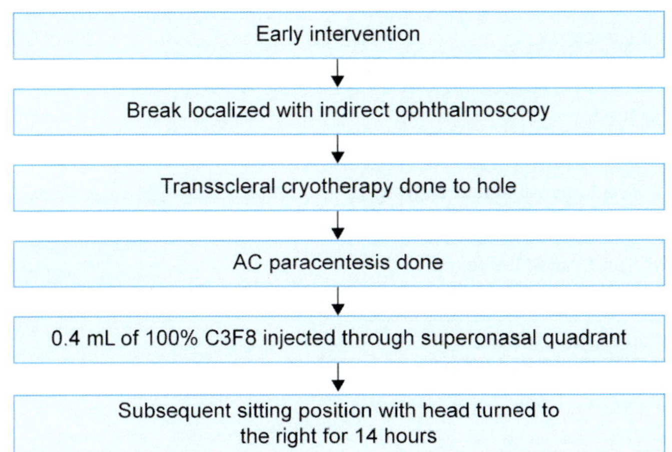

Thought Process

Decision	*Rationale*
Pneumoretinopexy	Superior break with surrounding shallow SRF
100% pure C3F8	Expansile gas for coverage of adequate area—smaller initial volume of gas can be injected for subsequent large area coverage, without sudden rise of IOP
Need for immediate prone	Ensure gas tamponades the macula first then milk toward the break
Positioning rationale	Subsequent positioning to ensure the area of the break is at the highest—for maximum tamponade effect at the site

OUTCOME MEASURE

On postoperative day 1, the patient had a flat posterior pole with shallow SRF around the break with gas bubble in situ. No air was noted in AC. IOP was 16 mm Hg.

At 8 weeks post-procedure, the retina was attached, BCVA was maintained at 6/18.

KEY POINTS

- Pneumoretinopexy is a less invasive technique that can be used as an effective management for redetachment in select vitrectomized eyes.
- Caution to be exercised in aphakic eyes to avoid gas causing a flat anterior chamber or migrating into the anterior chamber.

FURTHER READING

1. Mandelcorn E, Mandelcorn M, Manusow JS. Update on pneumatic retinopexy. Curr Opinion Ophthalmol. 2015;26:194-9.
2. Petrushkin HJ, Elgohary MA, Sullivan PM. Rescue pneumatic retinopexy in patients with failed primary retinal detachment surgery. Retina. 2015;35(9):1851-9.
3. Takeuchi J, Koto T, Inoue M. Rescue pneumatic retinopexy for recurrent retinal detachments due to superior retinal breaks following initial vitrectomy. Jpn J Ophthalmol. 2025. Online ahead of print.

CASE SCENARIO 5: MANAGEMENT OF GIANT RETINAL TEAR WITH DETACHMENT

Case Summary

A 12-year-old apparently healthy male presented with a drop in vision in the only seeing eye for 5 days. There was no history of trauma. No significant systemic condition. The left eye was phthisical with a history of old rhegmatogenous retinal detachment diagnosed 5 years back. On evaluation, BCVA of right eye was hand movements and IOP was 2 mm Hg. He was phakic with a clear lens. On fundus evaluation, he was noted to have a total retinal detachment with a giant retinal tear extending from 9 to 3 o'clock with rolled margins **(Fig. 11)**. An axial length of 29.18 mm was noted on B scan ultrasonography.

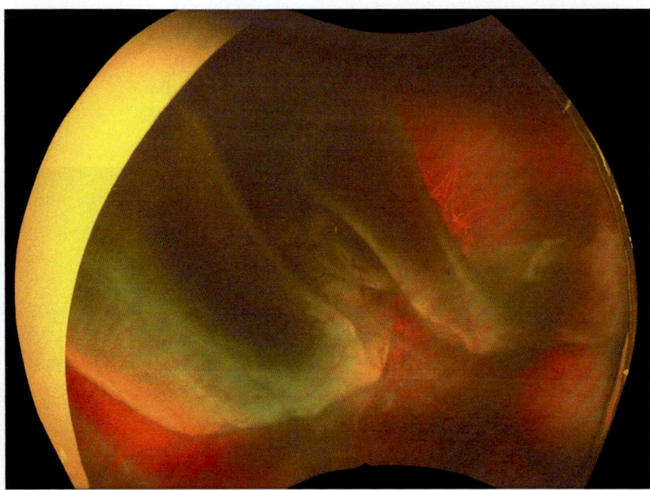

Fig. 11: Depicting ultra-widefield fundus photograph of right eye with a total retinal detachment with a giant retinal tear extending from 9 to 3 o'clock with in-rolling of margins. (Case 5)

Treatment Plan

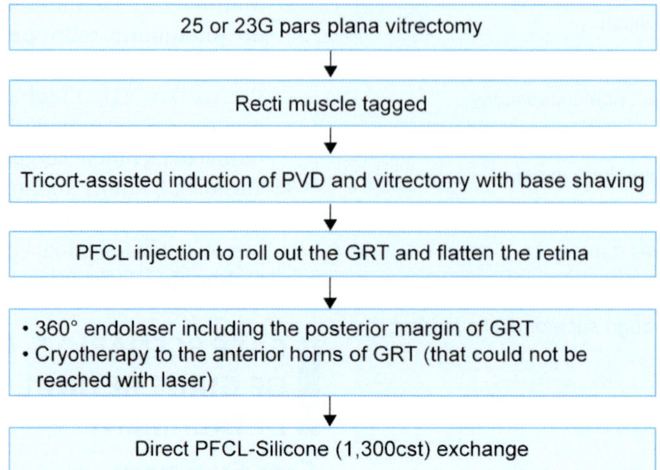

(GRT: giant retinal tear; PFCL: perfluorocarbon liquid; PVD: posterior vitreous detachment)

Thought Process

Decision	*Rationale*
Preserve phakic status	Clear lens with good view
Use of PFCL	• Unfolding the flap • High efficacy in displacing fluid from an anterior break
Direct PFCL-Silicone oil exchange	To avoid slippage of posterior edge of GRT if air is used
360° endolaser	To ensure any anterior microbreaks are covered
Cryo to the edges of GRT	Ensure adequate coverage to the GRT in a phakic patient if laser is not possible
Silicone oil (1,300 cst)	Long-term tamponade

(GRT: giant retinal tear; PFCL: perfluorocarbon liquid)

OUTCOME SUMMARY

Postoperative retina was attached **(Figs. 12 and 13)**.

The BCVA was counting fingers at 1 meters at 6 weeks post-operatively due to cataract with intraocular pressure of 12 mm Hg.

He underwent lensectomy with silicone oil removal after 4 months, BCVA recovered to 6/15 postoperatively. Intraocular pressure was normal.

KEY POINTS

- Early surgical intervention is compelling in cases of giant retinal tears owing to the rapid development of PVR in such eyes.

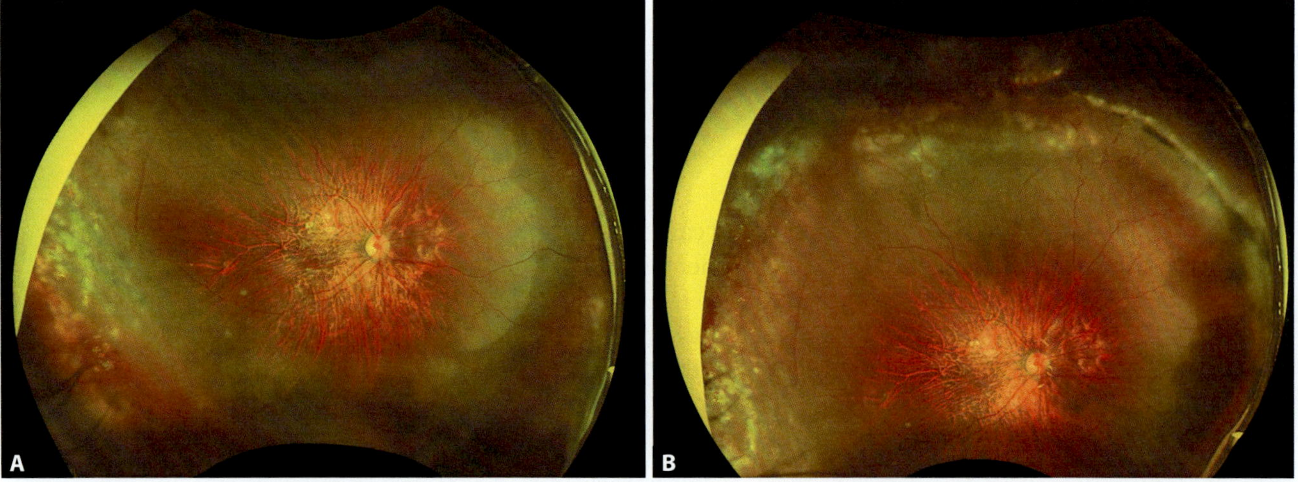

Figs. 12A and B: Postoperative day 4 ultra-widefield fundus photograph showing an attached retina with 360° laser marks. (Case 5)

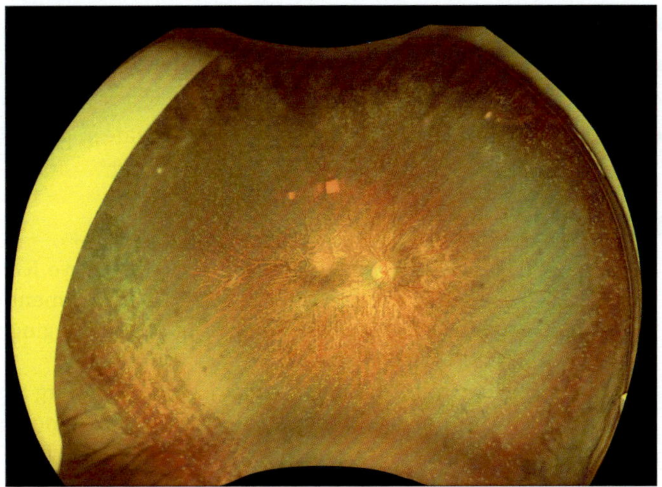

Fig. 13: 4th month postoperative fundus photograph showing an attached retina with 360° laser scars and oil emulsification. (Case 5)

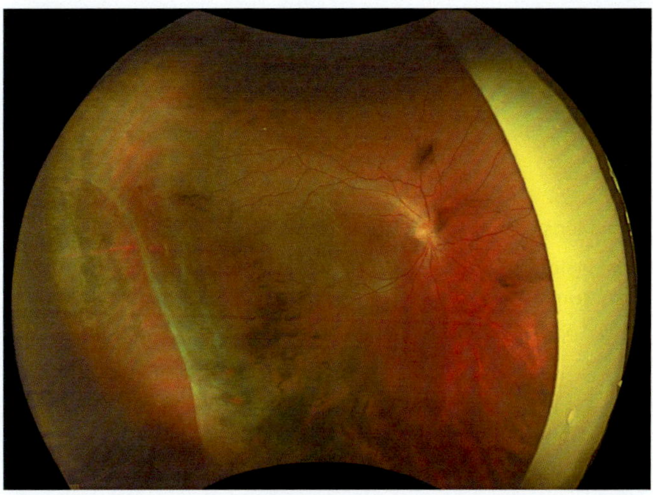

Fig. 14: Right eye ultra-widefield fundus photograph showing a temporal retinal dialysis with a subtotal retinal detachment and vitreous hemorrhage. (Case 6)

- Direct PFCL-oil exchange is quicker and minimizes the risk of flap slippage.

FURTHER READING

1. Choovuthayakorn J, Rajsirisongsri P, Patikulsila D, Nanegrungsunk O, Chaikitmongkol V, Seetasut S, et al. Characteristics and surgical outcomes of giant retinal tear associated rhegmatogenous retinal detachment. Sci Rep. 2024;14(1):19943.
2. Quiroz-Reyes MA, Quiroz-Gonzalez EA, Quiroz-Gonzalez MA, Lima-Gomez V. Systematic review of surgical techniques for treating giant retinal tears in adults: A current assessment of approaches and interventions. Lat Am J Ophthalmol. 2024;7:12.

CASE SCENARIO 6: COMBINED SB AND VITRECTOMY IN MANAGEMENT OF RRD WITH DIALYSIS

Case Summary

A 50-year-old male presented with floaters following a blunt trauma in the right eye due to recoil of a rubber band 3 months back.

He was noted to have a BCVA of 6/12 with a 180° angle recession and raised IOP (24 mm Hg). On fundus evaluation, he was noted to have a temporal retinal dialysis (6–10 o'clock) with shallow subtotal RD involving the macula and trace inferior vitreous hemorrhage **(Fig. 14)**. He was phakic with stable, clear lens.

Treatment Plan

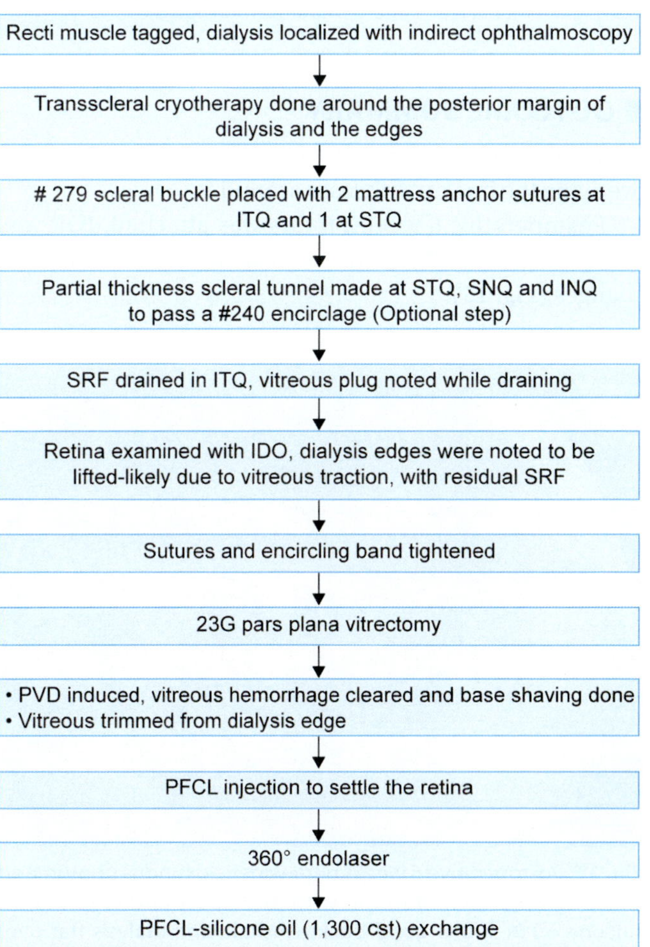

(PFCL: perfluorocarbon liquid; PVD: posterior vitreous detachment; SRF: subretinal fluid)

Thought Process

Decision	*Rationale*
SB attempted	Peripheral break (dialysis) with relatively clear view, shallow RD and phakic patient
Avoid lensectomy	Clear lens with good view
Conversion to vitrectomy	Vitreous in subretinal space limiting drainage of SRF, lifted dialysis edge
Use of PFCL	High efficacy in displacing fluid from an anterior break
Direct PFCL—silicone oil exchange	Low risk of slippage in a dialysis as opposed to GRT
Endolaser to posterior border of cryo	Risks of microbreaks within cryoed retina margins during vitrectomy maneuvers such as PVD extension
Silicone oil injection	• Surgeon preference • Early visual rehabilitation • Permits air travel

(GRT: giant retinal tear; PFCL: perfluorocarbon liquid)

OUTCOME SUMMARY

Retina was attached on postoperative day 1. Break was flat overlying the buckle with laser around it.

Postoperative 6 weeks, retina was attached, IOP was 14 mm Hg, and BCVA was 6/24 with early cataractous changes **(Fig. 15)**.

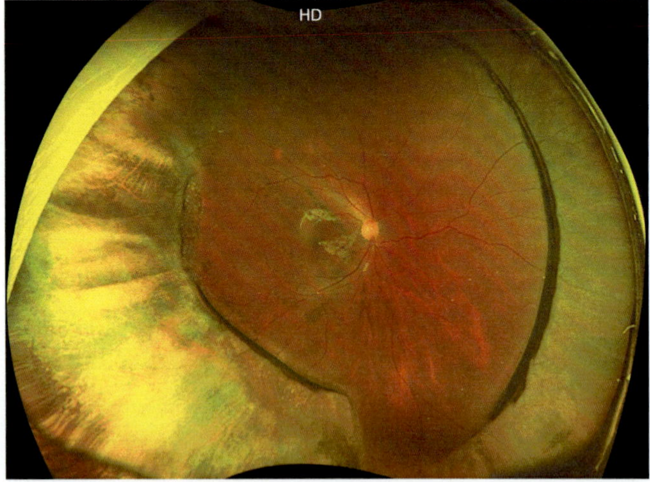

Fig. 15: Postoperative 6 weeks ultra-widefield fundus photograph showing an attached retina with 360° laser and cryo marks, silicone oil in situ, a good buckle indent, and dialysis flat over buckle indent. (Case 6)

KEY POINTS

- Scleral buckling is the preferred treatment in cases of retinal detachment with dialysis.
- Conversion to vitrectomy in case of inadequate support and inability to draw fluid in an inferior break.

FURTHER READING

1. Chang JS, Marra K, Flynn HW Jr, Berrocal AM, Arroyo JG. Scleral Buckling in the Treatment of Retinal Detachment Due to Retinal Dialysis. Ophthalmic Surg Lasers Imaging Retina. 2016;47(4):336-40.
2. Mahmoudzadeh R, Huang D, Salabati M, Awh K, Garg S, Hsu J, et al. Clinical Characteristics and Management Outcomes of Rhegmatogenous Retinal Detachments Due to Retinal Dialysis. J Vitreoretin Dis. 2021;5(5):405-11.

CASE SCENARIO 7: MANAGEMENT OF RECURRENT RRD AFTER SB

Case Summary

A 17-year-old male myope (–21 Diopter), operated with scleral buckle successfully in the left eye for multiple confluent superotemporal breaks with a total bullous retinal detachment 4 months prior, presented with recent onset flashes for few days. Patient had an INQ lattice degeneration which was previously treated **(Figs. 16A and B)**. 2 superior mattress anchor sutures had been placed on either side of superior rectus with a #240 encircling band all around and a superior #279 buckle.

The 6 weeks postoperative BCVA was 6/45 and macula was attached. BCVA was maintained at this presentation. IOP was 12 mm Hg with clear lens. The lattice in INQ had lifted with SRF extending posterior to the buckle **(Fig. 17)**.

Treatment Plan

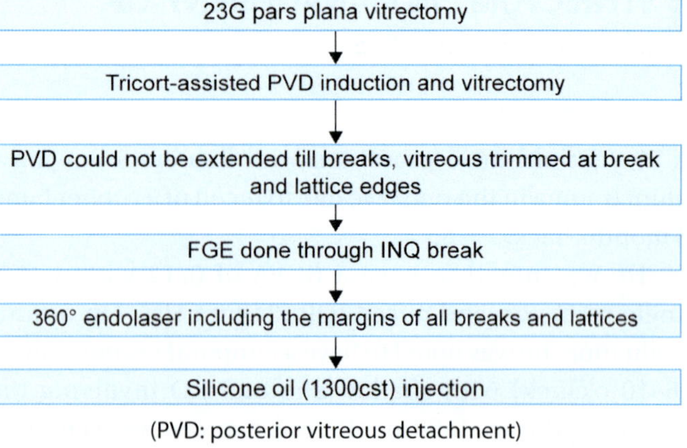

(PVD: posterior vitreous detachment)

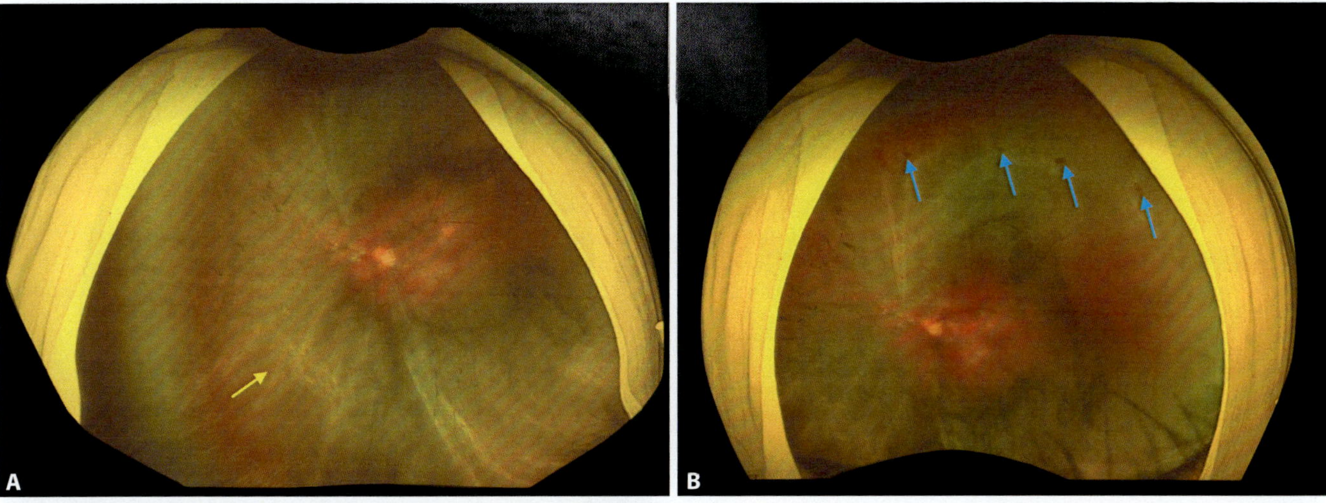

Figs. 16A and B: *First presentation (prior to scleral buckle):* Depicting left eye ultra-widefield fundus photograph showing a total retinal detachment with multiple superior breaks (blue arrows) and inferonasal lattice degeneration (yellow arrow). (Case 7)

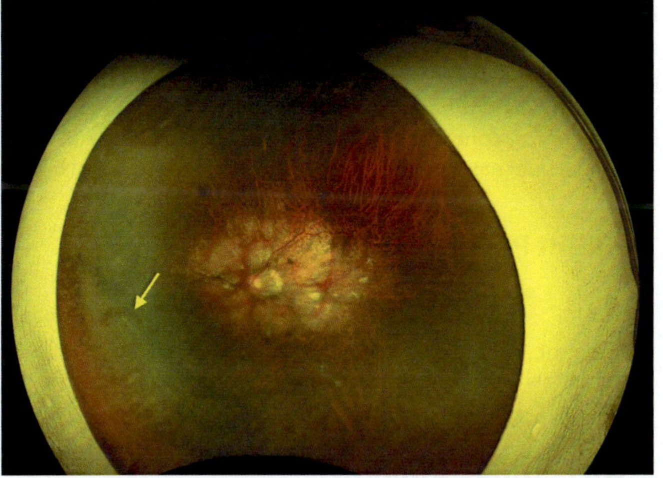

Fig. 17: *Second presentation (6 weeks postoperative to scleral buckle):* Left eye ultra-widefield fundus photograph showing a recurrent retinal detachment with an attached macula, and a fresh break at the edge of inferonasal lattice degeneration (yellow arrow). (Case 7)

Thought Process

Decision	*Rationale*
Tricort for PVD induction	To identify the posterior hyaloid in high myopes and ensure complete PVD due to high incidence of vitreoschisis in such eyes
Avoid lensectomy	Clear lens with good view, young patient
Vitreous trimming around the breaks	• PVD could not be induced beyond mid-periphery • Vitreous trimming done around the breaks to prevent any postoperative vitreous traction over the break
Avoid further retinotomy for drainage	Pre-existing break ensure that the existing buckle supports the residual vitreous
360° endolaser	To ensure any anterior microbreaks are covered
Silicone oil injection	Recurrent RD with inferior break

Contd...

Contd...

(PVD: posterior vitreous detachment)

OUTCOME SUMMARY

Retina was attached on postoperative day 1 **(Fig. 18)**.

Postoperative 6 weeks, retina was attached, IOP was 12 mm Hg, and BCVA was 6/36.

Lens was clear.

KEY POINTS

- Careful identification of posterior hyaloid using tricort to facilitate proper vitrectomy.
- The buckle helps to support uncut vitreous gel.
- Recurrent RD post-SB can be due to vitreous traction on previously treated supported breaks.

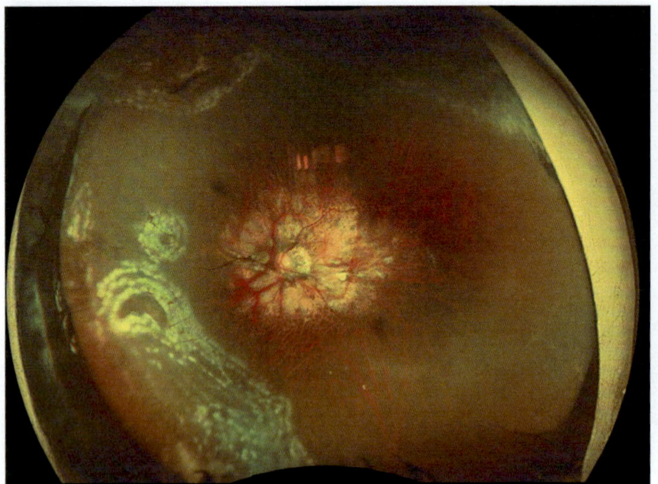

Fig. 18: Postoperative day 1 ultra-widefield fundus photograph showing an attached retina with silicone oil in situ, barrage laser marks around the break, lattice degeneration and 360°. (Case 7)

FURTHER READING

1. Mansouri A, Almony A, Shah GK, Blinder KJ, Sharma S. Recurrent retinal detachment: does initial treatment matter? Br J Ophthalmol. 2010;94(10):1344-7.
2. Wakabayashi T, Liu CK, Momenaei B, Nahar A, Yu J, Nguyen MK, et al.; Delayed Retinal Detachment Study Group. Delayed-Onset Recurrent Retinal Detachment More Than One Year After Pneumatic Retinopexy, Scleral Buckle, or Vitrectomy for Primary Rhegmatogenous Retinal Detachment Repair: Incidence, Characteristics, and Outcomes. Retina. 2025. Online ahead of print.

CASE SCENARIO 8: OBSERVATION AS A MANAGEMENT STRATEGY IN RRD

Case Summary

A 13-year-old female presented with drop in vision in the only seeing left eye.

Vision in the right eye was no light perception due to a chronic RD.

Left eye BCVA was 6/24 with IOP 12 mm Hg, the lens was clear.

Right eye had a total chronic retinal detachment. Left eye had 360° peripheral RD with macula spared and peripheral atrophic and avascular retina. No breaks/lattice were identified **(Figs. 19A and B)**.

Treatment Plan

To observe

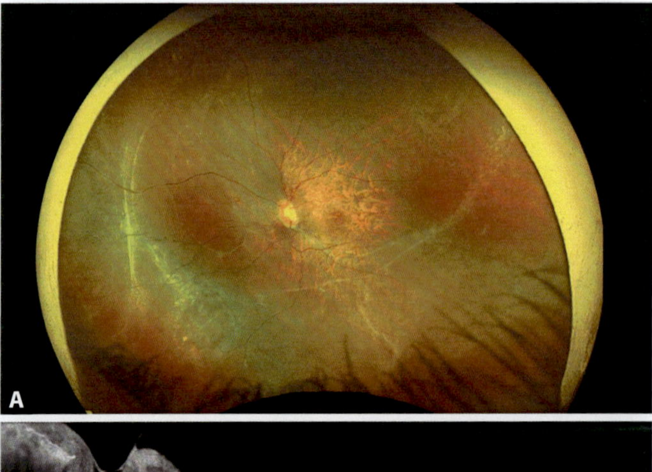

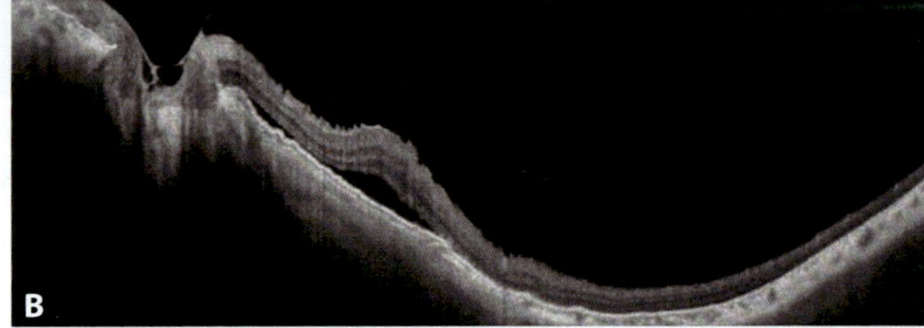

Figs. 19A and B: *At presentation:* Left eye ultra-widefield fundus photograph showing a subtotal chronic retinal detachment with multiple subretinal gliotic bands, macula attached and no breaks. Optical coherence tomography scan depicting a shallow subretinal fluid nasal to fovea with an attached fovea. (Case 8)

Thought Process

Decision	*Rationale*
To monitor progression	Long standing shallow RD with macula attached and no visible breaks

OUTCOME SUMMARY

At 4 months review, the condition was unchanged **(Fig. 20)**. Child was asked to come for regular follow-up.

KEY POINTS

- Discussion with family members of potential outcomes when deciding to observe or operate on a nonprogressive chronic RD is of utmost importance.
- Complications of vitrectomy in an eye with non-progressive RD, no break or PVD need to be considered.

FURTHER READING

1. Cohen SM. Natural history of asymptomatic clinical retinal detachments. Am J Ophthalmol. 2005;139(5):777-9.
2. Gan NY, Lam WC. Retinal detachments in the pediatric population. Taiwan J Ophthalmol. 2018;8(4):222-36.

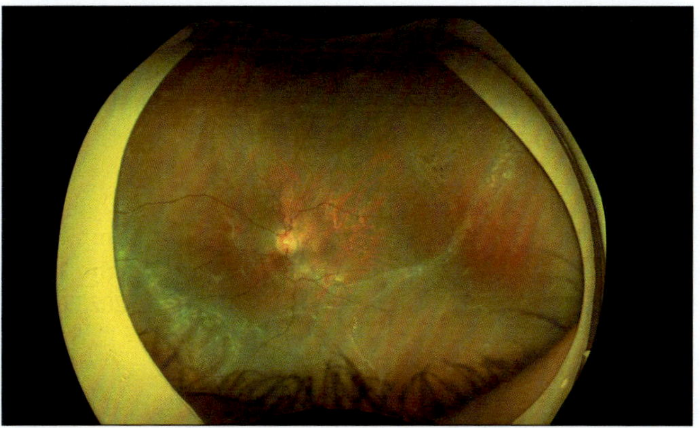

Fig. 20: After 4 months: Left eye ultra-widefield fundus photograph showing a 360° peripheral RD with macula attached and no peripheral breaks or lattices seen. (Case 8)

CASE SCENARIO 9: MANAGEMENT OF TRAUMATIC RRD

Case Summary

A 33-year-old male presented with left eye trauma with stone followed by scleral tear repair. He underwent lens matter aspiration with sulcus placed intraocular lens 4 months later. He was noted to have inferior RD then.

Patient presented 10 months post trauma for management.

BCVA was 1/60 with IOP 5 mm Hg, inferior iridodialysis, and IOL in situ (stable).

Retina showed a subtotal RD with thick epiretinal membrane at macula, subretinal gliosis, and an inferior retinal fold **(Fig. 21)**.

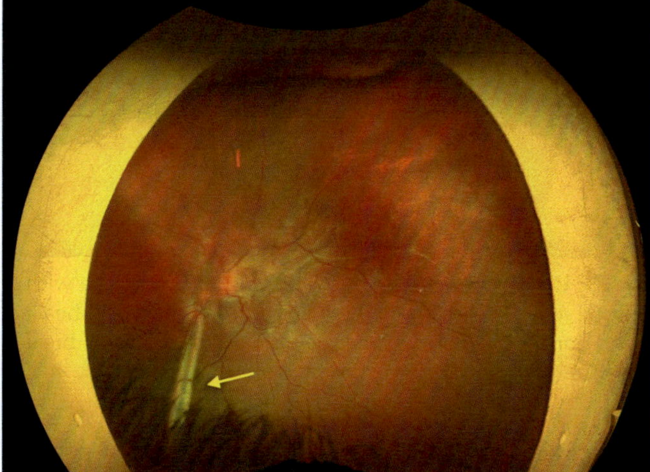

Fig. 21: Ultra-widefield fundus photograph of left eye with a subtotal retinal detachment with an inferior retinal fold (yellow arrow) and proliferative vitreoretinopathy epiretinal membranes. (Case 9)

Treatment Plan

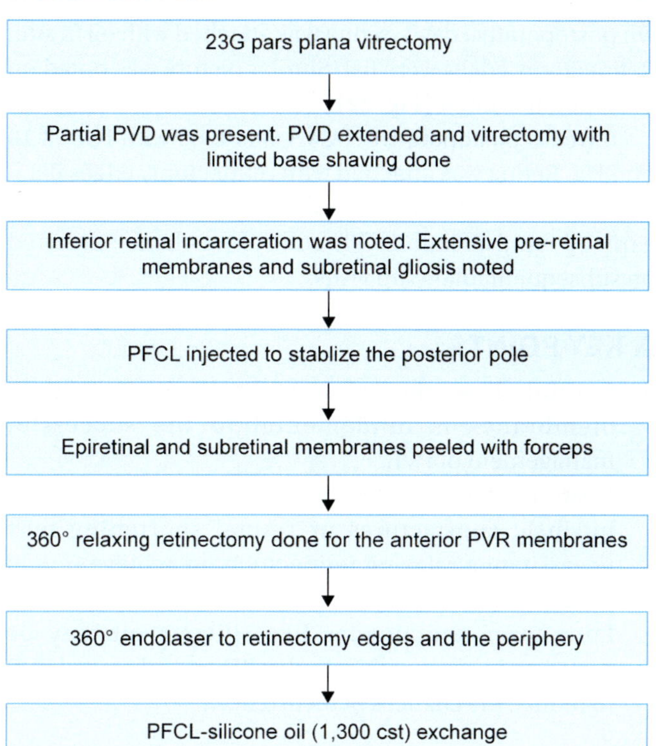

(PFCL: perfluorocarbon liquid; PVD: posterior vitreous detachment)

Thought Process

Decision	*Rationale*
Encircling band avoided	As retinectomy was planned, there was no need to support the vitreous base
Use of PFCL	To provide countertraction at posterior pole while extending PVD and making 360° retinectomy to avoid displacement of retina
360° retinectomy	In view of inferior retinal incarceration with folds and extensive peripheral membranes—to release the peripheral traction and counter the foreshortening of retina
Peeling subretinal and epiretinal membranes	To make the retina mobile, release stiffness for ease of attachment and to prevent early redetachment by contraction of these membranes
PFCL–silicone oil exchange	To avoid slippage of edge of retinectomy
Silicone oil (5,000 cst)	Long-term tamponade compared to gas

(PFCL: perfluorocarbon liquid; PVD: posterior vitreous detachment)

OUTCOME MEASURES

On postoperative day 1, retina was attached with oil in situ. Retinectomy edges were flat. Similar picture was noted on postoperative day 4 **(Fig. 22)**.

6 weeks postoperative, BCVA was 1/60 with IOP of 10 mm Hg. Retina was attached with retinectomy edges flat.

Patient had developed postoperative hypotony with early oil emulsification. Oil removal was hence deferred on subsequent follow-up visits.

KEY POINTS

- Careful dissection of epiretinal and subretinal membranes is fundamental to the successful management of PVR.
- Despite adequate membrane dissection, persistent intrinsic contractures or retinal shortening may necessitate a relaxing retinectomy to achieve retinal attachment.
- Long-term tamponades like silicone oil may be preferred in cases with complex RD and advanced PVR to reduce the chances of recurrence.

FURTHER READINGS

1. Ferro Desideri L, Artemiev D, Zandi S, Zinkernagel MS, Anguita R. Proliferative vitreoretinopathy: an update on the current and emerging treatment options. Graefes Arch Clin Exp Ophthalmol. 2024;262(3):679-87.
2. Ramamurthy SR, Dave VP, Chou HD, Ozdek S, Parolini B, Dhawahir-Scala F, et al. Retinotomies and retinectomies: A review of indications, techniques, results, and complications. Surv Ophthalmol. 2023;68(6): 1038-49.

CASE SCENARIO 10: MANAGEMENT OF RRD SECONDARY TO ACUTE RETINAL NECROSIS (ARN)

Case Summary

A 58-year-old one-eyed male with nil systemic comorbidities was on treatment for left eye acute retinal necrosis. He developed drop of vision 2 months later and was diagnosed to have a subtotal retinal detachment involving macula **(Fig. 23)**. He was on oral valacyclovir and steroids. Right eye had no light perception.

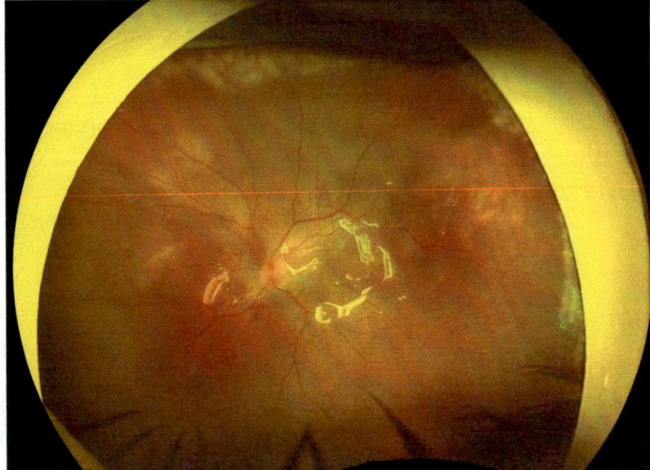

Fig. 22: Postoperative day 4 ultra-widefield fundus photograph showing an attached retina with 360° laser marks, silicone oil in situ. (Case 9)

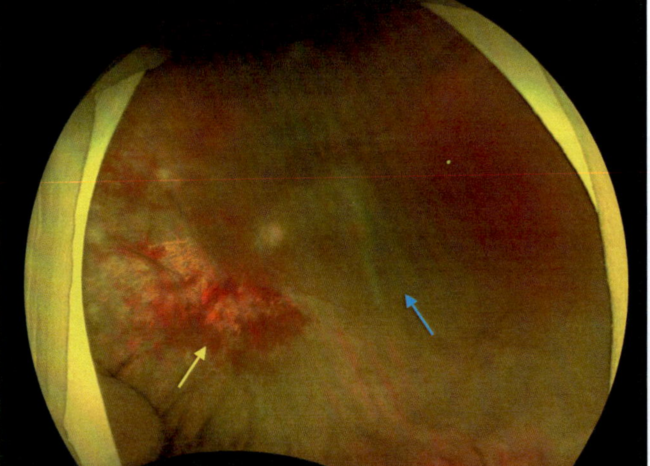

Fig. 23: Ultra-widefield fundus photograph of left eye with a subtotal retinal detachment (blue arrow) with peripheral healing ARN lesions (yellow arrow) and multiple peripheral small breaks. (Case 10)

Left eye was noted to have hand movements vision, intraocular pressure was 13 mm Hg, and a nuclear sclerosis of grade 1.

Valacyclovir tablets were continued, oral steroids were hiked up, and patient was taken up for surgical intervention.

Treatment Plan

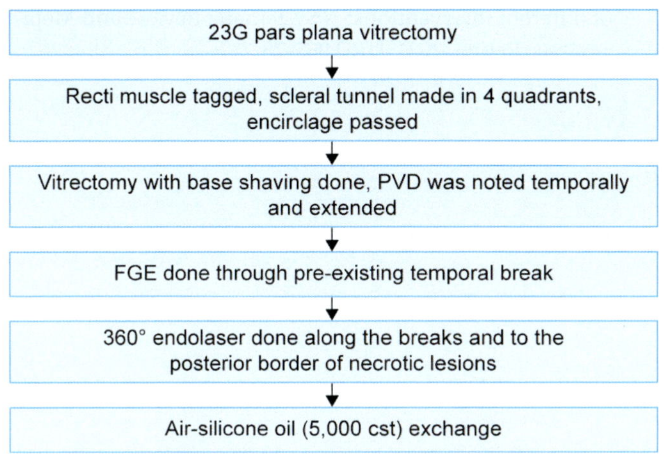

(PVD: posterior vitreous detachment)

Thought Process

Decision	*Rationale*
Encircling band	To provide support at vitreous base
Avoid lensectomy	Reasonably clear lens with good view
Hiking up oral steroids preoperative and intraoperative	To reduce inflammation in the postoperative period
Laser to the posterior border of ARN margins	High incidence of sieve like microbreaks within the retina affected by ARN
Silicone oil (5,000 cst)	Preferred in eyes with active infection and inflammation

OUTCOME MEASURES

On postoperative day 1 and 4, retina was attached with oil in situ with IOP 14 mm Hg **(Fig. 24)**. Patient was continued on tapering doses of oral steroids, and oral valacyclovir.

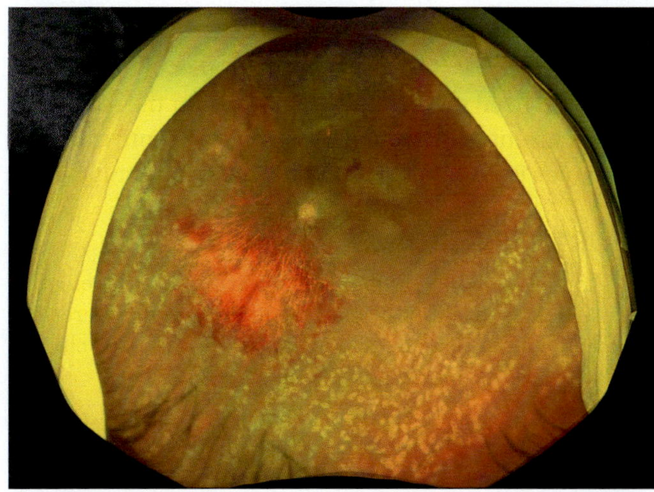

Fig. 24: Postoperative day 4 ultra-widefield fundus photograph showing an attached retina, 360° laser marks posterior to ARN margins and around the breaks with silicone oil in situ. (Case 10)

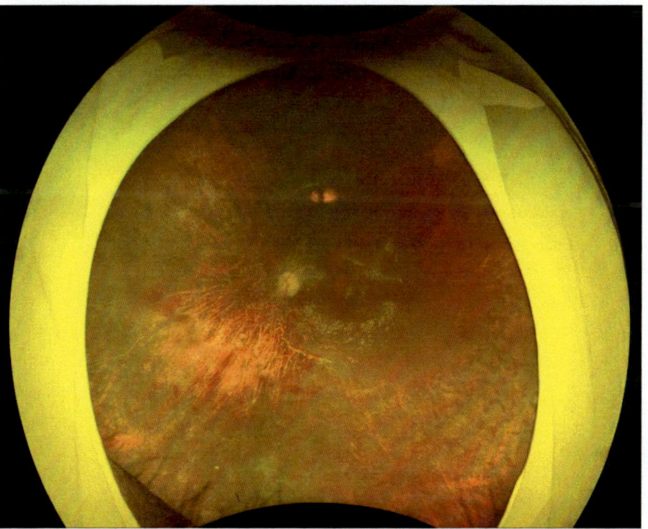

Fig. 25: Postoperative 6 weeks ultra-widefield fundus photograph showing an attached retina with 360° laser marks, silicone oil in situ and healed ARN lesions. (Case 10)

6 weeks postoperative, BCVA was 1/60 with IOP of 10 mm Hg. Retina was attached with ARN lesions healed **(Fig. 25)**.

KEY POINTS

- Eyes with viral retinitis have a high risk of developing RD and need to be closely monitored for the same.
- Concurrent management with systemic antivirals and steroids is essential for optimum surgical results.

FURTHER READING

1. Ahmadieh H, Soheilian M, Azarmina M, Dehghan MH, Mashayekhi A. Surgical management of retinal detachment secondary to acute retinal necrosis: clinical features, surgical techniques, and long-term results. Jpn J Ophthalmol. 2003;47(5):484-91.
2. Dave VP, Pappuru RR, Pathengay A, Tyagi M, Narayanan R, Jalali S. Vitrectomy with Silicone Oil Tamponade in Rhegmatogenous Retinal Detachment following Acute Retinal Necrosis: Clinical Outcomes and Prognostic Factors. Semin Ophthalmol. 2019;34(1):47-51.
3. Zhao XY, Meng LH, Zhang WF, Wang DY, Chen YX. Retinal detachment after acute retinal necrosis and the efficacies of different interventions: A Systematic Review and Meta-analysis. Retina. 2021;41(5):965-78.

CHAPTER 3

Decision Making in Surgical Management of Tractional Retinal Detachments

Chaitanya YVK, Deeksha Katoch

ALGORITHMIC APPROACH TO MANAGEMENT OF TRACTIONAL RETINAL DETACHMENT

Tractional retinal detachment

Preoperative considerations

- Visual acuity
- Duration of vision loss
- Lens status
- Media clarity
- Macular status
  - Structural
    - Attached
    - Threatened
    - Detached
  - Perfusion
    - Ischemic
    - Perfused
- PVD
  - Absent
  - Incomplete
  - Complete
- TRD
  - Vasucularity
  - Extent
    - Focal
    - Extensive
  - Location of traction
    - Predominantly anterior
    - Predominantly posterior
    - Combined (Napkin-ring)
- Systemic status
  - Glycemic control
  - Renal status
  - Anemia
  - Hypertension/CVS status
  - Antiplatelets/Anticoagulants
- Etiology

Ancillary investigations

Clear media:

- OCT (all cases)
  - Macular status
  - Integrity of ELM/EZ
  - DRIL
- FFA
  - Macular ischemia
  - Extent of peripheral CNP
  - Activity of neovascularization
- OCT angiography
  - FAZ enlargement
  - Deep capillary plexus loss

Poor fundus view:

- USG B+A scan

Preoperative anti-VEGF

Recommended (with early planned surgery):

- Broad, vascular, posterior FVP
- TRD with active neovascularization and vitreous hemorrhage

Not recommended:

- Predominantly fibrotic, avascular membranes
- Long-standing, stable TRD
- Surgery uncertain/delayed

Preoperative PRP

Recommended

Cataract surgery before or combined with vitrectomy

- Moderate to dense cataract
- Anterior or combined traction

Surgical considerations

Observation:

- Severe macular ischemia
- Chronic macula off TRD + retinal atrophy
- End-stage diabetic eye disease with no salvageable potential

Indications for surgery:

- Macula off TRD
- Macula threatening TRD
- Combined tractional-rhegmatogenous RD
- Recurrent VH with TRD
- TRD/VH with NVI

↓

- *Vitrectomy*
- Posterior hyaloid separation
- Membrane/FVP dissection
  - Segmentation/delamination
- Retina flattening (Fluid air exchange, if required)
- Endolaser
- Tamponade (if indicated)
- Postoperative anti-VEGF (if indicated)
- Positioning

Surgical considerations

Scleral encircIage

- Combined tractional rhegmatogenous RD
- Significant anterior traction
- Recurrent detachment after previous vitrectomy

ILM peeling

- Coexisting macular ERM

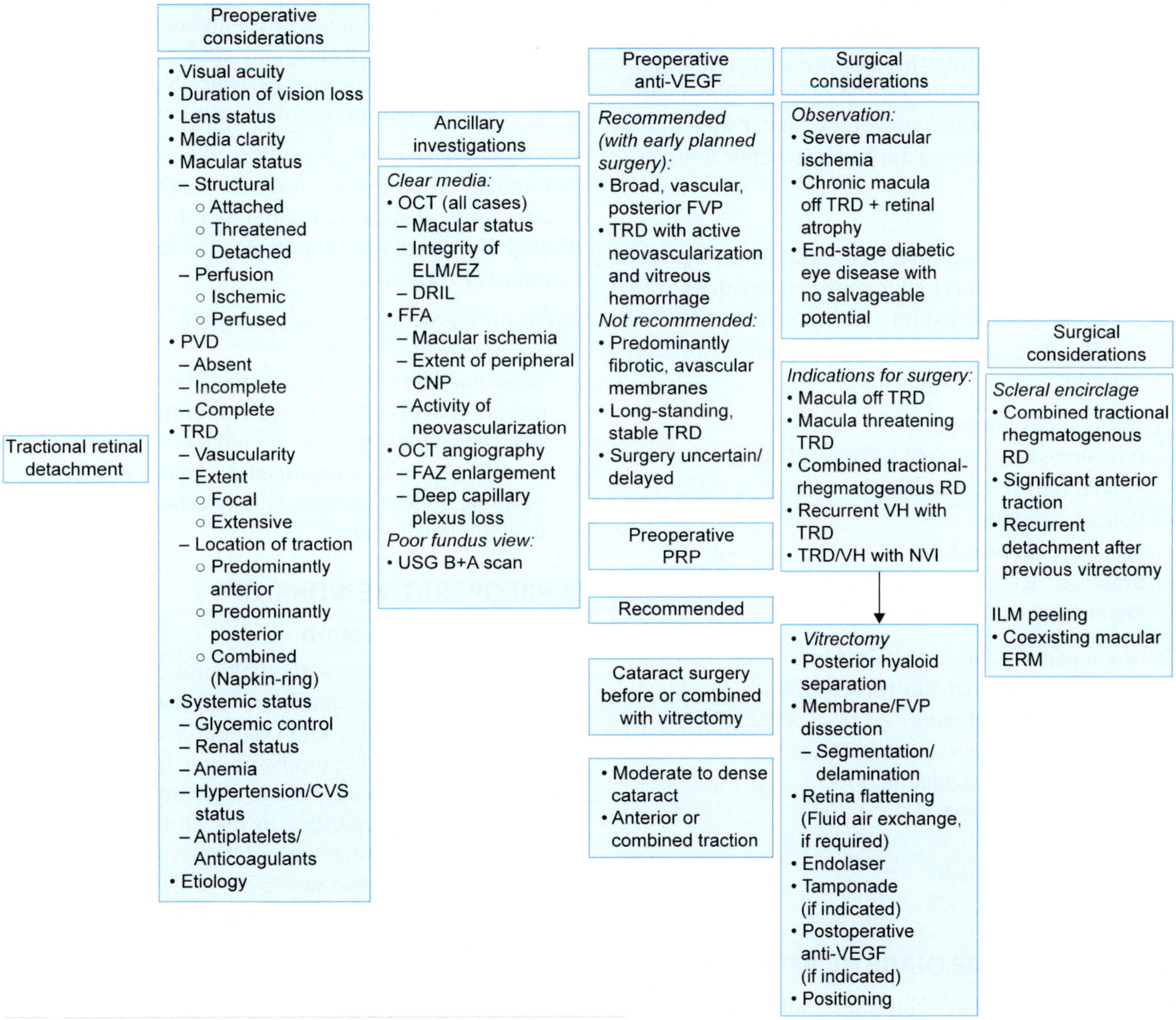

INTRODUCTION

Tractional retinal detachment (TRD) occurs when fibrovascular membranes on the retinal or vitreous surface exert contractile tractional forces that separate the neurosensory retina from the underlying retinal pigment epithelium (RPE). It is most commonly associated with retinal pathologies where chronic ischemia triggers vascular endothelial growth factor (VEGF)-driven neovascularization. The new vessels, along with proliferating glial cells and fibrous tissue, form adherent membranes that contract over time, creating traction on the retina. Unlike rhegmatogenous detachments, TRDs develop without retinal breaks, are concave or tent-like, relatively immobile and the management focuses on releasing the hyaloid and fibrovascular membranes surgically while preserving the fragile ischemic retina.[1]

ETIOLOGY

Tractional retinal detachment may develop as a consequence of various proliferative retinopathies, which can be broadly classified into two categories: (1) Those commonly affecting adults and (2) those more commonly affecting the pediatric population.[2]

Causes in adults include:

- Proliferative diabetic retinopathy (PDR)
- Retinal vein occlusion (RVO)
- Retinal vasculitis
- Sickle cell retinopathy
- Proliferative vitreoretinopathy (PVR)
- Penetrating ocular trauma

Causes in pediatric population include:

- Retinopathy of prematurity (ROP)
- Incontinentia pigmenti
- Familial exudative vitreoretinopathy (FEVR)
- Persistent fetal vasculature (PFV)
- Toxoplasma retinitis
- Toxocara retinitis
- Sickle cell retinopathy
- Trauma

PROLIFERATIVE DIABETIC RETINOPATHY

Kroll et al.[3] described the following classification which can influence surgical decision-making and carries prognostic value:

- *Stage A:* Proliferative changes are present, but there is no retinal detachment.
- *Stage B:* Vitreoretinal traction with shallow extra-macular detachment (macula not involved).
- *Stage C:* Partial detachment involving the macula.
- *Stage D:* Complete macular detachment.

The two principal anatomical indications for surgical intervention in TRD are detachment threatening the macula and detachment involving the macula.

Tractional retinal detachment threatening the macula: It is characterized by retinal elevation measuring ≥4 disk diameters, with part of the elevation located within 30° of the macular center. Alternatively, it may present as a smaller area of elevation (<4 disk diameters) associated with one or more vitreoretinal adhesions producing traction within 30° of the macula, typically in the presence of neovascularization or recent vitreous hemorrhage (VH).

Tractional retinal detachment involving the macula: Defined by vitreoretinal traction along the vascular arcades, optic disk, or tractional membranes extending through the fovea, resulting in macular detachment and consequent visual loss.

Based on the pattern of traction, the following types of TRD have been described:

- *Table-top TRD* presents as a broad, flat, and taut retinal elevation caused by diffuse vitreoretinal adhesions, often involving large areas including the macula.
- *Tent-like TRD* is a localized and peaked elevation resulting from focal vitreoretinal traction and is usually more limited in extent.

PREOPERATIVE WORK-UP

Systemic Optimization

In managing patients with PDR and TRD, systemic optimization is the first consideration. Achieving euglycemia and controlling systemic risk factors such as nephropathy and hypertension may help to stabilize retinopathy and reduce systemic morbidity.

- *Glucose levels:* According to the American Diabetes Association, the recommended perioperative target blood glucose is 80–180 mg/dL, while for critically ill patients the goal is a range of 140–180 mg/dL.[4]
- *Anesthesia considerations:* While most cases are operated under peribulbar anesthesia, patients with a history of coronary artery disease (CAD), stroke, or nephropathy.[5] It is recommended to prepare for monitored anesthesia care (MAC).
- *Anticoagulant therapy:* Evidence on perioperative management of anticoagulants and antiplatelets

in diabetic vitrectomy is conflicting. While some studies suggest increased risk of postoperative hemorrhage and reoperation if therapy is continued, others report no added risk. Decisions should be individualized, balancing ocular bleeding risk against systemic thromboembolic risk in consultation with the patient's physician. Perioperative continuation of anticoagulation or antiplatelet treatment may increase the risk of persistent postoperative vitreous cavity hemorrhage and the necessity for vitreous cavity lavage. Appropriate preoperative cessation of treatment appeared to reduce this risk; however, caution must be taken with regard to the systemic risk associated with cessation of therapy.

Preoperative Ocular Preparation

Cataract surgery: Simultaneous surgery has been reported to have slightly better visual outcomes, faster rehabilitation, and was safe. However increased risk of intraoperative miosis, posterior capsule rupture especially when the media is poor due to accompanying VH, increased postoperative inflammation and capsular opacification need to be borne in mind. It is an effective option, offering good anatomical and functional results in appropriately selected patients.[6]

Panretinal photocoagulation (PRP): PRP plays a key role in successful TRD surgery by limiting posterior pole detachment, stabilizing the periphery, and reducing the risk of iatrogenic breaks during membrane dissection. In extramacular TRDs, de novo or supplemental PRP helps to suppress neovascular activity, confine the detachment, and lower the risk of macular involvement. It is recommended to treat the attached retina with a safe margin of at least two disk diameters from the edge of traction to avoid worsening of contraction.

Anti-VEGF injection: Preoperative anti-VEGF is associated with reduced intraoperative bleeding, surgical time, iatrogenic retinal breaks, and the need for endodiathermy. Meta-analyses confirm that adjunctive anti-VEGF also lowers the risk of early postoperative vitreous cavity hemorrhage and reoperation.[7] Current evidence suggests that administering anti-VEGF 6–14 days prior to surgery offers the greatest benefit while minimizing the risk of progression of TRD.[8]

SURGICAL ARMAMENTARIUM AND SETUP

With the advent of small-gauge vitrectomy, the cutter itself now accomplishes most membrane dissection using lift-and-shave techniques, supported by wide-field viewing and valved cannula systems. High-speed small-gauge probes (≈10–20,000 cuts/min) with a port closer to the tip enable precise membrane segmentation and removal with minimal retinal traction, while their smaller diameter facilitates entry into narrow tissue planes and supports blunt dissection. For optimal surgical efficiency, the armamentarium must be organized with the following instruments and adjuncts:

Vitrectomy system	
Small gauge vitrectomy probes (25 and 27G)—up to 20,000 cuts/min, port close to the tip, beveled design	
Valved cannula-trocar system	To maintain stable chamber
High-resolution wide-field viewing system	
Chandelier illumination	For bimanual dissection
Dissection instruments	
ILM forceps Maxgrip forceps	For membrane peeling/ delamination
Delaminator	
Vertical/horizontal/curved scissors	For segmentation
Diamond dusted membrane scraper	For posterior hyaloid/to initiate planes
Finesse loop	
Adjuncts	
Triamcinolone acetonide	To stain vitreous to allow better visualization
Endolaser probes (straight/ flexible)	For PRP/to treat the breaks
Endodiathermy	For hemostasis
Endotamponade agents (SF6, C3F8, and silicone oil)	
Cryotherapy probe	For sclerotomy site

MICROSURGICAL TECHNIQUES

Port-site vitrectomy: Meticulous removal of vitreous from the superior sclerotomies should be done right at the beginning to minimize vitreous incarceration. This should be followed by clearing of retrolental space. In cases with partial PVD with elevated mid-peripheral vitreous, the hyaloid should be incised and the opening extended 360° to release anterior-posterior traction. Clear associated subhyaloid hemorrhage.

Posterior vitrectomy and membrane dissection: Posterior vitreous is trimmed using a high-cut-rate vitrector preferably used with low vacuum. Attempts to detach the posterior hyaloid should be made with caution, as this area is often tightly adherent. Intraocular forceps can be used to grasp the raised edge of the peripapillary fibrovascular proliferation (FVP) and gradually lift it after segmenting it from the surrounding adhesions to minimize the risk of iatrogenic break.

Segmentation: Dividing extensive FVP membranes into manageable islands. Tissue plane must be identified for safe introduction of instruments between fibrovascular membranes and retina. Cutter should be oriented in such a way that the port faces away from the retina. Dense FVP can be tackled by reducing the cut rates. Isolated nodes of proliferation are hence created which can then be removed.

Delamination: Delamination involves peeling the FVP and membranes off the retinal surface. Techniques for delamination include:

- *Fold back method:* Membranes are segmented and then removed by being folded back into cutter port while the bevel protects the retina.
- *Conformal delamination:* Orientation of the cutter follows the retinal contour and the beveled tip is applied to the edge of FVP.
- *Delaminator:* It helps to lift and separate tightly adherent FVP from the retinal surface, especially when dissection with scissors or the cutter risks creation of iatrogenic breaks and hemorrhage. The tip is gently slid between the membrane and the underlying retina to create or enlarge a dissection plane. Once the initial separation is achieved, the membrane can then be peeled with forceps or segmented with cutter.
- *Proportional reflux-assisted delamination:* Proportional reflux system available in some vitrectomy platforms has been described as a safe and controlled technique of enlarging the dissection plane.[9]
- *Bimanual dissection (scissors + forceps):* Useful when membranes are tightly adherent. Underlying retina should be protected by avoiding excessive spreading or force under membranes.

Internal limiting membrane (ILM) peeling: It is not always mandatory but can be considered in cases where the membrane scaffold may contribute to recurrent neovascularization or in detachments complicated by macular holes. Risks must be weighed, particularly in fragile retina.

Hemostasis: Once bleeding occurs, use cautery sparingly to coagulate bleeding vessels. Alternatively, gentle aspiration, increasing infusion pressure, or gentle tamponade with beveled tip of the cutter (especially for mild oozers) can be performed. Maintain awareness of disk perfusion—high infusion pressures may risk optic neuropathy or corneal edema, especially in eyes with compromised anterior segment health.

Endolaser (PRP): After all traction is relieved, laser photocoagulation is applied around retinal breaks. PRP extending to untreated peripheral ischemic areas (often aided by scleral depression) is done to reduce future neovascular drive and stabilize the retina.

Tamponade: When there are retinal breaks or a rhegmatogenous component, use gas or silicone oil tamponade. In cases without breaks, air may suffice—also helping with intraoperative visibility and reducing chance of postoperative hemorrhage.

Adjunctive anti-VEGF: It is recommended to administer anti-VEGF at the end of surgery to suppress any residual neovascularization and reduce the risk of postoperative vitreous cavity hemorrhage.

Wound closure: Secure port sites to avoid hypotony, which can exacerbate bleeding or worsen anatomical outcomes.

REFERENCES

1. Stewart MW, Browning DJ, Landers MB. Current management of diabetic tractional retinal detachments. Indian J Ophthalmol. 2018;66(12):1751-62.
2. Mishra C, Tripathy K. Retinal Traction Detachment. In: StatPearls [Internet]. Treasure Island (FL): StatPearls Publishing; 2025.
3. Kroll P, Rodrigues EB, Hoerle S. Pathogenesis and classification of proliferative diabetic vitreoretinopathy. Ophthalmologica. 2007;221(2):78-94.
4. American Diabetes Association. 14. Diabetes Care in the Hospital: Standards of Medical Care in Diabetes-2018. Diabetes Care. 2018;41(Suppl 1):S144-51.
5. Shaikh N, Kumar V, Ramachandran A, Venkatesh R, Tekchandani U, Tyagi M, et al. Indian J Ophthalmol. 2024;72(12):1704-13.
6. Moraru AD, Costin D, Moraru RL, Branisteanu DC. Outcomes of simultaneous vs. sequential pars plana vitrectomy and cataract surgery. Exp Ther Med. 2020; 20(6):183.
7. Zhao LQ, Zhu H, Zhao PQ, Hu YQ. A systematic review and meta-analysis of clinical outcomes of vitrectomy with or without intravitreal bevacizumab pretreatment for severe diabetic retinopathy. Br J Ophthalmol. 2011;95(9):1216-22.

8. Sun X, Wang X, Guo X, Wang M, Liu H. Combined use of anti-VEGF drugs before and during pars plana vitrectomy for severe proliferative diabetic retinopathy. Ophthalmol Ther. 2023;12(6):3133-42.
9. Jain S, Agarwal A, Aggarwal K, Gupta V. The role of proportional reflux during pars plana vitrectomy for tractional retinal detachments. Ophthalmic Surg Lasers Imaging Retina. 2019;50(2):113-5.

CASE SCENARIO 1: MANAGEMENT OF BILATERAL TRD WITH VH

Case Summary

A 62-year-old female, with history of type 2 diabetes, initially under regular review was lost to follow-up for 2 years and presented with severe diminution of vision in both the eyes (BE). She had visual acuity (VA) of hand movements in BE, fundus examination of right eye (RE) revealed partially treated PDR with laser scars, VH, and FVP involving the posterior pole **(Fig. 1A)**. Left eye (LE) had extensive FVP over the posterior pole with localized combined traumatic rhegmatogenous retinal detachment (T-RRD) **(Fig. 1B)**.

Treatment Plan

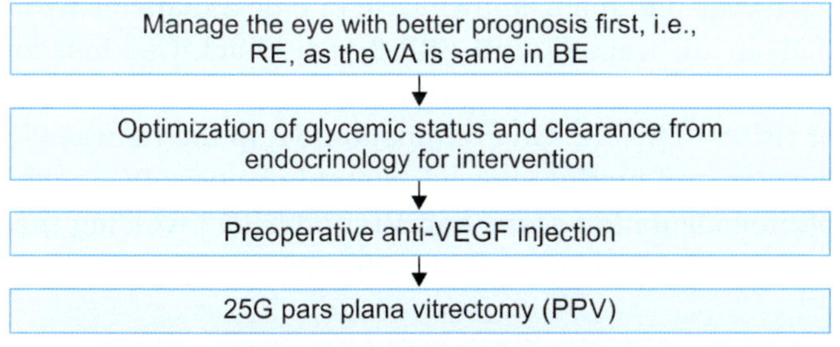

Surgical Steps

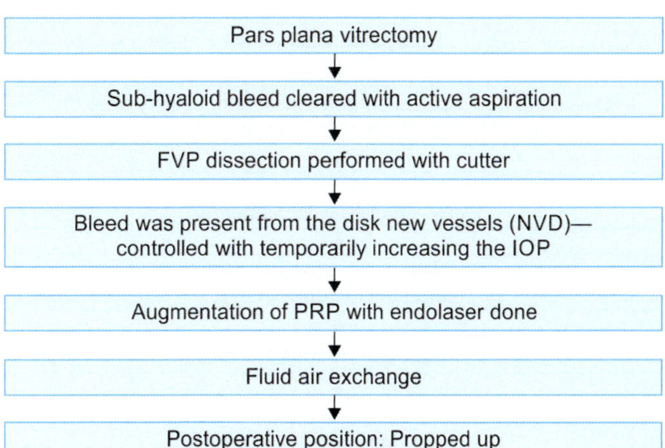

Thought Process

Decision	*Rationale*
Preoperative PRP	Easier induction of PVD, reduce vascularity of FVP
Preoperative anti-VEGF	To reduce intraoperative hemorrhage, easier surgical dissection of FVP, reduce postoperative vitreous cavity hemorrhage (POVCH)
Choice of tamponade	Complete traction release was achieved, and there was no significant intraoperative bleed, so air tamponade was chosen
Postoperative propped up	To aid inferior settling of any residual blood and optimize tamponade effect

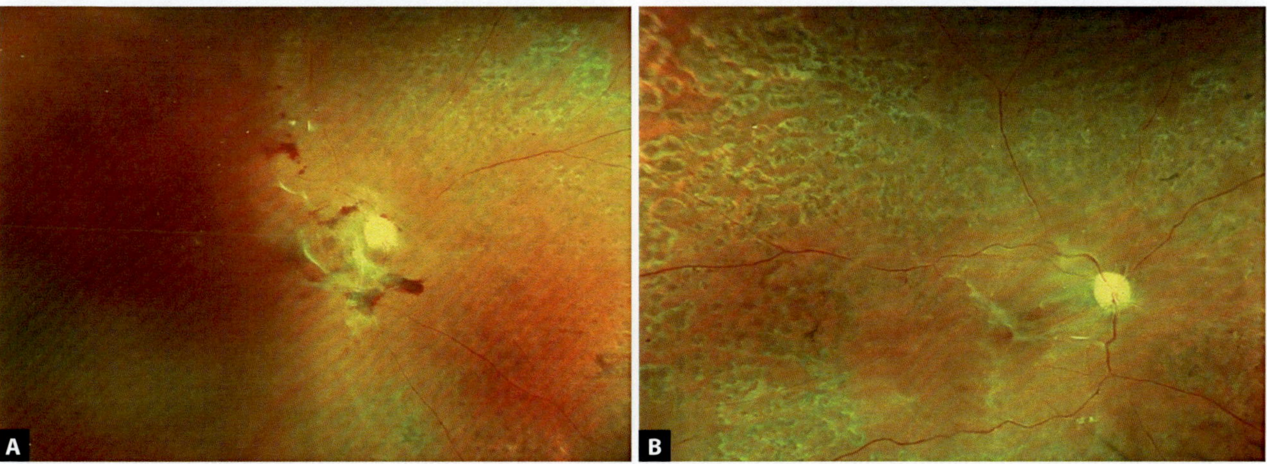

Figs. 1A and B: (A) Ultrawide field fundus photograph of RE showing partially treated PDR with vascular FVP and VH; (B) Postoperative photograph showing media grade I attached retina. (FVP: fibrovascular proliferation; PDR: proliferative diabetic retinopathy; RE: right eye; VH: vitreous hemorrhage)

Surgical Steps LE

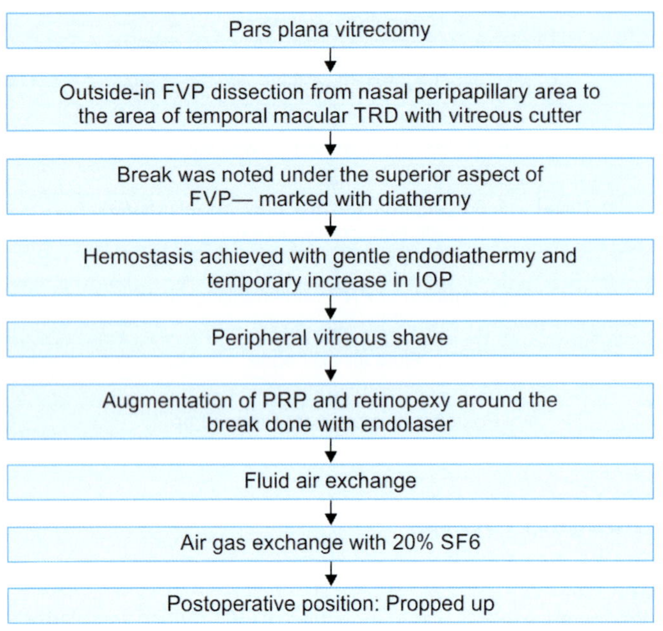

OUTCOME SUMMARY

Postoperative photographs RE and LE with clear media and attached retina **(Figs. 2A and B)**.

KEY POINTS

- In bilateral diabetic TRD with similar VA, the eye with less complex pathology should be prioritized to facilitate early functional recovery.
- Preoperative anti-VEGF, when combined with timely vitrectomy, facilitates safer FVP dissection by reducing intraoperative bleeding, but mandates vigilance for tractional progression.
- The choice of tamponade should be individualized based on adequacy of traction release and presence of retinal breaks.

FURTHER READING

1. McCullough P, Mohite A, Virgili G, Lois N. Outcomes and Complications of Pars Plana Vitrectomy for Tractional Retinal Detachment in People With Diabetes: A Systematic Review and Meta-analysis. JAMA Ophthalmol. 2023;141(2):186-95.
2. Zhao LQ, Zhu H, Zhao PQ, Hu YQ. A systematic review and meta-analysis of clinical outcomes of vitrectomy with or without intravitreal bevacizumab pretreatment for severe diabetic retinopathy. Br J Ophthalmol. 2011;95(9): 1216-22.

CASE SCENARIO 2: MANAGEMENT OF PDR WITH PREDOMINANTLY VASCULAR TRD

Case Summary

A 51-year-old, male, known case of type 2 diabetes with PDR in BE treated with PRP 3 years back was lost to follow-up and presented with sudden onset diminution of vision in his RE. On examination, VA in the RE was PL positive and fundus showed asteroid hyalosis, PDR with photocoagulation scars, and VH and TRD involving the macula with florid vascularity **(Fig. 3A)**.

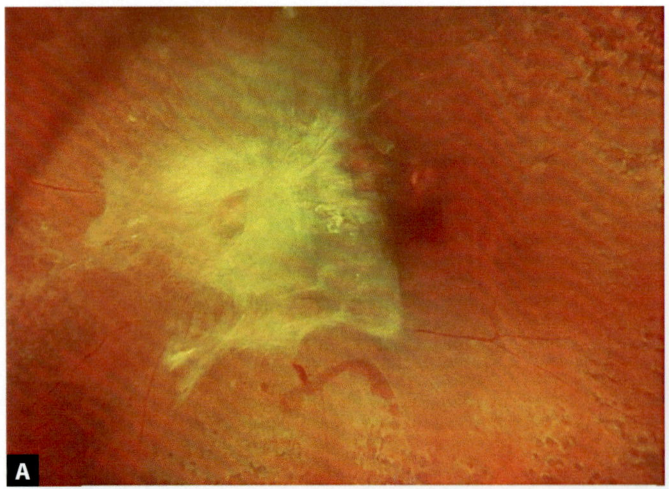

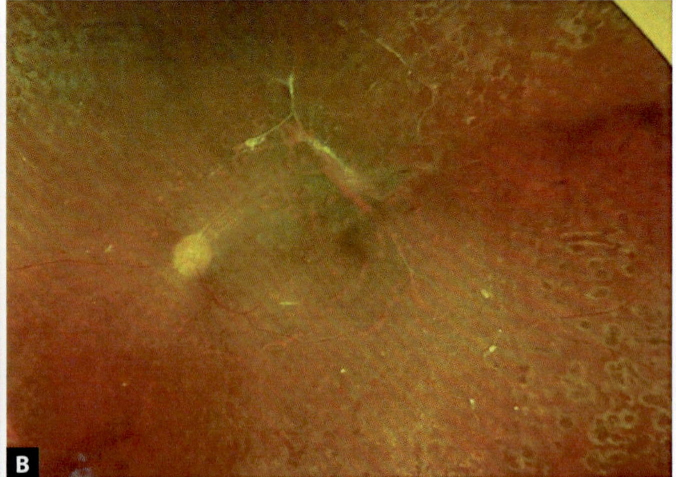

Figs. 2A and B: (A) Ultrawide field fundus photograph of LE depicting extensive FVP with prominent vascularity, combined T-RRD, and laser scars in the periphery; (B) Postoperative photograph showing media grade I attached retina. (FVP: fibrovascular proliferation; LE: left eye; T-RRD: traumatic rhegmatogenous retinal detachment)

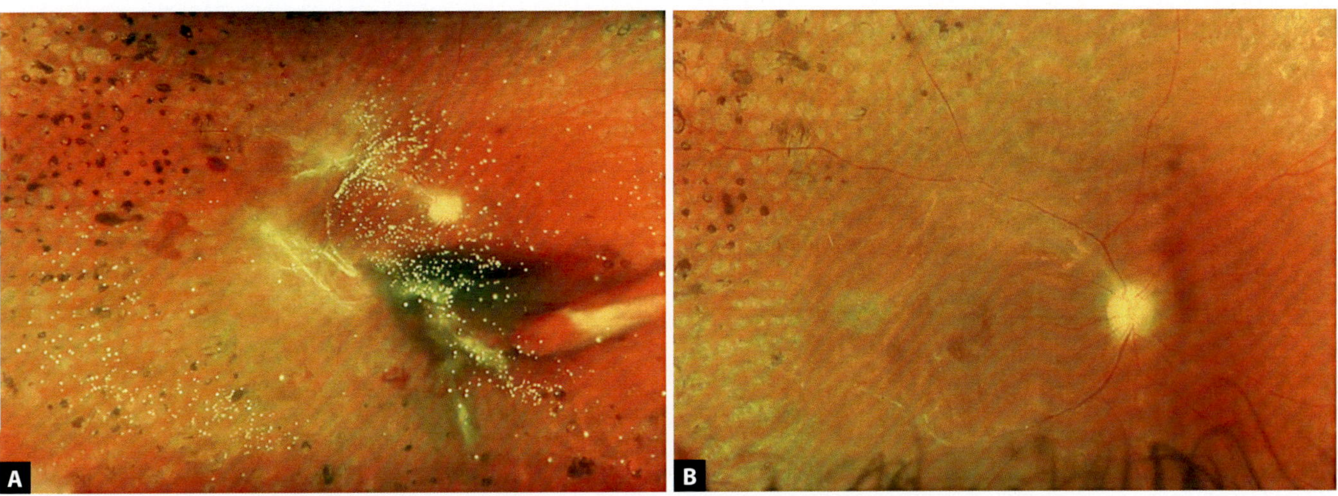

Figs. 3A and B: (A) Ultrawide-field fundus photograph of RE with asteroid hyalosis PDR, VH, and temporal macular TRD; and (B) Postoperative photograph showing media grade I, attached retina and PRP scars.

Treatment Plan

Optimisation of glycaemic status and clearance from endocrinology for intervention
↓
Augmentation of PRP
↓
Preoperative anti-VEGF injection
↓
25G PPV

Surgical Steps

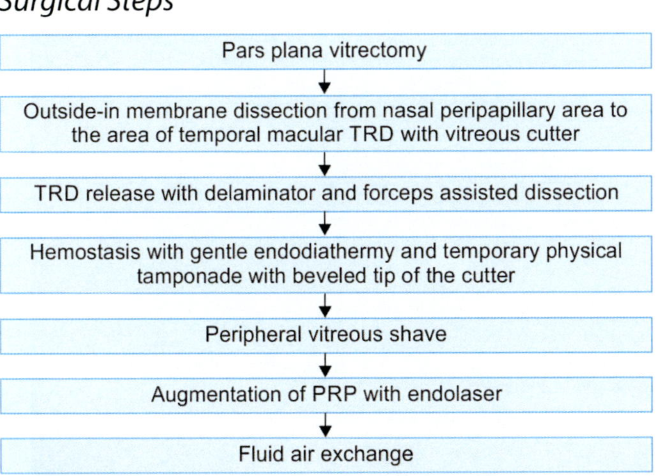

Thought Process

Decision	*Rationale*
Preoperative PRP augmentation	Easier induction of PVD, reduce vascularity of FVP
Preoperative anti-VEGF	To reduce intraoperative hemorrhage, easier surgical dissection of FVP, reduce postoperative vitreous cavity hemorrhage (POVCH)
Outside in delamination using vitreous cutter	Ease of creation of cleavage plane peripherally
Use of endodiathermy and mechanical tamponade with cutter tip	To immediately achieve hemostasis, prevention of clot formation
Air tamponade	Reduce chances of early post-operative vitreous cavity bleed

Contd...

Contd...

OUTCOME SUMMARY

Postoperative media was grade I, attached retina with adequate PRP scars **(Fig. 3B)**.

KEY POINTS

- Sudden visual loss in previously treated PDR should raise suspicion for acute vitreoretinal interface events such as VH with progressive macular traction.
- Outside-in delamination, initiated in relatively avascular peripapillary regions, provides a controlled and safer approach in eyes with dense, highly vascular FVP.
- Effective intraoperative hemostasis, combining endodiathermy and mechanical tamponade, is critical in reducing early POVCH and improving surgical visualization.

FURTHER READING

1. Chen YT, Radke NV, Amarasekera S, Park DH, Chen N, Chhablani J, et al. Updates on medical and surgical managements of diabetic retinopathy and maculopathy. Asia Pac J Ophthalmol (Phila). 2025;14(2):100180.
2. Liao A, Fortes B, Au A, Hou K. Management of diabetic tractional retinal detachments: surgical experiences from a large tertiary academic institution. Curr Opin Ophthalmol. 2025;36(3):177-81.

CASE SCENARIO 3: MANAGEMENT OF BILATERAL PDR WITH COMBINED TRACTIONAL-RHEGMATOGENOUS RD IN LE (MANAGED WITH GAS TAMPONADE) AND VH WITH TRD IN RE

Case Summary

A 41-year-old diabetic male with nephropathy, under regular follow-up for PDR with prior PRP and intravitreal anti-VEGF for macular edema, was lost to follow-up for 9 months. He presented with profound diminution of vision in BE, RE was CF @ ½ m and LE was HMCF. There was no iris neovascularization and fundus examination of both eyes showed treated PDR with VH, extensive FVP and TRD **(Fig. 4A)**.

Treatment Plan

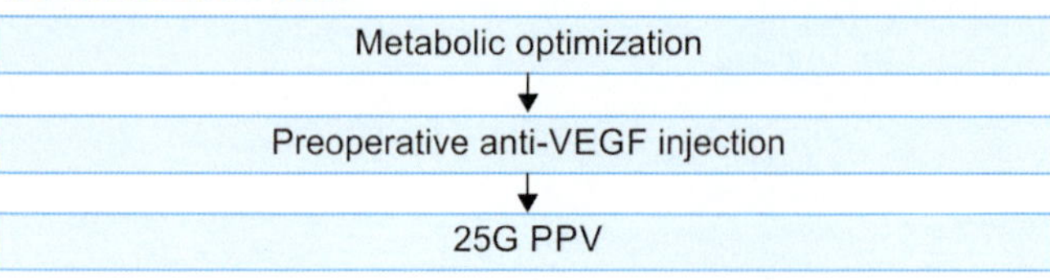

Surgical Steps LE

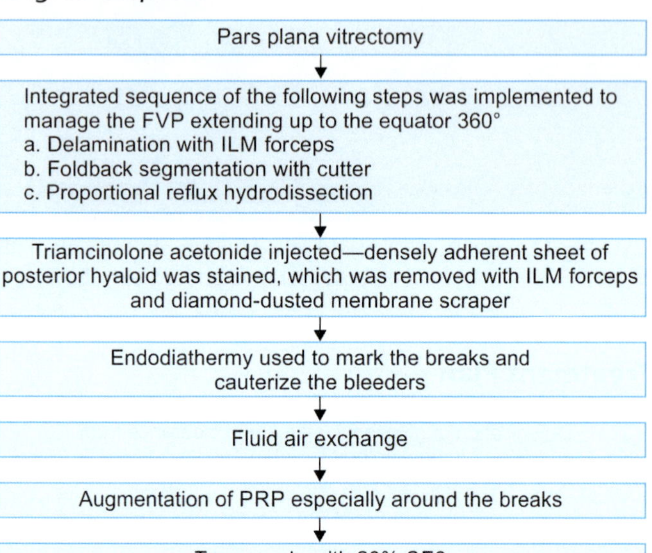

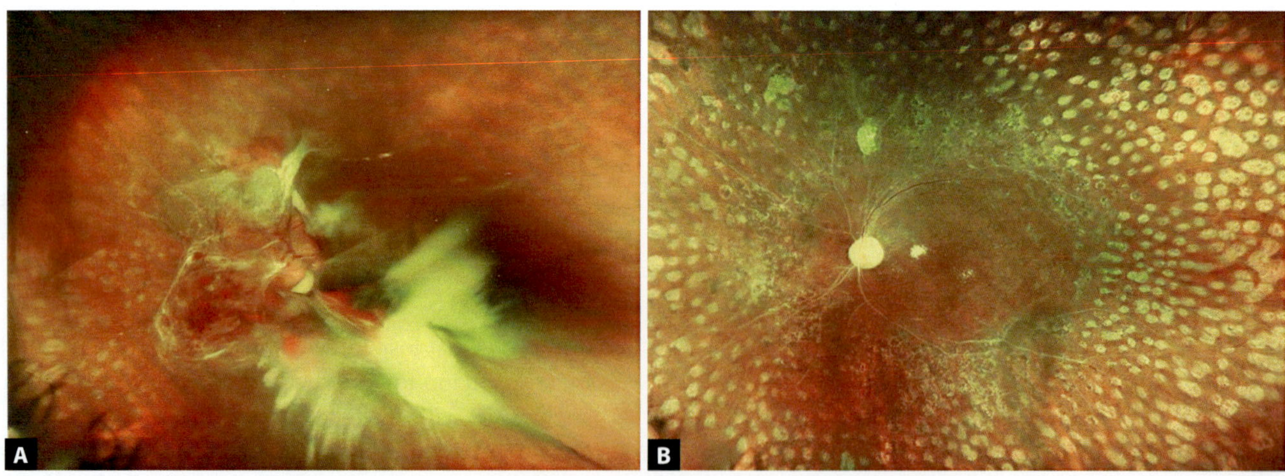

Figs. 4A and B: (A) Ultrawide field fundus photograph of the LE showing VH, extensive, predominantly vascular FVP involving the posterior pole and combined T-RRD, PRP, and scars present; (B) Postoperative photograph showing media grade I and attached retina. (FVP: fibrovascular proliferation; LE: left eye; PRP: panretinal photocoagulation; T-RRD: traumatic rhegmatogenous retinal detachment; VH: vitreous hemorrhage)

Postoperative Position

The patient was advised to assume prone position with an option to alternate with left lateral position (to effectively tamponade the break).

Thought Process

Decision	*Rationale*
Preoperative PRP	Easier induction of PVD, reduce vascularity of FVP
Preoperative anti-VEGF	To reduce intraoperative hemorrhage, easier surgical dissection of FVP, reduce postoperative vitreous cavity hemorrhage (POVCH)
Choice of tamponade	In view of adequate relief of traction and absence of inferior pathology, gas was chosen for internal tamponade

Surgical Steps RE

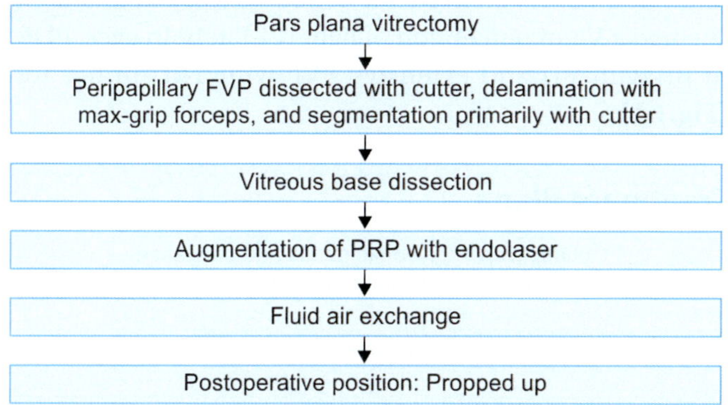

OUTCOME SUMMARY

Postoperative VA improved to 3/60 with media grade I, no loose blood, and attached retina with adequate PRP scars **(Fig. 4B)**.

KEY POINTS

- Circumferential (360°) FVP extending to the equator represents one of the highest-risk configurations in diabetic vitrectomy and requires a multimodal membrane dissection strategy rather than a single technique.
- Triamcinolone-assisted visualization of the posterior hyaloid is particularly valuable in eyes with dense, sheet-like adhesion, enabling safer and more complete traction relief.
- In combined RD with complete traction release and no inferior pathology, gas tamponade provides effective break support while avoiding the morbidity of long-term tamponade.

FURTHER READING

1. Gupta B, Wong R, Sivaprasad S, Williamson TH. Surgical and visual outcome following 20-gauge vitrectomy in proliferative diabetic retinopathy over a 10-year period, evidence for change in practice. Eye (Lond). 2012;26(4):576-82.
2. Shaikh N, Kumar V, Ramachandran A, Venkatesh R, Tekchandani U, Tyagi M, et al. Vitrectomy for cases of diabetic retinopathy. Indian J Ophthalmol. 2024;72(12):1704-13.

CASE SCENARIO 4: MANAGEMENT OF BRVO-RELATED TRD

Case Summary

A 66-year-old, female, poorly controlled hypertensive, presented with diminution of vision in her LE for 3 months. On examination, she had a VA of 1/60 in LE and fundus examination revealed superior combined traction rhegmatogenous retinal detachment with sclerosed vessels and scatter laser scars **(Fig. 5)**. Fundus fluorescein angiography (FFA) showed extensive capillary nonperfusion involving the superior retina and NVEs suggestive of superior BRVO-related combined RD.

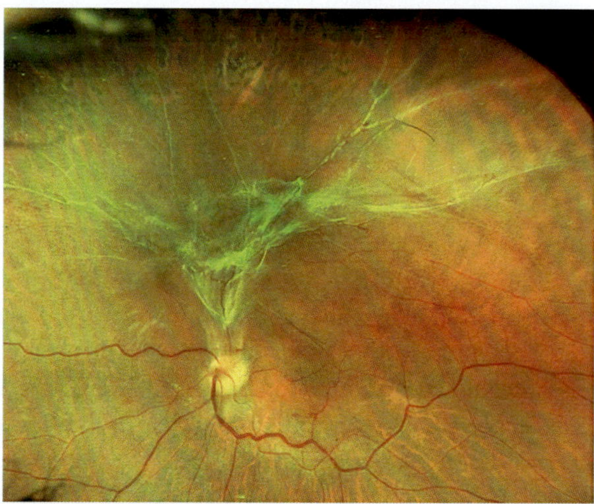

Fig. 5: Ultrawide field fundus photograph of the LE showing superior sclerosed vessels with combined RD and superior laser scars.

Treatment Plan

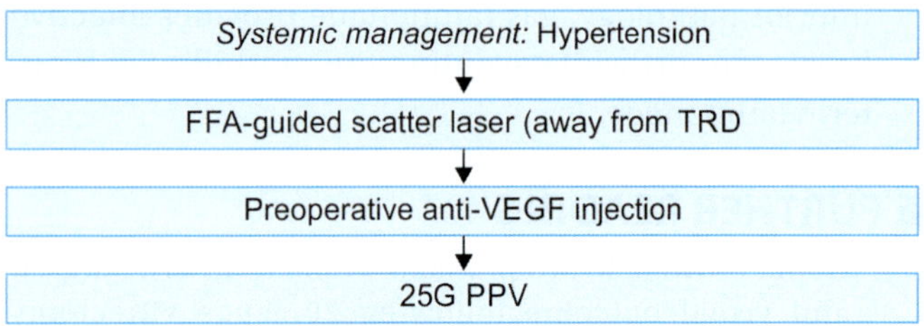

Surgical Steps

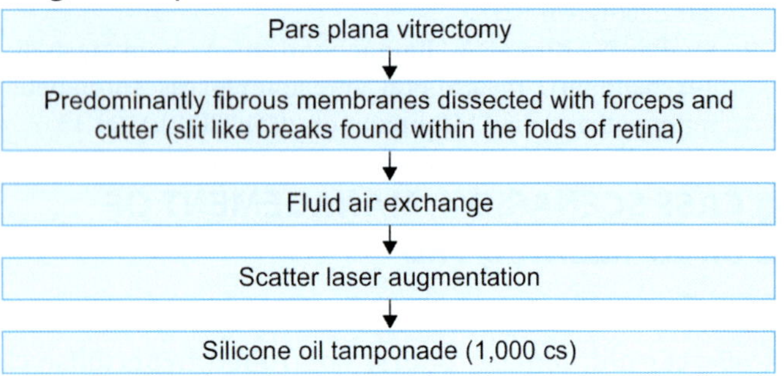

Thought Process

Decision	*Rationale*
Perform FFA	To determine the cause of combined RD and assess prognosis of intervention
Preoperative PRP augmentation	Easier induction of PVD, reduce vascularity of FVP
Preoperative anti-VEGF	To reduce intraoperative hemorrhage, easier surgical dissection of FVP, reduce POVCH
Injection of silicone oil	To provide long-term tamponade, prevent further neovascular growth

KEY POINTS

- BRVO-related TRD arises from chronic sectoral ischemia-driven neovascularization and should be distinguished from diabetic TRD due to its localized distribution and differing prognosis.
- FFA-guided assessment of capillary nonperfusion is critical in identifying the ischemic drive, planning laser placement away from tractional zones, and anticipating postoperative neovascular behavior.
- In combined RD associated with venous occlusion, long-term tamponade with silicone oil is often preferred to counter persistent ischemic stimulus and reduce the risk of recurrent traction or neovascular proliferation.

FURTHER READING

1. Ikuno Y, Ikeda T, Sato Y, Tano Y. Tractional retinal detachment after branch retinal vein occlusion. Influence of disc neovascularization on the outcome of vitreous surgery. Ophthalmology. 1998;105(3):417-23.

CASE SCENARIO 5: MANAGEMENT OF PDR WITH EXTENSIVE TRD

Case Summary

A 39-year-old, female, known diabetic for the last 9 years with poor glycemic control and history of diabetic foot (left) which required below-knee amputation presented with diminution of vision in BE for 3 months. On examination, she had a VA of perception of light (PL) in both eyes, PDR in BE with VH and extensive FVP with TRD in her RE **(Fig. 6A)**.

Treatment Plan

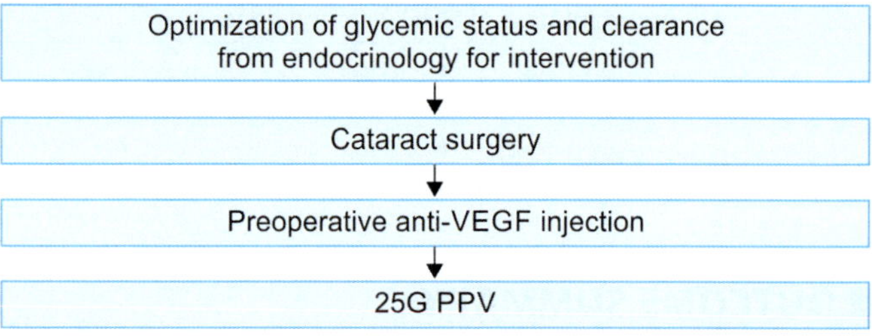

Surgical Steps

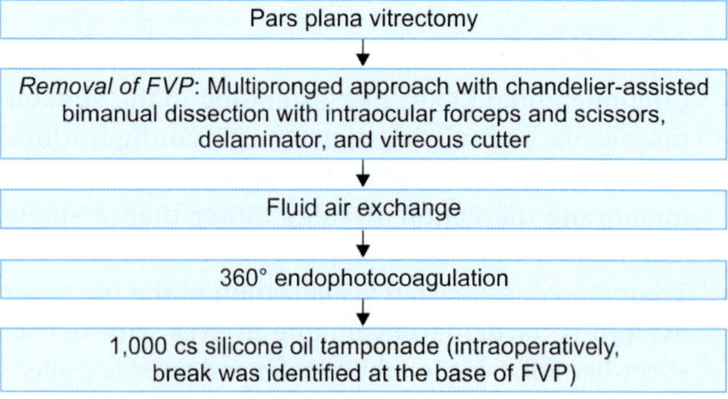

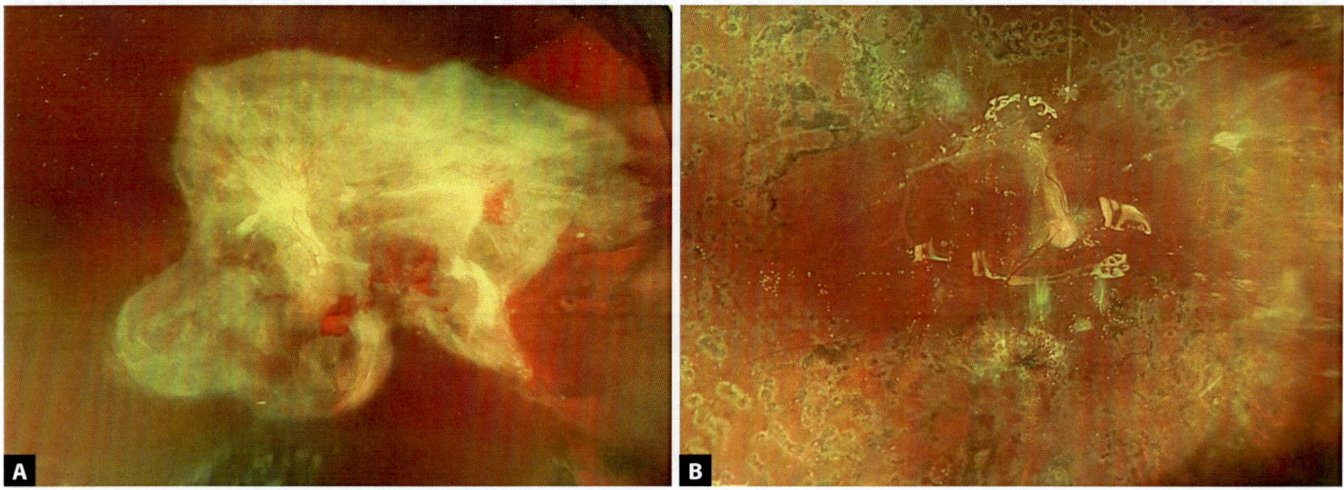

Figs. 6A and B: (A) Ultrawide field fundus photograph of RE depicting PDR with VH, extensive FVP; and TRD; (B) Postoperative photograph of RE with attached retina, PRP scars, silicone oil reflex. (FVP: fibrovascular proliferation; PDR: proliferative diabetic retinopathy; RE: right eye; PRP: panretinal photocoagulation; TRD: tractional retinal detachment; VH: vitreous hemorrhage)

Thought Process

Decision	*Rationale*
Preparatory cataract surgery	To improve the visualization of membranes during PPV
Preoperative anti-VEGF	To reduce intraoperative hemorrhage, easier surgical dissection of FVP, reduce postoperative vitreous cavity hemorrhage (POVCH)
Usage of Chandelier illumination	To facilitate bimanual dissection using a combination of forceps, scissors, delaminator, and beveled tip cutter
Injection of silicone oil	To provide long-term tamponade, prevent further neovascular growth

OUTCOME SUMMARY

Postoperative VA improved to counting finger close to face (CFCF) with attached retina under silicone oil **(Fig. 6B)**.

KEY POINTS

- Chandelier-assisted bimanual dissection is invaluable in extensive, densely adherent fibrovascular membranes, allowing controlled segmentation and delamination while minimizing iatrogenic retinal breaks.
- In eyes with extensive TRD, intraoperative breaks, and high ischemic drive, silicone oil provides durable tamponade and suppresses recurrent neovascularization when visual recovery is uncertain.

FURTHER READING

1. Shroff CM, Gupta C, Shroff D, Atri N, Gupta P, Dutta R. Bimanual Microincision Vitreous Surgery for Severe Proliferative Diabetic Retinopathy: Outcome in more than 300 eyes. Retina. 2018;38 (Suppl 1):S134-S145.

VIDEO LEGEND

Video 1: Tractional retinal detachment.

CHAPTER 4

Decision Making in Surgical Management of Exudative Retinal Detachments

Meenakshi Mahesh, Simakurthy Sriram, P Mahesh Shanmugam

ALGORITHMIC APPROACH TO MANAGEMENT OF EXUDATIVE RETINAL DETACHMENTS

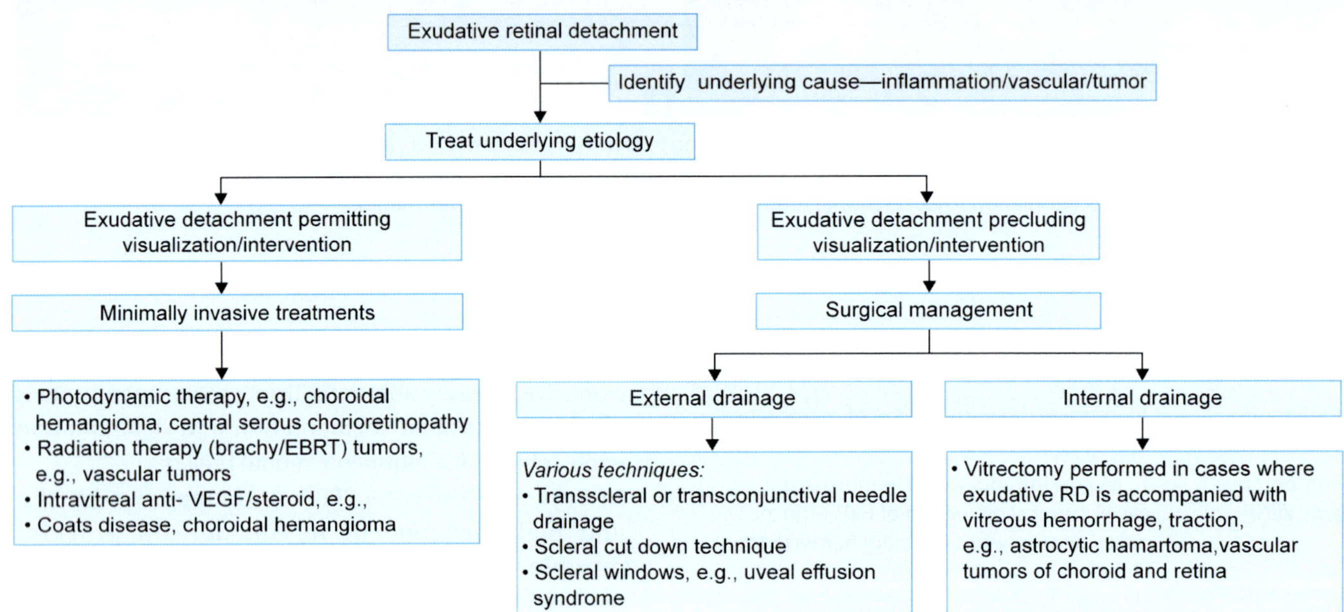

CASE SCENARIO 1: MANAGEMENT OF EXUDATIVE DETACHMENT IN COATS DISEASE

Coats disease, first described by George Coats in 1908, is a rare, idiopathic, nonhereditary retinal vascular disorder predominantly affecting young males, usually unilaterally. It is characterized by retinal telangiectasia, aneurysmal dilatations, and massive lipid exudation, which may progress to exudative retinal detachment (RD) and vision loss. The pathogenesis involves vascular endothelial growth factor (VEGF)-mediated breakdown of the blood-retinal barrier and subsequent exudation.

Indication

Exudative RD obscuring visualization/located immediately posterior to the lens precluding interventions such as laser photocoagulation.

Contraindications

- End-stage disease (stage 5) with phthisical or blind painless eye, where observation is preferred.
- Painful blind eye with neovascular glaucoma or phthisis, where enucleation is indicated.

Case Summary

A 6-year-old male child was brought by parents with complaints of poor vision in his left eye for last 8 months. Best-corrected visual acuity (BCVA) was 6/6 in the right eye and hand movements close to face (HMCF) in the left eye. Intraocular pressure was 16 mm Hg in the right eye and 24 mm Hg in the left eye. The right eye anterior segment and fundus examination was unremarkable. The left eye showed a shallow anterior chamber, clear lens, and an exudative RD just behind the lens with subretinal hard exudates and telangiectatic vessels **(Fig. 1)**.

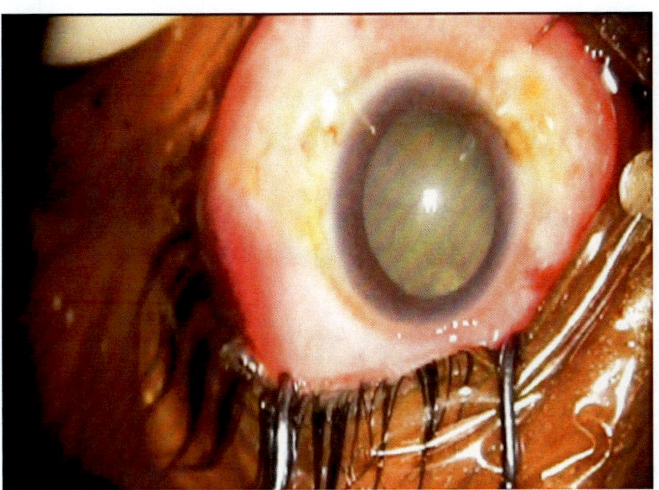

Fig. 1: Intraoperative snapshot showing exudative retinal detachment just behind the lens with subretinal yellowish exudates and telangiectatic vessels

B-scan ultrasonography showed a bullous RD with dot-like subretinal echoes due to subretinal exudates. No high amplitude mass lesion was noted in B-scan ultrasonography. There was no family history of similar ocular complaints. A clinical diagnosis of Coats disease with exudative RD was made, and external drainage of subretinal fluid (SRF) was performed under general anesthesia **(Figs. 2A to D)**.

Treatment Plan

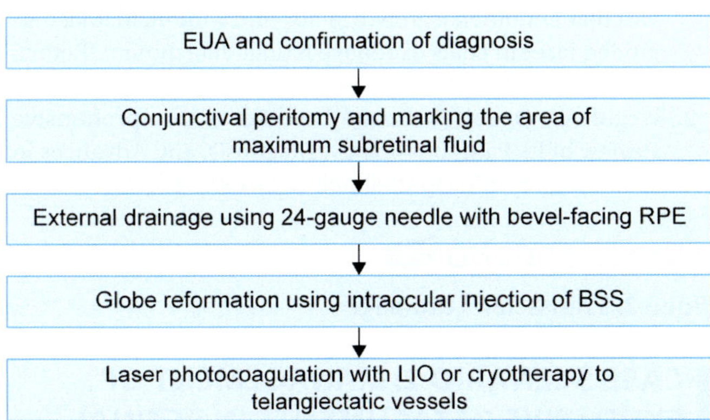

(BSS: balanced salt solution; EUA: examination under anesthesia; RPE: retinal pigment epithelium; LIO: laser indirect ophthalmoscopy)

Thought Process

Step	*Rationale*
Anesthesia	General anesthesia is usually preferred in pediatric age group
Peritomy and muscle tagging	• Helps to rotate globe to point of interest, i.e., site of external drainage, particularly in cases with scleral cut-down technique • Also, traction on muscles help in retention of globe contour during SRF drainage
Drainage	• Via needle—less traumatic, bevel should face surgeon and toward RPE when visualized internally • Via scleral cutdown—more traumatic than needle drainage, needs cauterization of choroid, but more likely to drain completely. Preferred in shallow RD wherein a needle drainage can cause iatrogenic retinal damage. • Alternatively, we can use laser drainage technique in scleral cut down, wherein laser cauterizes choroidal vessels
IOP maintenance	• Via intravitreal route or intracameral injection of saline helps to reform the globe pressure and provides a positive pressure to push subretinal fluid
Add-on procedures	• LIO done to telangiectasias helps to reduce the exudation • Green laser is preferred as the hemoglobin in the vascular malformations will absorb the same • Anti-VEGF/steroid injections at the end of the procedure help to counter the elevated VEGF levels in these cases

(IOP: intraocular pressure; LIO: laser indirect ophthalmoscopy; RD: retinal detachment; SRF: subretinal fluid; VEGF: vascular endothelial growth factor)

OUTCOME SUMMARY

Postoperatively, the retina was successfully reattached with regression of exudation and telangiectatic changes. The child's visual acuity improved to only counting fingers close to face at 3 months.

KEY POINTS

- In Coats disease, management depends on the stage and extent of exudation.
- External drainage is necessary in Coats disease in extreme RD or when the RD does not allow treatment of vascular malformations.

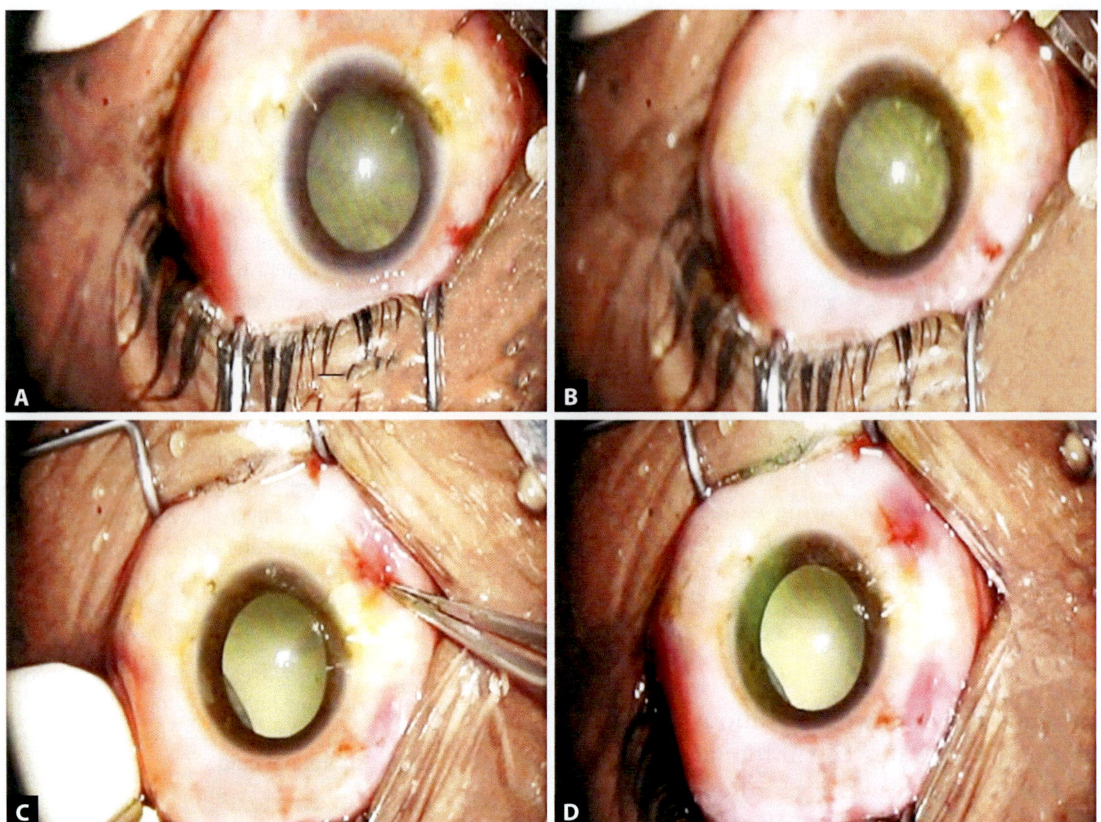

Figs. 2A to D: (A) At the beginning of surgery—exudative detachment just behind the lens; (B and C) Needle drainage at the site of maximum subretinal fluid; and (D) At the end of the procedure.

- External drainage avoids a retinotomy and is preferred. It can be transconjunctival or transscleral.
- In certain scenarios external drainage of subretinal fluid is combined with intravitreal injection of anti-VEGF/ steroid and laser photocoagulation of telangiectatic vessels.
- Possible complications include subretinal hemorrhage, residual detachment, proliferative vitreoretinopathy, recurrence of exudation, and secondary glaucoma.
- If an eye with Coats disease needs drainage, the visual prognosis in these eyes is poor due to extensive exudation, particularly submacular scar and poor retinal function due to long-standing RD. However, treating these eyes can prevent them from becoming totally blind and painful.
- Postoperatively, frequent follow-ups are warranted for need of additional laser photocoagulation for residual or new areas of telangiectasia or additional procedures such as repeat intravitreal injection of steroids/ anti-VEGF.

FURTHER READING

1. Stanga PE, Jaberansari H, Bindra MS, Gil-Martinez M, Biswas S. Transscleral drainage of subretinal fluid, anti-vascular endothelial growth factor, and wide-field imaging-guided laser in coats exudative retinal detachment. Retina. 2016;36(1):156-62.
2. Ucgul AY, Özdek Ş. Coats' Disease: A Comprehensive Review of Its Pathophysiology, Diagnosis, and Advances in Treatment. Semin Ophthalmol. 2025;40(6):458-73.

VIDEO LEGEND

Video 2: Transscleral drainage

CASE SCENARIO 2: MANAGEMENT OF EXUDATIVE DETACHMENTS IN RETINAL HEMANGIOBLASTOMA

Retinal hemangioblastoma (retinal capillary hemangioma) is a rare and benign vascular tumor commonly associated with von Hippel–Lindau (VHL) disease, and an autosomal dominant hereditary disorder. Clinically, it appears as a pinkish-orange nodular mass with dilated, tortuous feeder, and draining vessels. Leakage from these vessels can lead to intraretinal and subretinal exudation, resulting in vision-threatening complications such as macular edema or exudative RD. In contrast, choroidal hemangioma is a benign vascular tumor of the choroid, typically appearing as an orange-red and dome-shaped lesion associated with serous RD. It may occur as a circumscribed form or as part of systemic conditions such as Sturge–Weber syndrome.

Indication

Bullous RD not allowing for laser treatment of tumor

Contraindications

- Tumors with significant tractional/combined exudative/tractional and rhegmatogenous RD
- Tumors which are visible enough to allow laser treatment/photodynamic therapy (PDT)

Case Summary

A 17-year-old male patient presented with gradually progressive blurred vision in his left eye for last 6 months. Best-corrected visual acuity (BCVA) was 6/6 in the right eye and hand movements close to face (HMCF) in the left eye. Intraocular pressure was 12 mm Hg in the right eye and 24 mm Hg in the left eye. The right eye was unremarkable. Left eye showed a reddish-orange mass lesion at posterior pole with exudative RD with subretinal hard exudates **(Fig. 3)**. A clinical diagnosis of peripapillary hemangioblastoma with exudative RD was made. As PDT was unavailable, surgical external drainage of the SRF was performed under binocular indirect ophthalmomicroscopic (BIOM) visualization. After reduction of SRF, laser photocoagulation was applied to the tumor **(Fig. 4)**, followed by an intravitreal injection of triamcinolone.

Treatment Plan

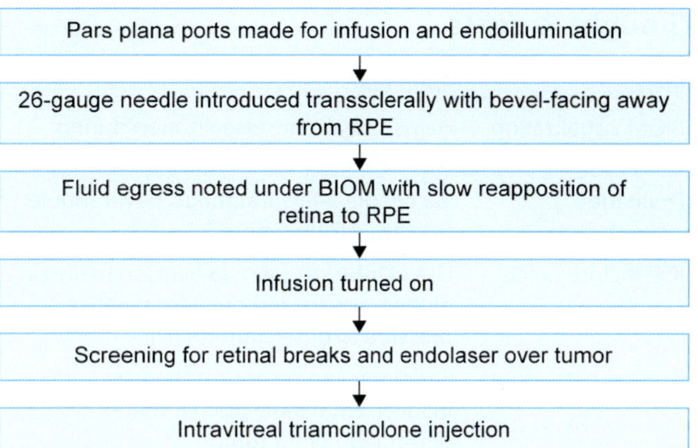

(BIOM: binocular indirect ophthalmomicroscopy; RPE: retinal pigment epithelium)

Learning points of the technique: The needle mounted on the syringe is held in the dominant hand of the surgeon and the needle is used to depress on the sclera, visualizing the depressed mound internally. The needle tip is gently moved to the area of maximum SRF, monitored by the movement of the depression mound (as one would do localization of the break in scleral buckling surgery). Once the needle tip is in the correct place, the needle is

Fig. 3: Intraoperative snapshot showing orange-red mass lesion at posterior pole with exudative retinal detachment.

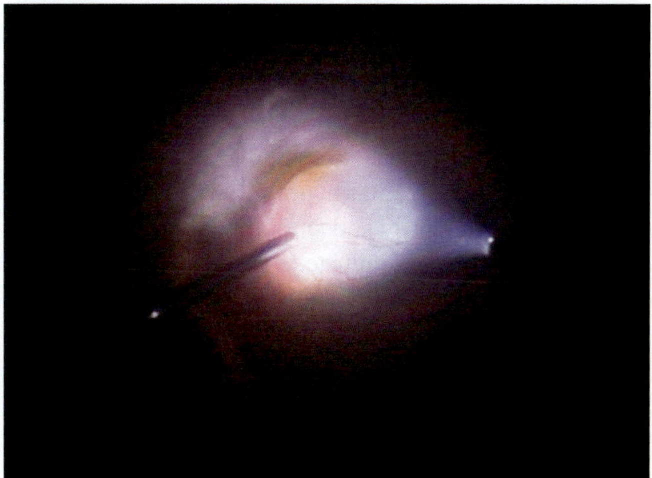

Fig. 4: Intraoperative snapshot after external drainage of subretinal fluid showing orange-red peripapillary hemangioblastoma.

tangentially inserted through the sclera. The tip of the metallic needle entering the subretinal space can be seen and once the bevel is within the eye, further advancement of the needle is not necessary.

As the SRF egresses the eye, the retina can be seen to drape the surface of the needle—the needle is then gently eased out along the same path of insertion.

Thought Process

Step	*Rationale*
BIOM visualization	Helps in real-time visualization during drainage
Drainage	Via needle—less traumatic, bevel should face away from retina
IOP maintenance	Use of infusion cannula helps to maintain globe pressure and provides positive pressure to push subretinal fluid
Add-on procedures	Endolaser can be done if there is inadvertent needle drainage site perforation or for tumor

(BIOM: binocular indirect ophthalmomicroscopy; IOP: intraocular pressure)

OUTCOME SUMMARY

Postoperatively, the retina was successfully reattached; however, the visual acuity continues to be guarded due to long-standing RD.

KEY POINTS

- *Optimal needle orientation:* The needle bevel should always be directed away from the retina to minimize the risk of retinal incarceration or inadvertent retinal break formation.
- *Controlled drainage:* Maintaining intraocular pressure with an infusion cannula prevents choroidal detachment and ocular hypotony. The needle should be withdrawn slowly and smoothly to avoid tractional injury during fluid drainage.
- *Immediate tumor-directed therapy:* Once the exudative detachment is drained and the retina reattaches, tumor-targeted treatment—such as laser photocoagulation or PDT—can be performed in the same session.
- Combined vitrectomy-assisted drainage may be preferable for extensive, posteriorly located, or recurrent lesions where external drainage alone may be insufficient.

FURTHER READING

1. Huang Y, Hu W, Huang X. Retinal hemangioblastoma in a patient with Von Hippel-Lindau disease: A case report and literature review. Front Oncol. 2022;12:963469.
2. Shields CL, Honavar SG, Shields JA, Cater J, Demirci H. Circumscribed choroidal hemangioma: Clinical manifestations and factors predictive of visual outcome in 200 consecutive cases. Ophthalmology. 2001;108(12):2237-48.

VIDEO LEGEND

Video 3: Needle drainage under BIOM

CASE SCENARIO 3: MANAGEMENT OF EXUDATIVE DETACHMENT IN UVEAL EFFUSION

Background

A scleral window is a lamellar sclerectomy, created to enhance the uveoscleral outflow, and reducing scleral resistance to the outflow. This method was first described by Gass et al. in 1983.[1] Some authors described vortex vein decompression or unroofing the veins during sclerectomy. This could, however, lead to vein amputation or hemorrhage. The presence of large flaps during vein decompression was thought to produce better results. Multiple groups have, thereafter, described positive long-term results with this procedure.[2] Usage of topical mitomycin C has been described to prevent recurrent fibrosis or blockage of the outflow path. With regard to nanophthalmic eyes, adequate precautions should be ensured and the risks involved clearly discussed. Most authors suggest scleral windows before or during cataract or other intraocular surgeries to prevent uveal effusion, expulsive hemorrhage or aqueous misdirection.

Indications

- Uveal effusion secondary to:
  - Nanophthalmos
  - With angle closure disease
  - Refractory choroidal effusion
- To prevent choroidal detachment or hemorrhage after glaucoma surgery in a high-risk eye
- Glaucoma management in uncontrolled IOP, aphakic eyes, some cases of uveitic and congenital glaucoma

Contraindication

Eyes with thinned out sclera—myopes, previous scleral inflammation with thinning or trauma.

Case Summary

A 47-year-old man presented with history of decreased vision in both eyes for 2 weeks. He had a history of headache and tinnitus. He was diagnosed to have Vogt–Koyanagi–Harada (VKH) elsewhere but noticed minimal improvement of vision with intravenous methylprednisolone (IVMP). Best corrected visual acuity was 6/9 N8 and 6/24 N10 in right and left eye, respectively. Fundus examination showed disc hyperemia and occasional vitreous cells in both eyes. The right eye also showed RPE: retinal pigment epithelium (RPE) changes temporal to the macula, with SRF. The left eye had subretinal fibrin, inferior exudative RD and peripheral choroidal detachment **(Figs. 5A and B)**. Optical coherence tomography (OCT) of both eyes showed pachychoroid (700 and 800 μ in right and left eye, respectively) **(Figs. 6A and B)**. Axial length of both eyes was around 23 mm, on B scan. Fluorescein angiography (FFA) showed focal inkblot leaks, suggestive of central serous chorioretinopathy (CSR) **(Figs. 7A to D)**, for which focal laser was done. 1-week post-laser, the right eye showed resolution of SRF. However, there was a significant increase in the height of bullous detachment which was almost touching the lens in the left eye, along with peripheral choroidal detachment **(Figs. 8A and B)**. Type II UES was the working diagnosis. Hence, a four-quadrant scleral window with surgical decompression of vortex veins and trans-scleral SRF drainage was performed. Histopathology of the scleral tissue was suggestive of increased alcian blue uptake of scleral tissue due to increased glycosaminoglycans, indicating thickened sclera **(Figs. 9A and B)**.

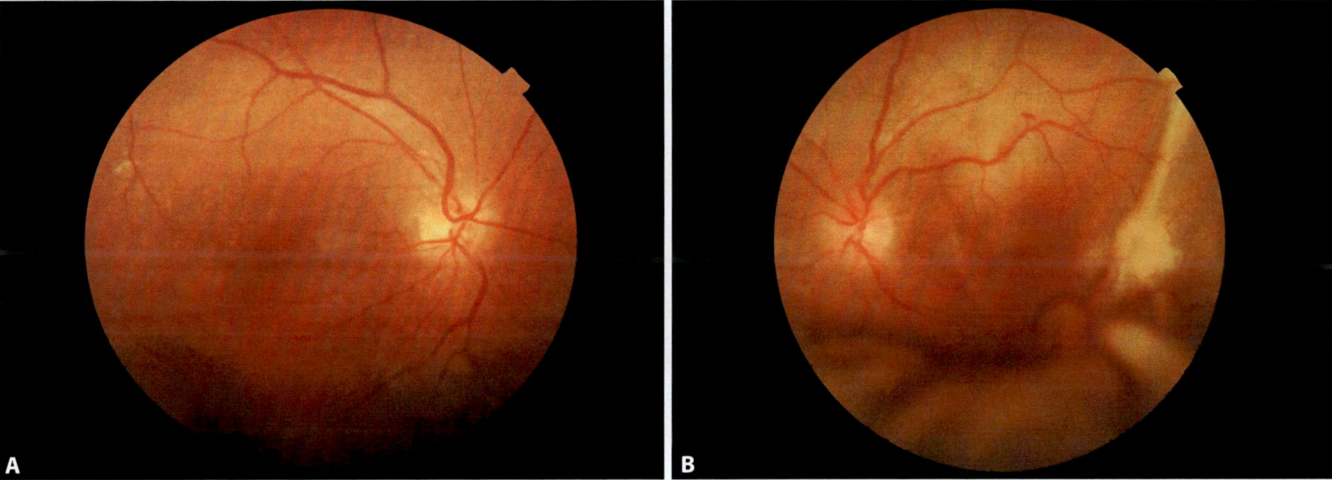

Figs. 5A and B: (A) Fundus photograph of the right eye showing minimal disk hyperemia, RPE changes temporal to the macula and SRF; (B) Fundus photograph of the left eye showing minimal disk hyperemia, subretinal fibrin and inferior exudative retinal detachment. (RPE: retinal pigment epithelium; SRF: subretinal fluid)

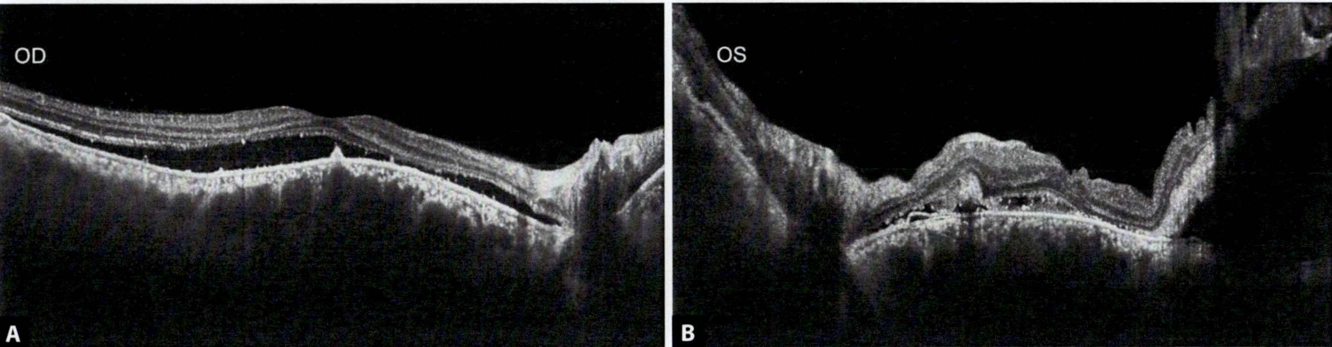

Figs. 6A and B: (A) OCT of the right eye showing vitreous cells, shallow SRF and PED with pachychoroid; (B) OCT of the left eye showing vitreous cells, subretinal fibrin and SRF, with pachychoroid. (OCT: optical coherence tomography; PED: pigment epithelial detachments; SRF: subretinal fluid)

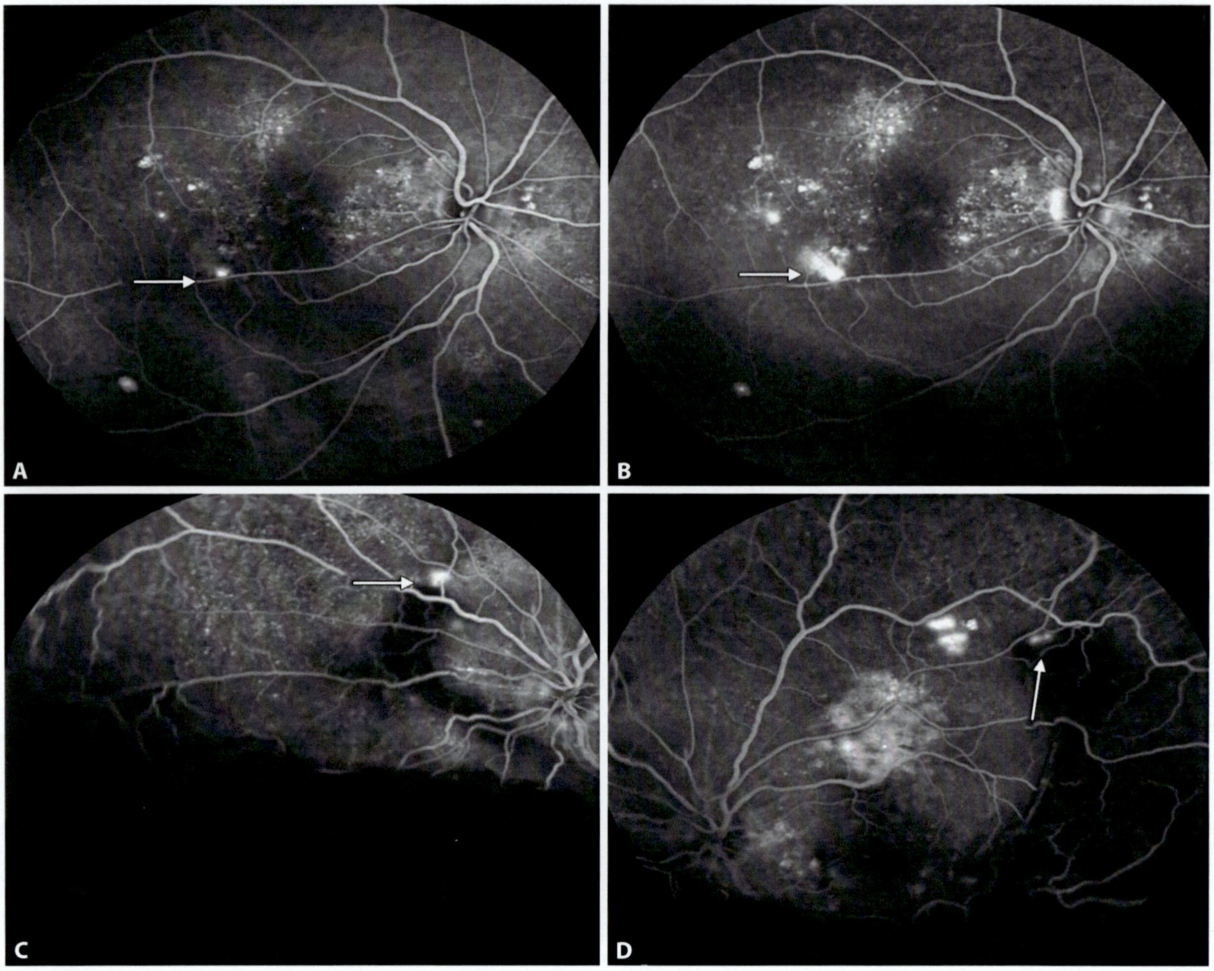

Figs. 7A to D: Fundus fluorescein angiography (FFA) of the right and left eye showing focal leaks, increasing in intensity and size in late frames.

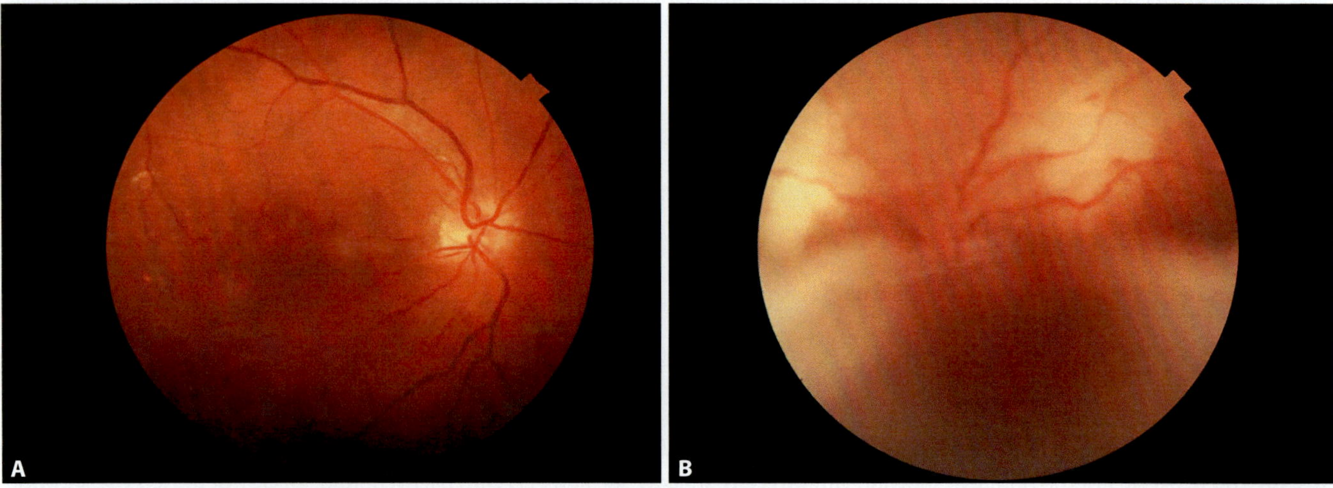

Figs. 8A and B: 1-week postfocal laser—right eye shows resolution of the SRF; (B) 1-week postfocal laser—left eye—increase in height of bullous retinal detachment, anteriorly touching lens, along with 360° choroidal detachments.

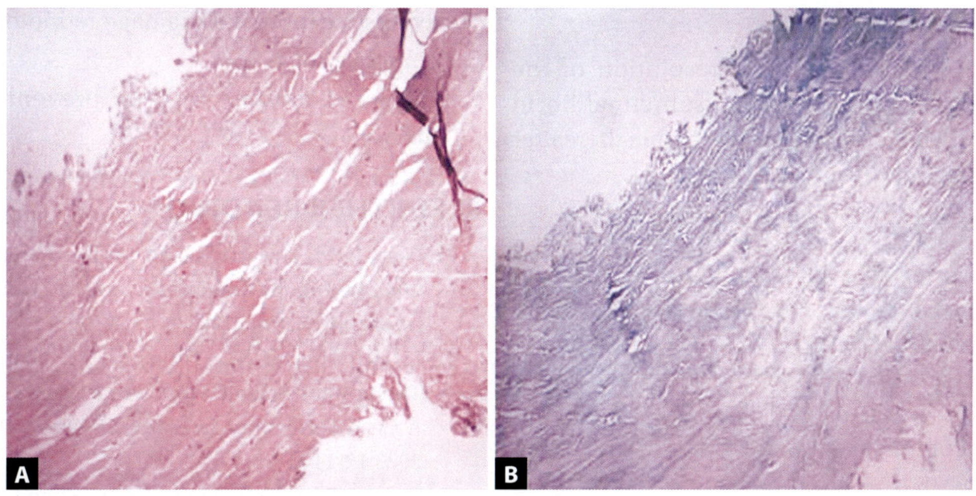

Figs. 9A and B: Histopathological examination (HPE) showing increased Alcian blue uptake of scleral tissue suggesting increased amount of glycosaminoglycans indicating thickened sclera.

Treatment Plan

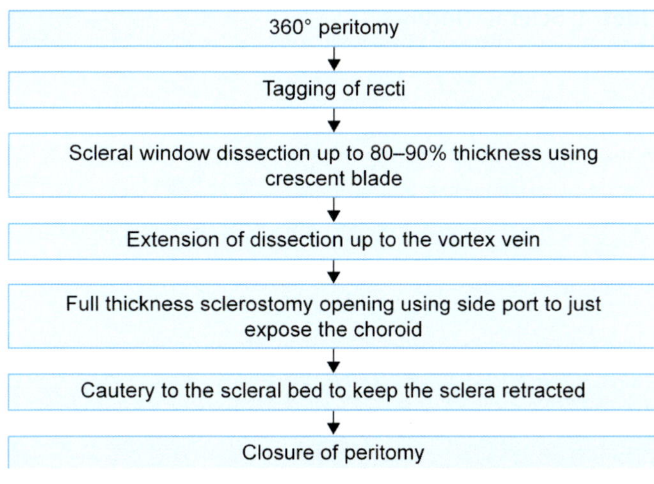

Thought Process

Step	*Rationale*
Peritomy and tagging of recti	Essential to provide adequate posterior exposure during the surgery
Scleral window dissection	• Number of quadrants decided based on the severity of the effusion • 80–90% thickness of the sclera • 4–6 mm area • Anterior edge 1–2 mm behind recti insertion • Can also be full thickness, and left open with choroidal show and continued drainage
Extension of dissection up to the vortex vein	• Careful deroofing of the vein to avoid vein amputation and hemorrhage • Is found to be useful when combined with large scleral flaps

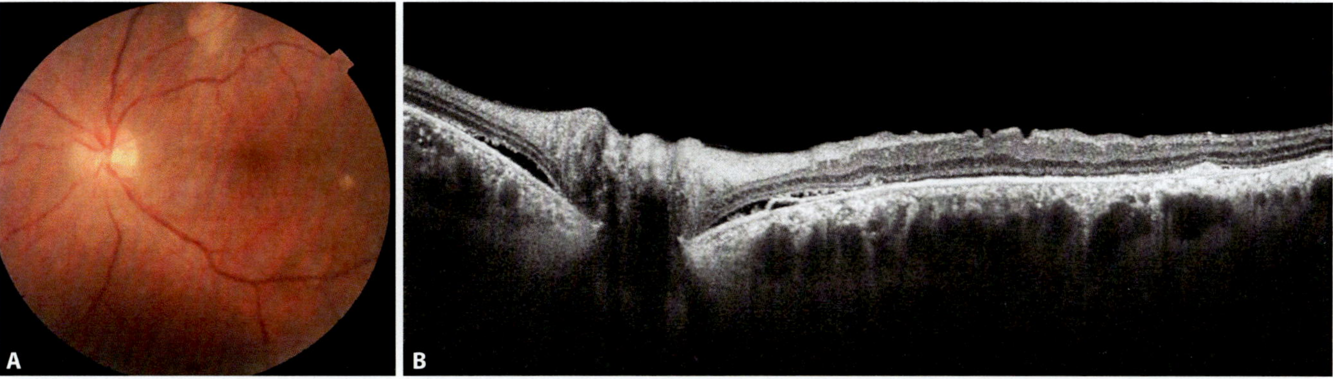

Figs. 10A and B: Postoperative fundus photograph and OCT of the left eye at 1-week postoperative showing near complete resolution of the SRF. (OCT: optical coherence tomography; SRF: subretinal fluid)

OUTCOME SUMMARY

On follow-up, there was near total resolution of the exudative detachments, with minimal subretinal fibrin **(Figs. 10A and B)**. The patient remained stable thereafter and is on follow-up.

KEY POINTS

- Adequate preoperative assessment, with accurate axial length measurement, is a very important step in surgical planning.
- Meticulous dissection to obtain the correct thickness and plane of dissection
- Following the contour of the globe, to avoid inadvertent perforation
- Careful dissection along the vortex veins to avoid intraoperative bleeding

ADDITIONAL STEPS IN SPECIAL SCENARIOS

1. Transscleral drainage of fluid with simultaneous fluid injection to aid in further subretinal fluid drainage, avoids creation of a drainage retinotomy, and related complications
2. Usage of mitomycin-C to prevent blockage and fibrosis

FURTHER READING

1. Gass JDM. Uveal effusion syndrome: a new hypothesis concerning pathogenesis and technique of surgical treatment. Retina. 1983.
2. Li HH, Hunter KC, Thomson AC, Hunter AA. Medical Therapy and Scleral Windows for Uveal Effusion Syndrome: A Case Series and Literature Review. Ophthalmol Ther. 2023;12(1):35-53.
3. Yang N, Jin S, Ma L, Liu J, Shan C, Zhao J. The pathogenesis and treatment of complications in nanophthalmos. J Ophthalmol. 2020;2020:6578750.

VIDEO LEGEND

Video 4: Scleral windows

CHAPTER 5

Decision Making in Surgical Management of Combined Retinal Detachments

Arkaprava Pradhan, Pramod S Bhende

ALGORITHM FOR MANAGEMENT OF COMBINED RETINAL DETACHMENT

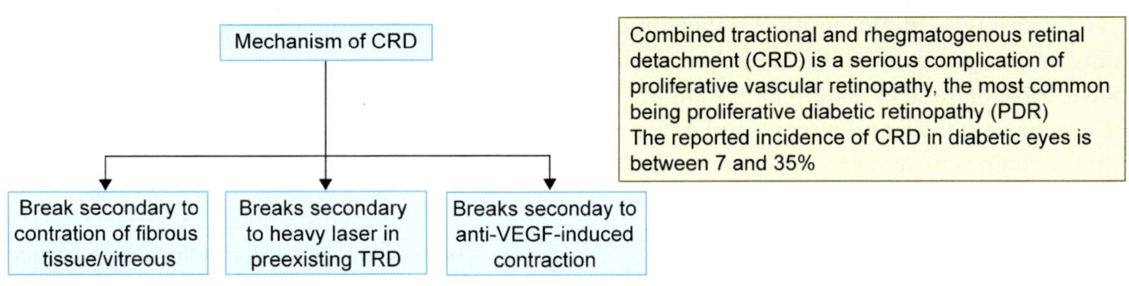

Combined tractional and rhegmatogenous retinal detachment (CRD) is a serious complication of proliferative vascular retinopathy, the most common being proliferative diabetic retinopathy (PDR)
The reported incidence of CRD in diabetic eyes is between 7 and 35%

(CRD: combined retinal detachment; TRD: tractional retinal detachment; VEGF: vascular endothelial growth factor)

CONFIGURATION OF RETINAL DETACHMENT

- Mobile retina with convex configuration like rhegmatogenous retinal detachment (RD) but incomplete posterior vitreous detachment (PVD) and a tiny single oval break adjacent to fibrovascular proliferation (FVP)/area of vitreoretinal (V-R) traction *(most common)*
- Flap tears (anteroposterior traction)
- Slit or round break without flap/operculum (tangential traction)
- Thick preretinal FVP, retinal folds, vitreous hemorrhage/opacities which may preclude detection of break preoperatively

The CRD can rapidly reach up to ora serrata but usually limited to preexisting laser scars. The retina in CRD is usually thin and atrophic (suggestive of old RD) with overlying FVP of variable severity. It needs to be differentiated from tractional schisis.

SURGICAL APPROACHES

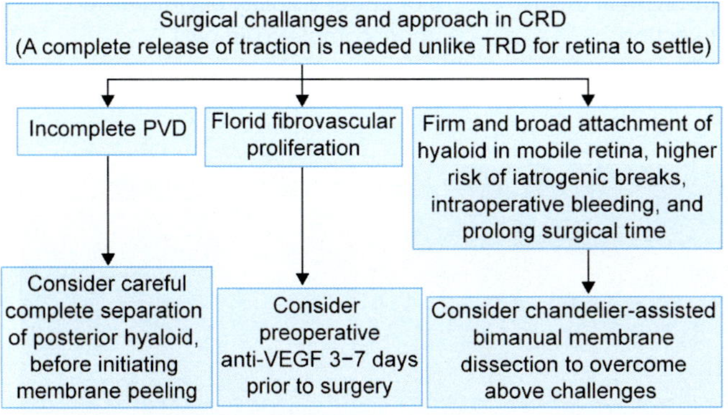

(CRD: combined retinal detachment; PVD: posterior vitreous detachment; TRD: tractional retinal detachment; VEGF: vascular endothelial growth factor).

- *Segmental buckle or encirclage:* In eyes with residual peripheral traction, depending on the extent, either segmental buckle or 360° encirclage can be used to counteract the traction.
- *Relaxing retinotomy/retinectomy:* If there is unrelieved traction even after complete membrane peeling (MP) or in eyes with localized firmly adherent membranes, not amenable to peeling, occasionally focal retinectomy or retinotomy may be necessary.
- *Using perfluorocarbon liquid (PFCL):* PFCL can occasionally be used in CRD surgery to hold back the posterior retina while working anteriorly. It is important to clear the posterior pole membranes before injecting PFCL. It can also be used to

displaced thick subretinal fluid (SRF) out in vitreous cavity.

- *Combined cataract surgery:* If there is significant cataract limiting the fundus view for membrane surgery or if there is inadvertent lens touch during surgery, the lens removal can be combined with vitrectomy. Phacoemulsification with in the bag intraocular lens (IOL) implantation is the preferred choice. Multifocal IOL should be avoided in these eyes.
- *Fluid air/gas exchange (FGE) and internal tamponade:* Once the traction is completely relieved and retina is mobile, FGE with internal drainage of SRF, either through preexisting or iatrogenic retinal break, helps retina to settle down. Most of these eyes have long-standing RD and SRF can be very thick and viscous and may need longer time to drain it out and flatten the retina. Though long-acting gas (SF6 or C3F8) is preferred, the choice of internal tamponade depends on number and location of the break/s, status of the retina, status of the other eye, patient's travel options, and possible compliance.
- *Laser PHC:* All the breaks need to be treated with laser. Also, fill in pan-retinal photocoagulation can be completed during the same sitting.

CASE SCENARIO 1: UTILITY OF ANTI-VEGF IN MANAGEMENT OF CRD

Case Summary

A 47-years-old male, known diabetic, reported with drop in vision in both eyes over 2 months. At presentation, his vision was 6/24 and 6/18 in the right and left eye, respectively. Right eye had PDR with CRD, threatening macula and extending up to mid-periphery and almost no PVD. The florid FVP was extending along both the arcades and the disc with retinal break along superotemporal arcade **(Figs. 1A and B)**. The left eye had lasered PDR.

Treatment Plan

Intravitreal ranibizumab was administered in the right eye 3 days preoperatively to reduce the vascularity and the risk of intraoperative bleeding

↓

25G pras plana vitrectomy was done

↓

Tricort was used to make sure that vitreous was removed completely

↓

25G MVR was used to make a nick in posterior hyaloid to get cleavage plain

↓

Chandelier illumination was used for bimanual dissection to remove extensive membrane on mobile, detached retina

↓

Intraocular forceps and scissors were used to remove all the membrane

↓

25G cutter with lower cut rate (as mechanical scissors) was used to remove thick membranes

↓

Hemostasis was achieved with direct pressure on the bleeding point using cutter tip and with intermittently increasing intraocular pressure (IOP)

↓

Fluid gas exchange with internal SRF drainage was done through preexisting break to reattach the retina

↓

Barrage laser was done around the break along with pan retinal photocoagulation

↓

Silicone oil was used as internal tamponade

↓

Small blood clot was left on the disc

Thought Process

Action	*Rationale*
Presurgery intravitreal anti-VEGF injection	To reduce vascularity of FVP and the risk of intraoperative bleeding
Intravitreal tricort injection	For better visibility of vitreous for more complete removal

Contd...

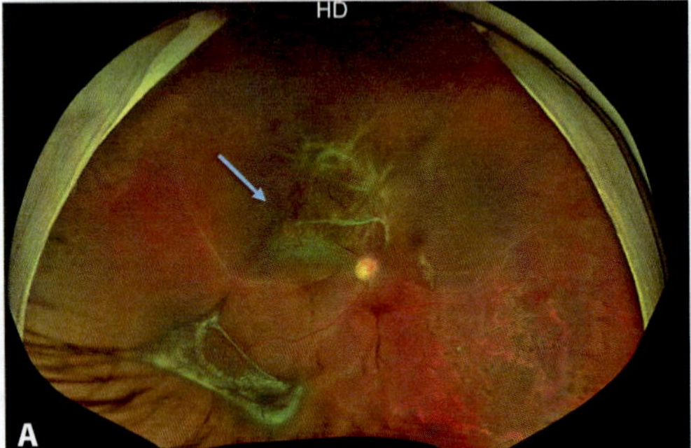

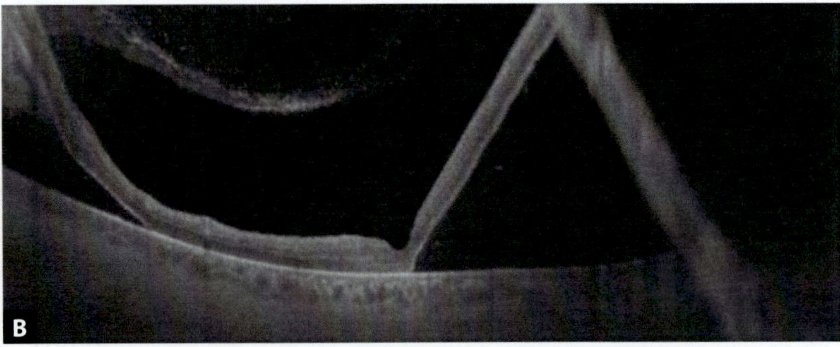

Figs. 1A to B: Preoperative OPTOS and OCT. (A) Combined retinal detachment in the right eye (Break - Blue arrow); (B) Retinal detachment approaching macula.

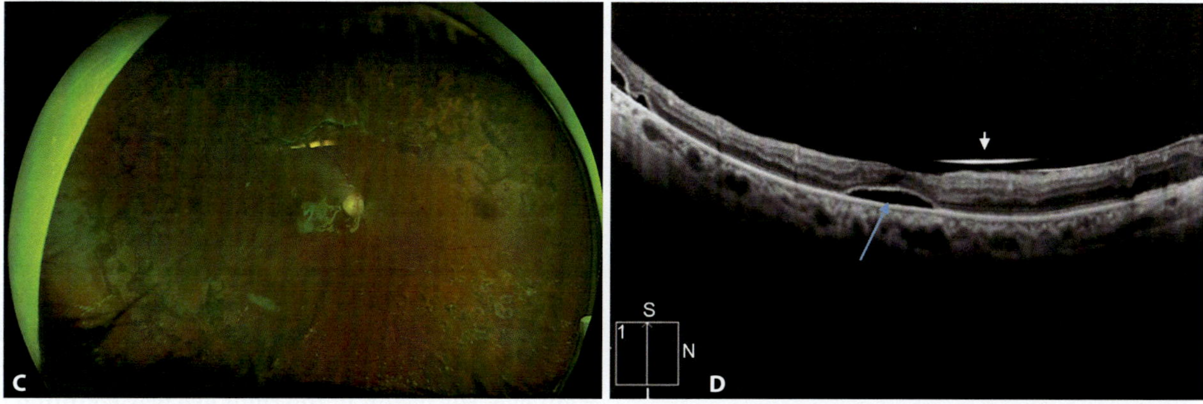

Figs. 1C to D: Postoperative OPTOS and OCT at 6 weeks. (C) Attached retina in silicone oil-filled eye; (D) Retina attached, small SRF pocket at fovea. *Note:* Small SRF pocket (blue arrow) and silicone oil meniscus (white arrow)

Contd...

Action	*Rationale*
MVR to nick posterior hyaloid face	To get cleavage plane
Chandelier illumination and bimanual dissection using intraocular forceps and scissors	Ease and better control for membrane surgery with mobile, detached retina
MIVS cutter with reduced cut rate and shaving mode	Using cutter as automated scissors
FGE with internal SRF drainage	To reattach the retina for retinopexy (Laser)

(FGE: fluid gas exchange; FVP: fibrovascular proliferation; SRF: subretinal fluid; MIVS: microincision vitrectomy surgery; MVR: microvitreoretinal; VEGF: vascular endothelial growth factor)

OUTCOME SUMMARY

- 6 weeks postsurgery, right eye had attached retina, 6/9, N6 vision, and IOP was 14 mm Hg **(Figs. 1C and D)**.
- The patient is waiting for silicone oil removal (SOR).

KEY POINTS

- Early and timely intervention leads to good outcome.
- Presurgery intravitreal anti-VEGF injection helps to reduce vascularity and thereby reduces the chances of intraoperative bleeding and iatrogenic complications.
- In eyes with mobile retina and florid proliferation, bimanual dissection using chandelier illumination is very helpful.
- Smaller gauge (25 G or 27 G) instruments are better for membrane surgery.
- In eyes with no or incomplete PVD and taut flat posterior hyaloid, sharp instrument like MVR blade or needle may help to initiate the dissection.

FURTHER READING

1. Bonnar J, Tan CH, McCullough P, Wright DM, Williamson T, Lois N; IRB-RRD Study Group. Scleral Buckle, Vitrectomy, or Combined Surgery for Inferior Break Retinal Detachment: Systematic Review and Meta-Analysis. Ophthalmol Retina. 2023;10:837-47.
2. Cruz-Iñigo YJ, Berrocal MH. Twenty-seven-gauge vitrectomy for combined tractional and rhegmatogenous retinal detachment involving the macula associated with proliferative diabetic retinopathy. Int J Retina Vitreous. 2017;3:38.

CASE SCENARIO 2: BIMANUAL SURGERY IN MANAGEMENT OF CRD

Case Summary

A 43-year-old male, known diabetic and already had laser PRP and intravitreal anti-VEGF injections for PDR, reported with sudden drop in vision in both eyes of 1-month duration **(Fig. 2A)**. Ultrasonography was suggestive of subhyaloid hemorrhage in both eyes. Right eye also had RD.

Treatment Plan

25G, three port pars plana vitrectomy was done to clear vitreous hemorrhage

↓

As there were extensive preretinal membranes, chandelier illumination placed in ITQ next to infusion cannula, for bimanual dissection

↓

Intraocular forceps and intraocular scissors were used to remove all the membranes

↓

Hemostasis was achieved with the direct pressure on the bleeding point with the help of cutter and with FGE

↓

Subretinal fluid was drained through the superotemporal break

↓

Laser was done around the break and PRP completed

↓

Silicone oil was exchanged with air as an internal tamponade

Thought Process

Action	*Rationale*
Presurgery ultrasonography	To assess V-R relationship in an eye with hazy media to plan the surgery steps
Chandelier illumination placed in ITQ	For unrestricted ocular mobility during surgery and ease of bimanual dissection in an eye with mobile retina
Direct but gentle pressure on the bleeding point with cutter	To help hemostasis without raising IOP
Silicone oil injection	As a long-term internal tamponade

(IOP: intraocular pressure; V-R: vitreoretinal)

OUTCOME SUMMARY

- At 6 weeks, retina was attached with clear vitreous cavity and 6/36. N18 vision. IOP was 14 mm Hg.
- SOR combined with cataract surgery was done 4 months after the primary surgery. At last follow-up, vision improved to 6/24, N12. Retina was attached **(Fig. 2B)**.

KEY POINTS

- Minimize the use of diathermy as there is a risk of iatrogenic break.
- Direct gentle pressure on the bleeding point with the help of cutter can stop the bleeding and reduce the risk of compromising of optic disc perfusion with high IOP.
- Plan the location of chandelier for better illumination during MP.
- With port optimization, cutter can be used as a multifunction instrument. However, in eyes with mobile retina, scissor may give better control and minimizes the risk of iatrogenic break/s.

FURTHER READING

1. Thompson JT, de Bustros S, Michels RG, Rice TA, Glaser BM. Results of vitrectomy for proliferative diabetic retinopathy. Ophthalmology. 1986;93(12):1571-4.

CASE SCENARIO 3: MANAGEMENT OF MACULAR HOLE WITH CRD

Case Summary

A 46-year-old male with retinal perivasculitis and had sectoral laser for the same in past presented with full thickness macular hole and CRD **(Figs. 3A and B)** in the right eye. His vision in the right eye was counting finger close to face (CFCF).

Treatment Plan

Encircling band was placed to counter peripheral traction

↓

25G pras plana vitrectomy was done. Chandelier illumination was placed at 7 o'clock meridian through a 25G sclerotomy

↓

Iatrogenic break was noted during membrane removal in superotemporal quadrant

↓

Corneal epithelium was debrided for better visualization

↓

Brilliant blue-assisted ILM peeling was done for the macular hole

↓

Limited retinectomy was done in superotemporal quadrant to relieve the traction caused by FVP

↓

Subretinal fluid was drained through the superotemporal break

↓

Laser was done around the break and cryopexy was done for the anterior margin of the break

↓

Encircling band indentation was adjusted and silicone oil was exchanged with air

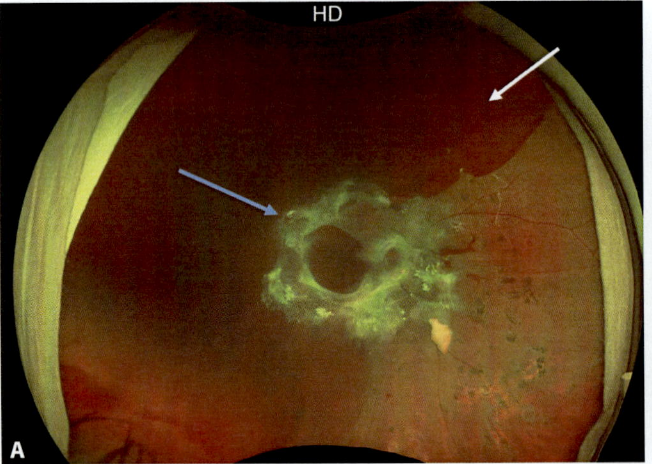

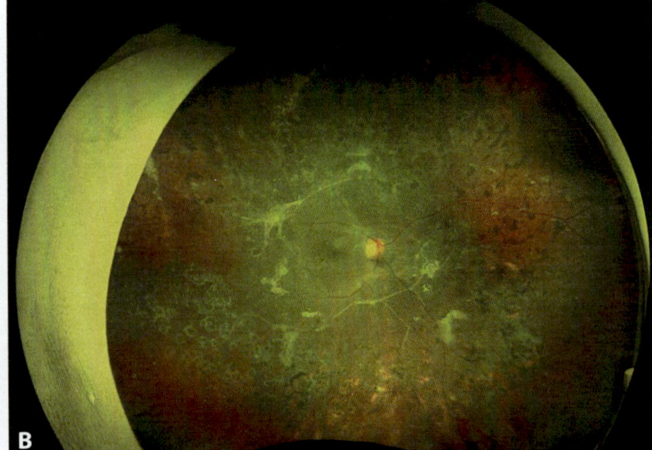

Figs. 2A and B: Preoperative and postoperative fundus. (A) Subhyaloid hemorrhage (white arrow) and TRD with break underneath (blue arrow); (B) After silicon oil removal and cataract surgery.

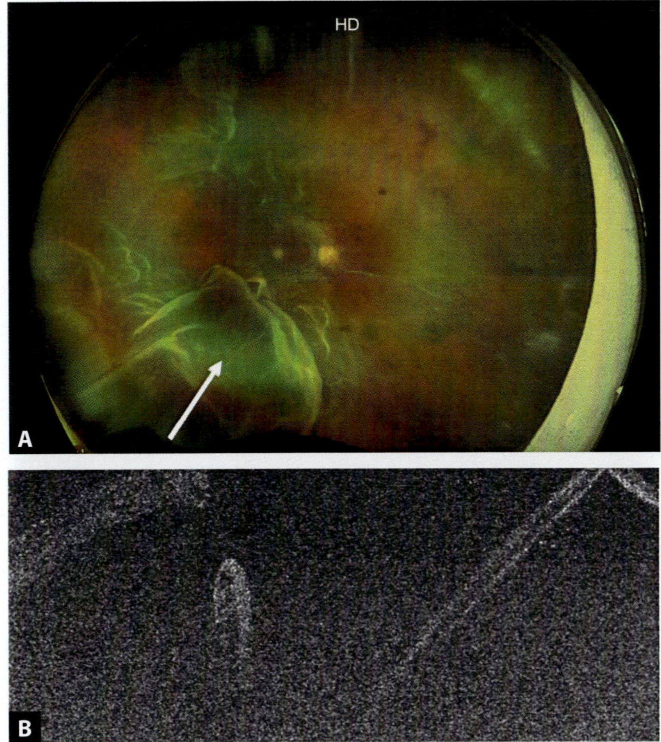

Figs. 3A and B: Preoperative fundus and OCT. (A) Bullous retinal detachment (white arrow); (B) Macular hole with retinal detachment.

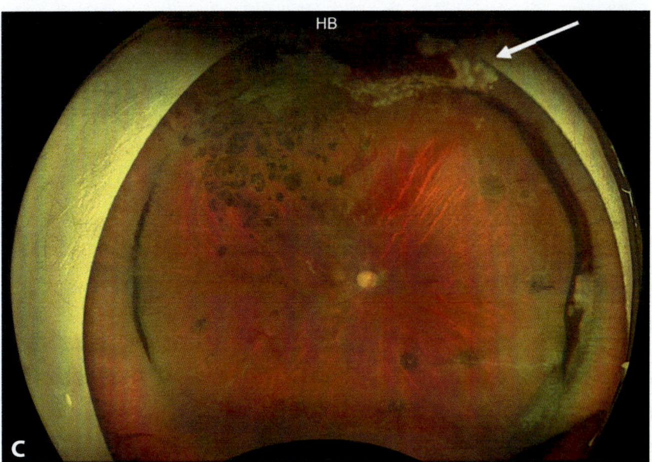

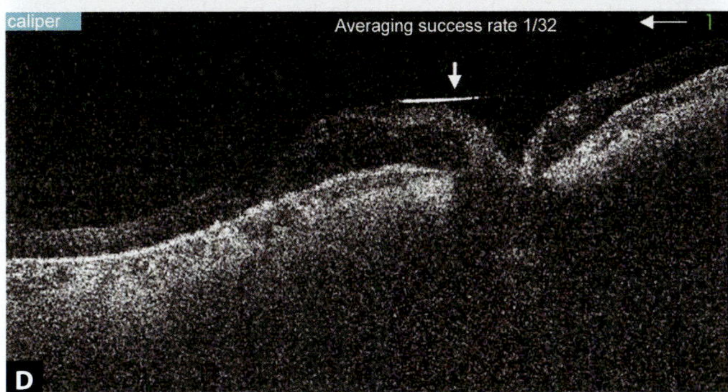

Figs. 3C and D: Postoperative fundus. (C) Laser marks around RR edge (white arrow); (D) Closed macular hole with attached retina silicone oil reflex (arrow).

Thought Process

Action	*Rationale*
Encircling band	Young patient with clear lens and retinal perivasculitis. To counter peripheral residual traction without sacrificing clear lens
Chandelier illumination and bimanual dissection	Ease and better control during membrane surgery for extensive proliferation
Corneal epithelium debridement	Should be avoided in a diabetic eye as far as possible but occasionally may need for better visualization
Intravitreal brilliant blue green injection	To assist ILM peeling
Retinectomy with excision of FVP	To relieve residual traction caused by FVP as FVP was firmly adherent to the retina

(FVP: fibrovascular proliferation; ILM: internal limiting membrane)

OUTCOME SUMMARY

At 1-year follow-up, right eye retina was attached and macular hole was closed. Vision was only CF, due to dense cataract. IOP was 10 mm of Hg. The patient is waiting for SOR + cataract surgery **(Figs. 3C and D)**.

KEY POINTS

- In young adults with perivasculitis, encircling band is useful to support the peripheral residual traction without causing anterior segment ischemia.
- Though technically difficult, ILM peeling can be done in eyes with CRD and full thickness macular hole.
- Occasionally localized retinectomy is needed to relieve the traction.
- In phakic eyes with peripheral break/s, it is difficult to do laser, without lens touch. The anterior margin of the break/s can be treated with cryopexy and laser for the posterior margin.

FURTHER READING

1. Bonnar J, Tan CH, McCullough P, Wright DM, Williamson T, Lois N; IRB-RRD Study Group. Scleral Buckle, Vitrectomy, or Combined Surgery for Inferior Break Retinal Detachment: Systematic Review and Meta-Analysis. Ophthalmol Retina. 2023;10:837-47.
2. Iyer SSR, Regan KA, Burnham JM, Chen CJ. Surgical management of diabetic tractional retinal detachments. Surv Ophthalmol. 2019;64(6):780-809.

3. Newman DK. Surgical management of the late complications of proliferative diabetic retinopathy. Eye. 2010;24(3):441-9.
4. Stewart MW, Browning DJ, Landers MB. Current management of diabetic tractional retinal detachments. Indian J Ophthalmol. 2018;66(12):1751-62.

CASE SCENARIO 4: MANAGEMENT OF CRD WITH TRACTIONAL RETINOSCHISIS

Case Summary

A 70-year-old male presented with reduced vision in the right eye for 5 months. His vision was 6/36, N24. Fundus examination revealed vitreous hemorrhage and CRD like configuration involving macula but break was not seen **(Fig. 4A)**. Left eye underwent PRP for PDR.

Treatment Plan

Intravitreal ranibizumab was administered 4 days prior to surgery in the right eye

↓

25G MIVS was used

↓

Attachments to peripheral vitreous were cut from the central FVP to release transvitreal and anteroposterior traction

↓

Tractional retinoschisis with densely adherent posterior hyaloid was noted along inferotemporal arcade. With 25 G chandelier at 7 o'clock, and forceps in one hand and cutter (with low cut rate) in the other, MP was done using bimanual technique

↓

Hemostasis was achieved with the help of raised IOP. The IOP was gradually decreased to normal range to ensure that there is no active bleeder

↓

Though retina was mobile, no obvious retinal break was seen even with thorough and repeated inspection under high magnification

↓

Fill in PRP was done. No internal tamponade was given

Thought Process

Action	*Rationale*
Presurgery intravitreal anti-VEGF injection	To reduce the risk of intraoperative bleeding
Truncation of cone	To release transvitreal and anteroposterior traction
Chandelier illumination	For bimanual surgery for densely adherent PHF and tractional retinoschisis
Transient increase in intraocular pressure	For hemostasis
No internal tamponade	Only retinoschisis but no obvious break was seen

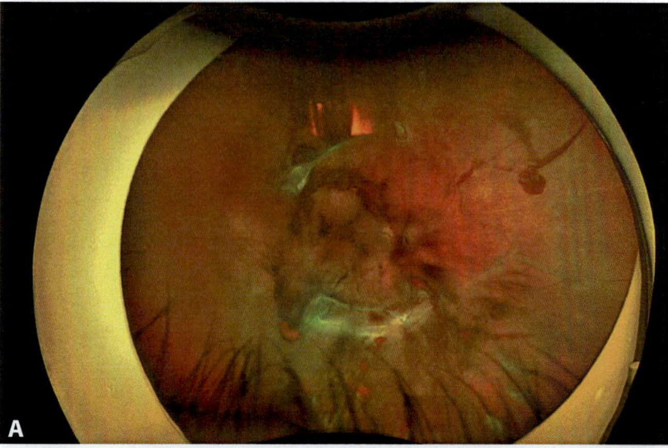

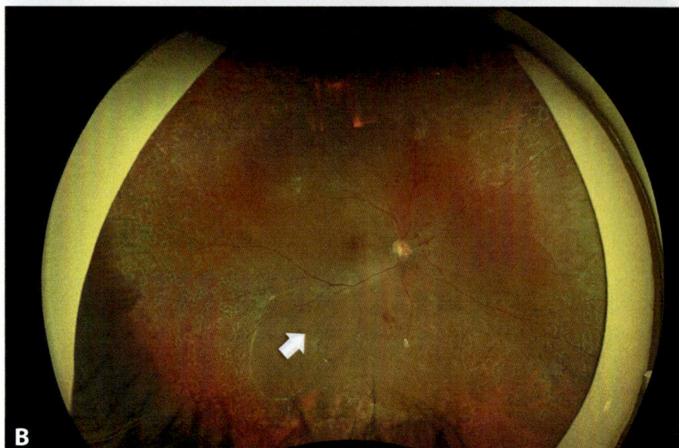

Figs. 4A and B: Preoperative and postoperative fundus. (A) Combined RD involving macula with vitreous hemorrhage; (B) Attached macula but persistent retinoschisis.

OUTCOME SUMMARY

- *1-week postsurgery:* Localized retinal elevation was noted.
- *At 6 weeks postsurgery:* Right eye vision improved to 6/18, N6. IOP was 16 mm of Hg. The persistent schitic retina was noted, though the height was reduced and macula was attached **(Fig. 4B)**.

KEY POINTS

- The configuration of RD can be misleading. There is a need to differentiate TRD/CRD from tractional schisis.
- It is important to relieve the bridging transvitreal and anterior-posterior traction.
- 25 G cutter with low cut rate and shaving mode, acts as automated scissors.
- After MP, thorough inspection of retina is necessary to ensure that there is no preexisting or iatrogenic retinal break/s.

- After achieving the hemostasis, gradual lowering of the IOP helps to get sustained hemostasis and to minimize the risk of early postoperative bleeding.
- There is no need of internal tamponade if there is no break.

FURTHER READING

1. Aaberg TM, Abrams GW. Changing indications and techniques for vitrectomy in management of complications of diabetic retinopathy. Ophthalmology. 1987;94(7):775-9.
2. Eliott D, Hemeida T. Diabetic traction retinal detachment. Int Ophthalmol Clin. 2009;49(2):153-65.
3. Smiddy WE, Flynn HW. Vitrectomy in the Management of Diabetic Retinopathy. Surv Ophthalmol. 1999;43(6):491-507.

CASE SCENARIO 5: MANAGEMENT OF IATROGENIC BREAK IN CRD WITH MACULAR HOLE

Case Summary

A 28-year-old female, known diabetic, presented with diminution in vision in right eye for 15 days. Her vision was 3/60 in the right eye and fundus examination reveals RD with full thickness macular hole **(Fig. 5A)**. Left eye had vitrectomy for vitreous hemorrhage 4 years back.

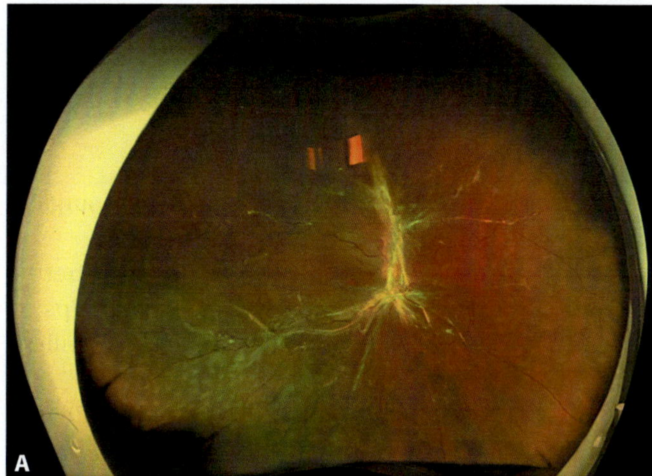

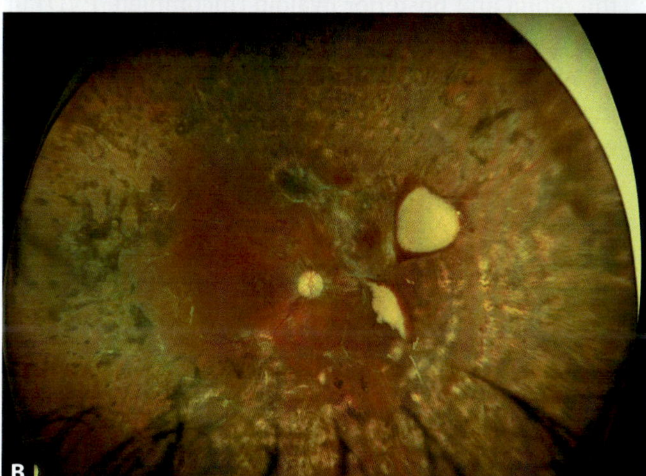

Figs. 5A and B: Preoperative and postoperative fundus. (A) Combined RD with full thickness macular hole; (B) Retina was attached and macular hole was closed.

Treatment Plan

Bimanual surgery was planned. Four sclerotomies were made with chandelier at 7 o'clock

↓

With limbal side port, posterior synechiolysis was done under viscoelastic cover

↓

There was an incomplete PVD. Truncation was initiated superonasally along the edge of FVP

↓

During MP, iatrogenic retinal break occurred and retina becomes bullous

↓

Subretinal fluid was drained through iatrogenic break to reduce the RD height to complete the MP.

↓

Macular hole size reduced after all the traction was relieved, but proceeded with conventional BBG assisted ILM peeling

↓

Retina settled with FGE and drainage of SRF through iatrogenic break. Fill in PRP and laser was done around the iatrogenic break

↓

Silicone oil was used as an internal tamponade

Thought Process

Action	*Rationale*
Posterior synechiolysis	For pupillary dilatation and better view of the fundus during surgery
Truncation of cone	To release anterior-posterior traction
SRF drainage through mid-surgery	To reduce the height of detached retina to create space for membrane surgery
Silicone oil injection	For long-term internal tamponade

(SRF: subretinal fluid)

Outcome Summary

- Early postoperative period: Preretinal hemorrhage was noted.

- At 2 months follow-up, right eye vision improved to 6/60, N36 and retina was attached with closed MH **(Fig. 5B)**.

KEY POINTS

- Decide about bimanual surgery early and plan surgical steps accordingly.
- Good pupillary dilatation is needed for better intraoperative fundus view. Synechiolysis helps to enlarge pupillary size. If needed, mechanical pupillary expanders can be used.
- Finding the plane for dissection is the key. We initiated truncation superonasally, as there was a gap between the retina and posterior hyaloid (incomplete PVD) in that quadrant.
- In eyes with bullous detachment, SRF drainage gives more working space and reduces retinal mobility for ease of MP.
- Preferably avoid SRF drainage through macular hole.
- As most macular holes in this setting are stretch holes, reduced macular hole size after MP indicates adequate release of traction. ILM peeling, however, ensures complete removal of residual premacular vitreous and membrane.

FURTHER READING

1. Cruz-Iñigo YJ, Berrocal MH. Twenty-seven-gauge vitrectomy for combined tractional and rhegmatogenous retinal detachment involving the macula associated with proliferative diabetic retinopathy. Int J Retina Vitreous. 2017; 3:38.
2. Eliott D, Hemeida T. Diabetic traction retinal detachment. Int Ophthalmol Clin. 2009;49(2):153-65.
3. Meleth AD, Carvounis PE. Outcomes of vitrectomy for tractional retinal detachment in diabetic retinopathy. Int Ophthalmol *Clin*. 2014;54(2):127-39.

CASE SCENARIO 6: UTILITY OF PFCL IN MANAGEMENT OF CRD

Case Summary

A 42-year-old male presented with diminution in vision in both the eyes of 6 months' duration. His vision was 2/60 and 3/60 in right and left eyes, respectively. Right eye had TRD involving macula **(Fig. 6A)**. OCT confirms premacular membrane and macular detachment **(Fig. 6B)**. Left eye already had surgery for TRD due to PDR.

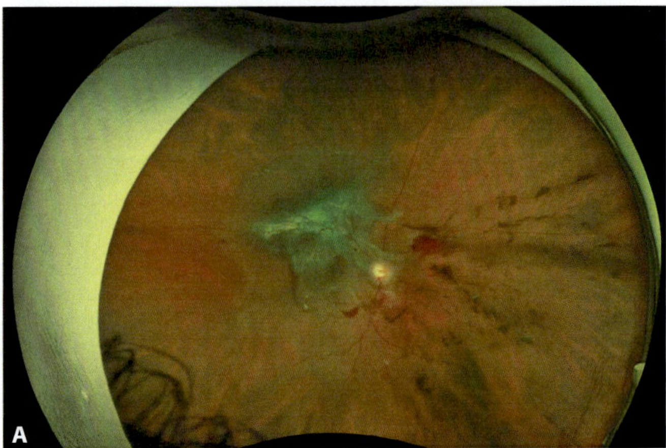

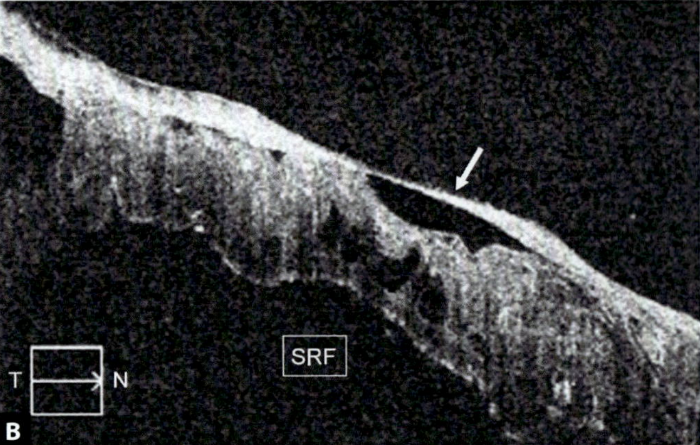

Figs. 6A and B: Preoperative fundus and OCT. (A) Traction involving the macula; (B) OCT: Traction involving the macula preretinal proliferation (white arrow).

Treatment Plan

With presurgery intravitreal anti-VEGF injection, 25G bimanual pars plana vitrectomy was performed

↓

Vitreoschisis was identified, extending 1–2 disk areas beyond the visible edge of FVP

↓

MP completed using bimanual technique with forceps and cutter under chandelier illumination

↓

Two very small breaks were noted in superonasal quadrant at the edges of FVP

↓

After marking the breaks with endodiathermy, endodrainage was attempted through the preexisting break. Retina could not be settled completely as SRF was very thick and viscous. PFCL was used to squeeze the SRF out and flatten the retina

↓

Breaks were lasered under PFCL

↓

PFCL-air exchange was done and silicone oil was used as an internal tamponade

Thought Process

Action	*Rationale*
Presurgery intravitreal anti-VEGF injection	To reduce the risk of intraoperative bleeding
Bimanual surgery with forceps and cutter under chandelier illumination	For better control during membrane surgery
PFCL injection	To squeeze out thick vicious SRF and flatten the retina

(PFCL: perfluorocarbon liquid; SRF: subretinal fluid; VEGF: vascular endothelial growth factor)

OUTCOME SUMMARY

- *Early postoperative period:* Persistent localized RD and preretinal hemorrhages were noted at posterior pole.
- At 5 weeks, right eye vision improved to 3/60. Few cystic space were noted at macula. Breaks were flat and well-covered with laser scars. Peripheral retina was attached, but residual SRF was present at posterior pole **(Fig. 6C)**. At 6 months follow-up, vision improved further to 6/60, N36 but SRF has also increased on OCT **(Fig. 6D)**. No obvious break was seen. The eye was oil-filled with improved vision and there was no visible break, so decided not to intervene and review the patient after 3 months.

KEY POINTS

- Important to differentiate between TRD, tractional schisis and CRD as RD configuration can be misleading and tiny break/s may be hidden under the FVP.
- Important to understand the concept of vitreoschisis or second membrane to identify the correct plane for membrane dissection.
- Vitrectomy cutter with low cut rate can be used as an automated scissor for MP.
- After achieving hemostasis, gradually lower the IOP, to get sustained hemostasis.
- PFCL is not routinely used in PDR surgery. But, in an exceptional situation like this, PFCL can help to squeeze the viscous SRF out and flatten the retina.
- Thick and viscous SRF may take very long time to get absorbed. If there is no communicating break, these eyes can be safely watched.

Postoperative OCT (5 weeks)

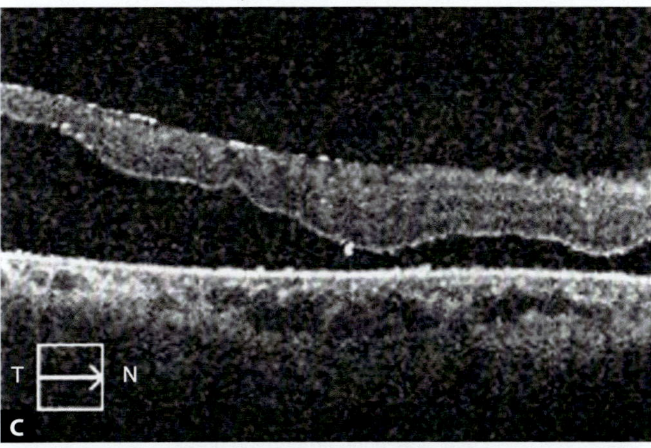

Postoperative OCT (6 months)

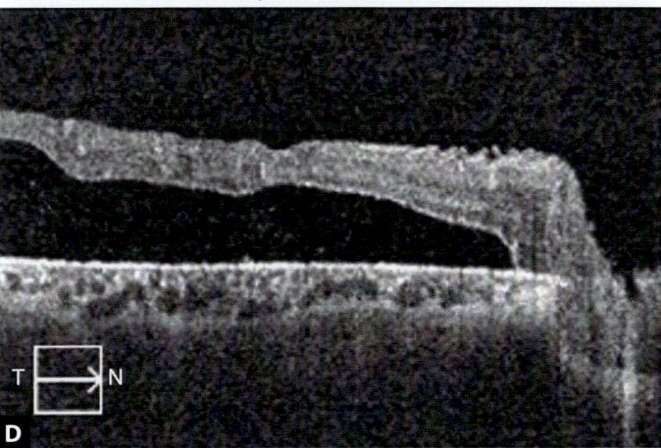

Figs. 6C and D: Postoperative OCT: (C) Thinned out macula with persistent SRF; (D) Persistent SRF, 6 months postsurgery (increased than before).

FURTHER READING

1. Aaberg TM, Abrams GW. Changing indications and techniques for vitrectomy in management of complications of diabetic retinopathy. Ophthalmology. 1987;94(7):775-9.
2. Meleth AD, Carvounis PE. Outcomes of vitrectomy for tractional retinal detachment in diabetic retinopathy. Int Ophthalmol *Clin*. 2014;54(2):127-39.
3. Newman DK. Surgical management of the late complications of proliferative diabetic retinopathy. Eye. 2010;24(3):441-9.

CASE SCENARIO 7: MANAGEMENT OF CHRONIC SUBRETINAL FLUID POST-CRD SURGERY

Case Summary

A 53-year-old male presented with diminution in vision in the left eye for 2 months. The left eye vision was 6/24, N6 and had CRD involving macula **(Fig. 7A)**. Right eye was operated before for diabetic TRD.

Treatment Plan

25G pars plana vitrectomy was done

↓

PVD was induced and preretinal membranes were removed. Break was noted along superotemporal quadrant

↓

Hemostasis was achieved with the help of direct pressure with the cutter tip and by intermittently raising the IOP

↓

Fluid air exchange was done and SRF was drained through the preexisting break, to reattach the retina. Laser was done around the break

↓

14% of C3F8 gas was exchanged with air as an internal tamponade

Thought Process

Action	*Rationale*
PVD induction	There was incomplete PVD and PVD induction helped to get correct plane for dissection
Fluid air exchange with internal SRF drainage	To reattach the retina
C3F8 injection	For internal tamponade of superior quadrant break

OUTCOME SUMMARY

- *Early postoperative period:* Localized subretinal fluid was noted at posterior pole.
- *At 4 months postsurgery:* Vision was 6/60, N36 (less than presurgery vision). Persistent SRF was noted at posterior pole. It took almost 16 months for SRF to resolve completely **(Figs. 7B to D)**. Vision dropped further to 3/60 even though retina was fully attached. There was a significant cataract.

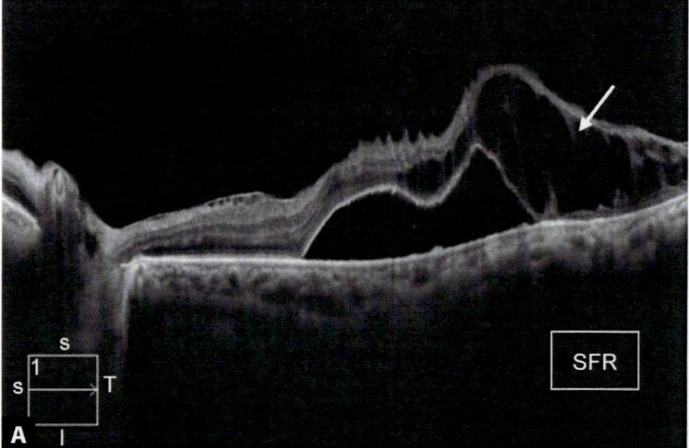

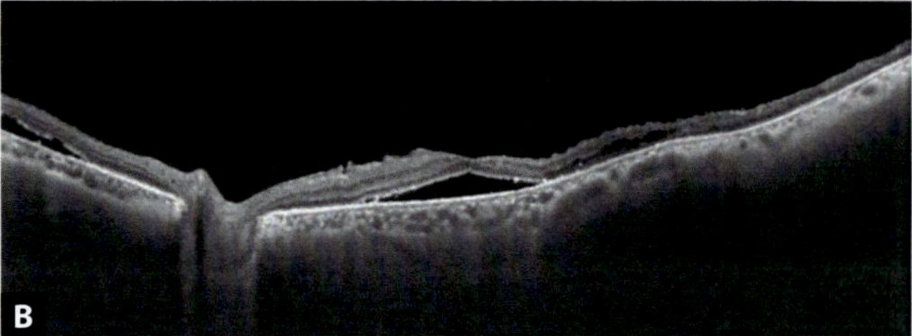

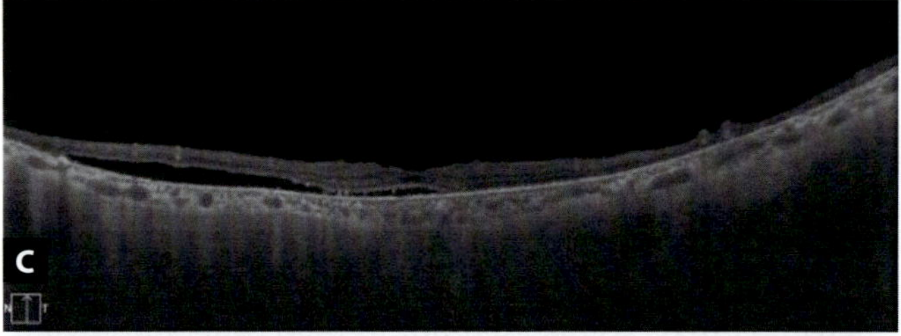

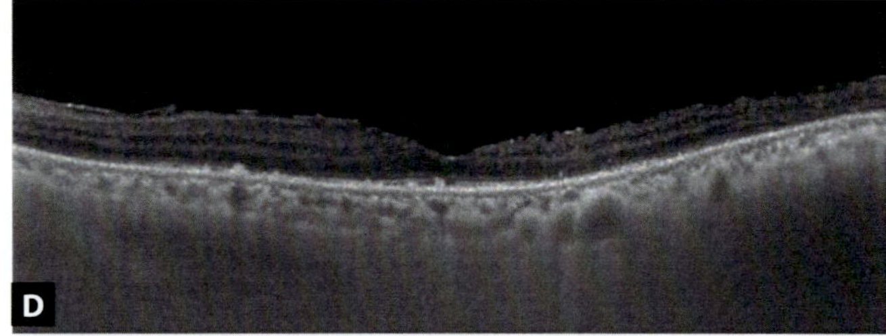

Figs. 7A to D: Preoperative OCT: (A) TRD involving macula and retinoschisis (white arrow). Serial postoperative OCT; (B) 4 months after surgery; (C) 10 months after surgery; (D) 16 months after surgery.

KEY POINTS

- Though clinical picture was like TRD, intraoperatively break could be identified.
- Break/s at the base of FVP can easily be missed preoperatively and needs thorough evaluation intraoperatively to identify those.
- C3F8 gas would be the preferred choice as a tamponade, however, the choice of tamponade depends on number and location of the breaks.
- Thick and viscous SRF in chronic detachments may take longer time to get absorbed. If there is no communicating break, these eyes can safely be watched.

FURTHER READING

1. Yang CM. Surgical treatment for diabetic retinopathy: 5-year experience. J Formosan Med Assoc. 1998;97(7): 477-84.

2. Yang CM, Su PY, Yeh PT, Chen MS. Combined rhegmatogenous and traction retinal detachment in proliferative diabetic retinopathy: clinical manifestations and surgical outcome. Canad J Ophthalmol. 2008;43(2):192-8.

CASE SCENARIO 8: CATARACT SURGERY COMBINED WITH CRD MANAGEMENT

Case Summary

A 33-year-old male presented with diminution in vision in both the eyes for 3 months. His vision was 2/60 in both the eyes. The right eye had posterior subcapsular cataract, nonresolving vitreous hemorrhage and subhyaloid hemorrhage with underlying RD **(Fig. 8A)**. Combined cataract extraction and vitrectomy was planned.

Treatment Plan

Intravitreal ranibizumab was administered in the right eye, 3 days preoperatively

↓

Before making sclerotimies, phacoemulsification was done. Capsular bag was filled with viscoelastic substance. It was decided to implant IOL after vitrectomy

↓

A 25G vitrectomy system was used. Vitrectomy was done to clear vitreous hemorrhage

↓

There was incomplete PVD with very taught PHF. MVR was used to make the initial cut in elevated temporal posterior hyaloid and truncation was done with gradually lifting the PHF, clock hour by clock hour, using suction of the cutter and then trimming it all around 360°

↓

Subhyaloid blood was cleared using suction mode of vitrector and with proportional reflux

↓

FVP superior to optic disc was removed with cutter. Retina was elevated with a preexisting break noted under the FVP. The break was marked with diathermy

↓

Hemostasis was achieved with the help of direct pressure with cutter and intermittently raising the IOP

↓

Monofocal IOL was implanted in the capsular bag and viscoelastic substance in AC was washed out.

↓

Fluid air exchange was done. Internal drainage of SRF was done through the break to reattach the retina

↓

PRP was done with laser around the preexisting retinal break

↓

C3F8 was exchanged with air as an internal tamponade

Thought Process

Action	*Rationale*
Phacoemulsification	To clear media during surgery. The patent had significant posterior subcapsular cataract.
MVR for initial cut in PHF	To create a plane for dissection in an eye with incomplete PVD
Proportional reflux	For safe and quick removal of settled preretinal blood
Diathermy to mark the break	Easy to identify the break (for laser) after FGE and reattachment of the retina
IOL implantation	Monofocal IOL is preferred in eyes with posterior segment pathology

(FGE: fluid gas exchange; IOL: intraocular lens; MVR: microvitreoretinal; PHF: posterior hyaloid face; PVD: posterior vitreous detachment)

OUTCOME SUMMARY

- *1-week postoperative:* Retina was attached. Preretinal hemorrhage was noted along inferior arcade.
- Vision in the right eye improved to 6/24, N6, 5 months after the surgery. IOP was 16 mm of Hg **(Fig. 8B)**. But, there was gross cystoid macular edema on OCT (subfoveal thickness - 787 μm) **(Fig. 8C)**. Injection ozurdex was planned.

KEY POINTS

- Eyes with vitreous hemorrhage and underlying RD need early surgery, especially if there is no history of prior laser PRP.
- Cataract surgery can be combined with vitrectomy, if necessary. IOL can be implanted before or after vitrectomy as per surgeons' discretion. Monofocal IOL is preferred.
- Irrespective of configuration of RD, always rule out preexisting break/s. Mark all the break/s (preexisting and iatrogenic, if any) with diathermy before fluid air exchange.
- There is a need for prolonged follow-up for recurrent hemorrhage, reproliferation and CME. Appropriate treatment can be administered, if needed.

FURTHER READING

1. Su XJ, Qi YX, Zhang J. Vitrectomy combined with intraocular lens implantation for the treatment of diabetic retinopathy complicated with cataract. Guoji Yanke Zazhi (Int Eye Sci). 2019;19(3):477-80.

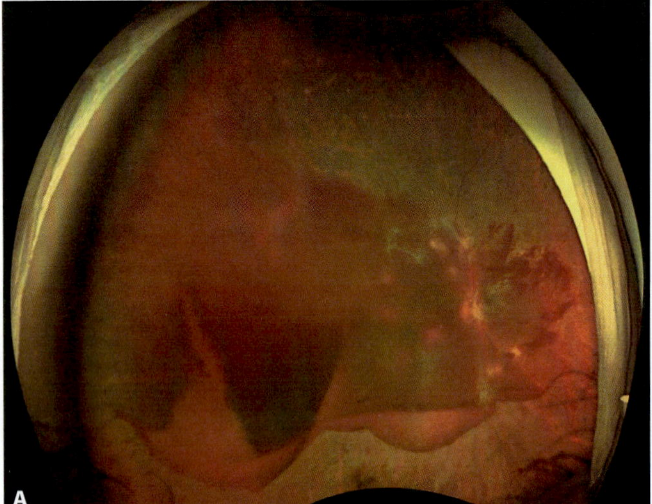

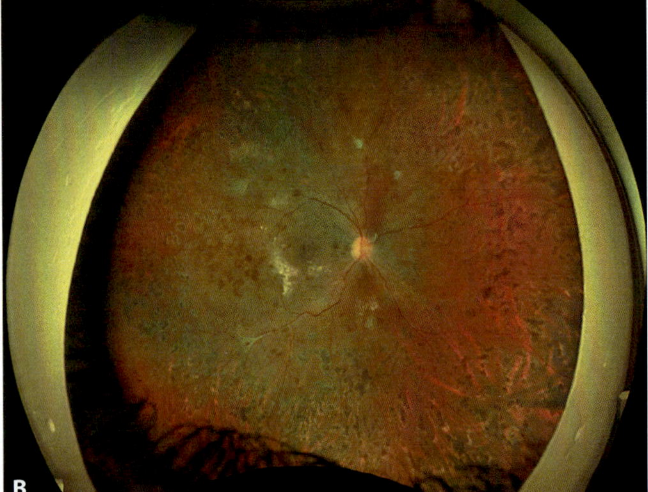

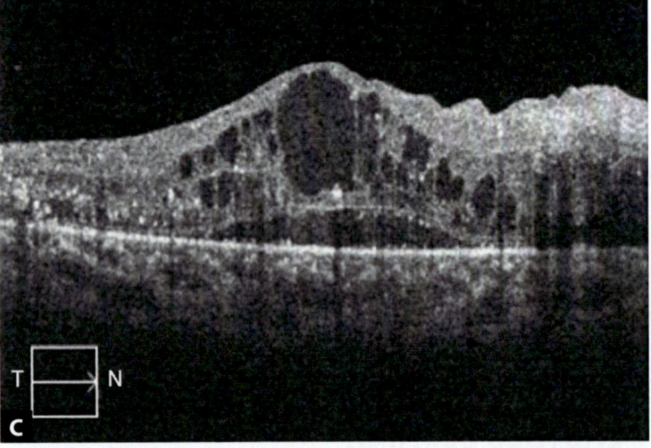

Figs. 8A to C: Preoperative and postoperative fundus: (A) Traction at posterior pole with vitreous and subhyaloid hemorrhage; (B) Retina attached (5 months postsurgery); (C) Postoperative OCT showing cystoid macular edema and sensory RD.

2. Xiao K, Dong YC, Xiao XG, Liang SZ, Wang J, Qian C, et al. Effect of Pars Plana Vitrectomy With or Without Cataract Surgery in Patients with Diabetes: A Systematic Review and Meta-Analysis. Diabetes Ther. 2019;10:1859-68.

CASE SCENARIO 9: MANAGEMENT OF RECURRENT DETACHMENT IN CRD

Case Summary

A 41-year-old male presented with recent drop in vision in the right eye. He had two prior vitrectomies for PDR in the right eye, 4 and 3 months back respectively. There was nasal and inferior retinal detachment under silicone oil. Two large breaks were noted inferonasally. Macula was attached **(Fig. 9A)**. His vision was 6/18, N6 in the right eye. The left eye was blind.

Surgical Steps

Silicone oil was removed with active suction

↓

Perisilicone membranes were removed with cutter

↓

LPFC was injected over posterior pole to keep the posterior retina and macula attached during MP

↓

There was subretinal silicon oil. Active suction was used to bring the oil in vitreous cavity and was then removed out

↓

Preretinal membranes were cleared with forceps. Inferonasal retinectomy was done to release the traction and to mobilize contracted retina. LPFC was filled just beyond the retinectomy edge to flatten the retina

↓

Laser was done along the posterior edge of the retinectomy. Cryotherapy was done for the anterior margin of the retinectomy

↓

Direct LPFC: Silicon oil exchange was done

Thought Process

Action	*Rationale*
PFCL injection	To prevent macular detachment and to stabilize posterior retina during membrane surgery and then to reattach the retina after complete release of traction
Retinectomy	To mobilize the contracted retina for reattachment
Cryopexy	For peripheral edge of the anterior breaks. Sometimes it is difficult to reach these locations with endolaser

(PFCL: perfluorocarbon liquid)

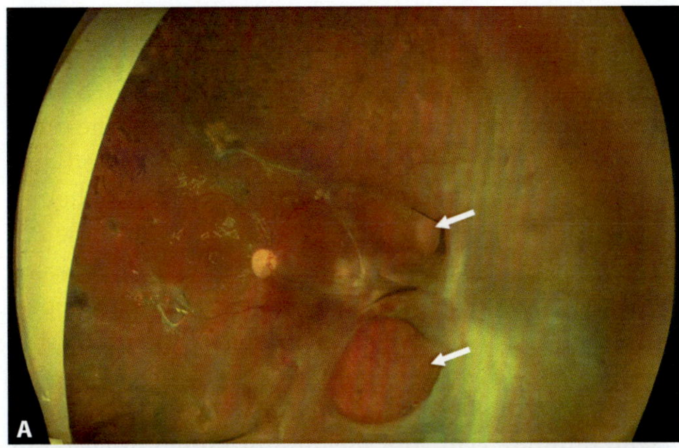

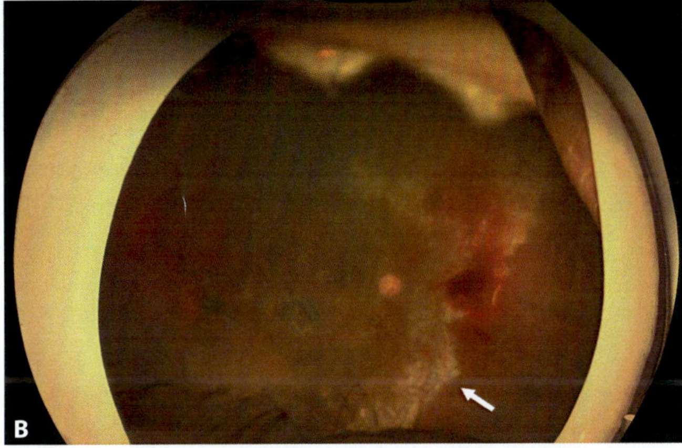

Figs. 9A and B: (A) Preoperative fundus: Nasal retinal detachment in silicon oil-filled eye. Retinal breaks marked with white arrows; (B) Postoperative (1 week) fundus: Nasal retinectomy (white arrow) with laser marks.

OUTCOME SUMMARY

- At last follow-up, retina was attached **(Fig. 9B)** and IOP was 14 mm Hg. The vision was dropped marginally, probably due to worsening of cataract.
- The patient is awaiting silicone oil removal and cataract surgery.

KEY POINTS

- Postvitrectomy PDR eyes with recurrent RD, usually presents more like a rhegmatogenous RD with PVR and need to manage accordingly.
- Presence of subretinal silicone oil indicates severe contraction of the retina and invariably needs relaxing retinotomy/retinectomy.
- Meticulous removal of perisilicone oil membranes is necessary for better anatomical and functional success.
- Injection of PFCL before initiating the MP helps to keep macula attached and also stabilizes mobile retina for ease of membrane surgery.
- Relaxing retinectomy, though is the last option, may be needed to relieve the traction and to reattach the retina, in select eyes.
- In a phakic eye, it may be difficult to laser anterior edge of peripheral tear/s. Trans-scleral cryopexy can be useful in this situation. It also minimizes the risk of lens touch.

FURTHER READING

1. Cruz-Iñigo YJ, Berrocal MH. Twenty-seven-gauge vitrectomy for combined tractional and rhegmatogenous retinal detachment involving the macula associated with proliferative diabetic retinopathy. Int J Retina Vitreous. 2017;3:38.
2. Idrees S, Sridhar J, Kuriyan AE. Proliferative Vitreoretinopathy: A Review. Int Ophthalmol Clin. 2019;59(1):221-40.
3. Newman DK. Surgical management of the late complications of proliferative diabetic retinopathy. Eye. 2010;24(3):441-9.
4. Stewart MW, Browning DJ, Landers MB. Current management of diabetic tractional retinal detachments. Indian J Ophthalmol. 2018;66(12):1751-62.

SUMMARY KEY POINTS

- In select cases, preoperative anti-VEGF helps to decrease the vascularity for easy membrane dissection and to reduce the risk of intra- and postoperative bleeding.
- In eyes with CRD, mobility of the underlying retina significantly increases the risk of iatrogenic breaks as MP is more difficult due to lack of countertraction. It is important to have proper preoperative planning, selection of instrumentation and willingness to modify the steps intraoperatively, if necessary, for better final outcome.
- 25 G or 27 G cutter is better, as port optimization and beveled tip helps easy access between retina and membrane.
- Vitreous cutter with very low cut-rate and shaving mode, behaves like an automated scissor.
- To approach correct plane for dissection, understanding the concept of vitreoschisis is important during diabetic vitrectomy.
- Complete removal of posterior hyaloid is necessary to mobilize the retina. In eyes with taut PHF, MVR blade can be used to create an edge to lift the PHF.

- Intravitreal injection of triamcinolone can help to visualize the cortical vitreous better for easier and more complete removal of vitreous.
- "Inside-out" approach is better when dealing with mobile retina. The dissection is initiated at the optic nerve head and then extended toward the periphery where disc acts as fulcrum.
- The decision to support the vitreous base with encircling band should be considered, if there is residual peripheral traction, but with caution. As anterior segment ischemia may ensue in these eyes with already compromised perfusion.
- Chandelier illumination can be used through a fourth port, if planning bimanual membrane dissection. Another option is lighted infusion. It typically obviates the need for an additional sclerotomy. However, care should be taken during the vitrectomy, as the vacuum of the cutter may outpace the inflow. Once the bimanual dissection is completed, the lighted infusion can be switched back to the traditional infusion.
- Hemostasis can be achieved by increasing the IOP for a moment during surgery. In diabetic patients, the optic nerve head circulation is already compromised and higher IOP for longer duration can worsen ischemic damage leading to overall poorer functional outcome. So, other methods of hemostasis, like direct gentle pressure on the bleeding point with a cutter or any blunt-tipped instrument can be a safer option to achieve hemostasis.
- Although gas is generally preferred, the choice of endotamponade (gas/silicon oil) depends upon the number, size, and location of retinal breaks, the possible risk of postoperative bleeding and the status of the fellow eye.
- Advances in surgical technology and techniques have significantly improved anatomical outcomes. But, final visual prognosis often depends on disc and macula status, chronicity, and systemic factors like diabetes control.

CHAPTER 6

Decision Making in Scleral Buckle Surgeries

Manoj Shettigar, Padmaja Kumari Rani

SCLERAL BUCKLE IN RRD MANAGEMENT

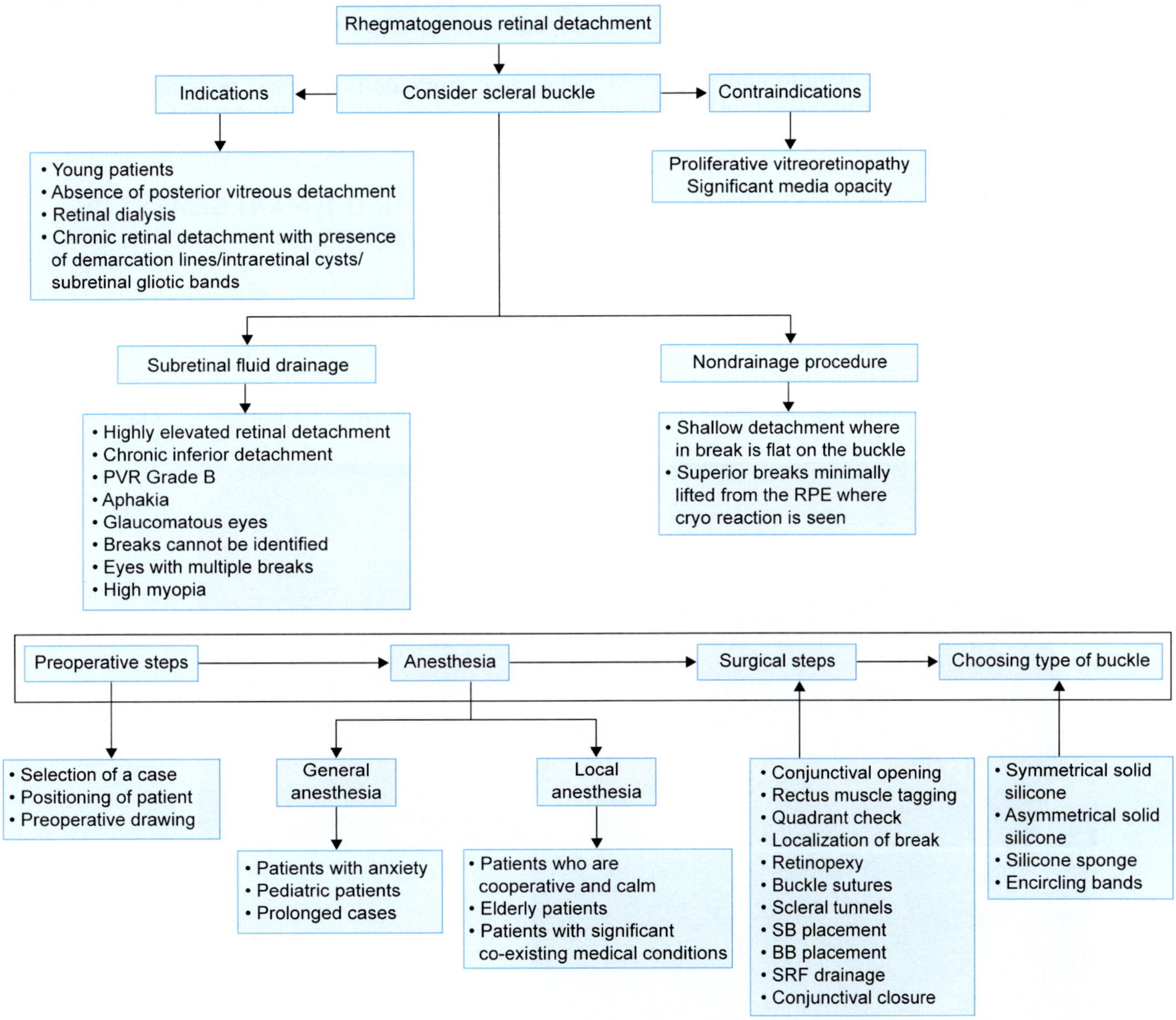

Rhegmatogenous retinal detachment

Consider scleral buckle

Indications

- Young patients
- Absence of posterior vitreous detachment
- Retinal dialysis
- Chronic retinal detachment with presence of demarcation lines/intraretinal cysts/ subretinal gliotic bands

Contraindications

Proliferative vitreoretinopathy
Significant media opacity

Subretinal fluid drainage

- Highly elevated retinal detachment
- Chronic inferior detachment
- PVR Grade B
- Aphakia
- Glaucomatous eyes
- Breaks cannot be identified
- Eyes with multiple breaks
- High myopia

Nondrainage procedure

- Shallow detachment where in break is flat on the buckle
- Superior breaks minimally lifted from the RPE where cryo reaction is seen

Preoperative steps → Anesthesia → Surgical steps → Choosing type of buckle

Preoperative steps

- Selection of a case
- Positioning of patient
- Preoperative drawing

Anesthesia

General anesthesia

- Patients with anxiety
- Pediatric patients
- Prolonged cases

Local anesthesia

- Patients who are cooperative and calm
- Elderly patients
- Patients with significant co-existing medical conditions

Surgical steps

- Conjunctival opening
- Rectus muscle tagging
- Quadrant check
- Localization of break
- Retinopexy
- Buckle sutures
- Scleral tunnels
- SB placement
- BB placement
- SRF drainage
- Conjunctival closure

Choosing type of buckle

- Symmetrical solid silicone
- Asymmetrical solid silicone
- Silicone sponge
- Encircling bands

Rhegmatogenous retinal detachment (RRD) is an important cause of visual impairment, and surgical management remains the gold standard of care. Among the various surgical modalities—scleral buckling (SB), pars plana vitrectomy (PPV), and pneumoretinopexy—SB continues to be the gold standard for the repair of primary RRD. Introduced by Custodis in 1949, SB involves creating an indentation of the sclera to close retinal breaks and relieve vitreoretinal traction. The procedure is often combined with cryotherapy at the site of retinal breaks, preventing liquefied vitreous from entering the subretinal space and allowing the retinal pigment epithelium to pump out subretinal fluid effectively.

Scleral buckling retains a unique and important role even in selected cases of tractional or combined retinal detachments (RDs), such as those seen in familial exudative vitreoretinopathy (FEVR) or combined RDs where fibrovascular membranes extend to the periphery, limiting safe dissection during vitrectomy.

Numerous studies—both prospective and retrospective—have compared PPV, SB, and combined PPV + SB approaches in managing RRD. Evidence from randomized clinical trials suggests that SB achieves superior anatomical and functional outcomes in phakic eyes, while PPV may offer advantages in pseudophakic eyes. The primary anatomical success rate with SB exceeds 90%, making it a highly effective and durable intervention. In addition to its anatomical success, SB is cost-effective. Studies have shown that the average cost per procedure is approximately $400 for SB, compared to $1,000 for PPV. Moreover, the mean number of hospital visits (9 vs. 6) and resurgeries tend to be higher in the PPV group than in the SB group, further underscoring the economic and logistical advantages of SB.

Despite advancements in vitreoretinal surgery, SB remains a time-tested, reliable, and effective technique—especially for younger and phakic patients. A successful scleral buckle surgery requires careful preoperative planning, meticulous surgical technique, and close postoperative follow-up, all of which contribute to excellent long-term anatomical and visual outcomes.

CASE SCENARIO 1: MANAGEMENT OF RETINAL DIALYSIS

Case Summary

A 55-year-old male presented with defective vision for 8 months **(Fig. 1A)**. Examination revealed a large retinal dialysis located at the level of the third-order retinal venules (approximately 5 mm from the ora serrata) **(Figs. 1B and C)**.

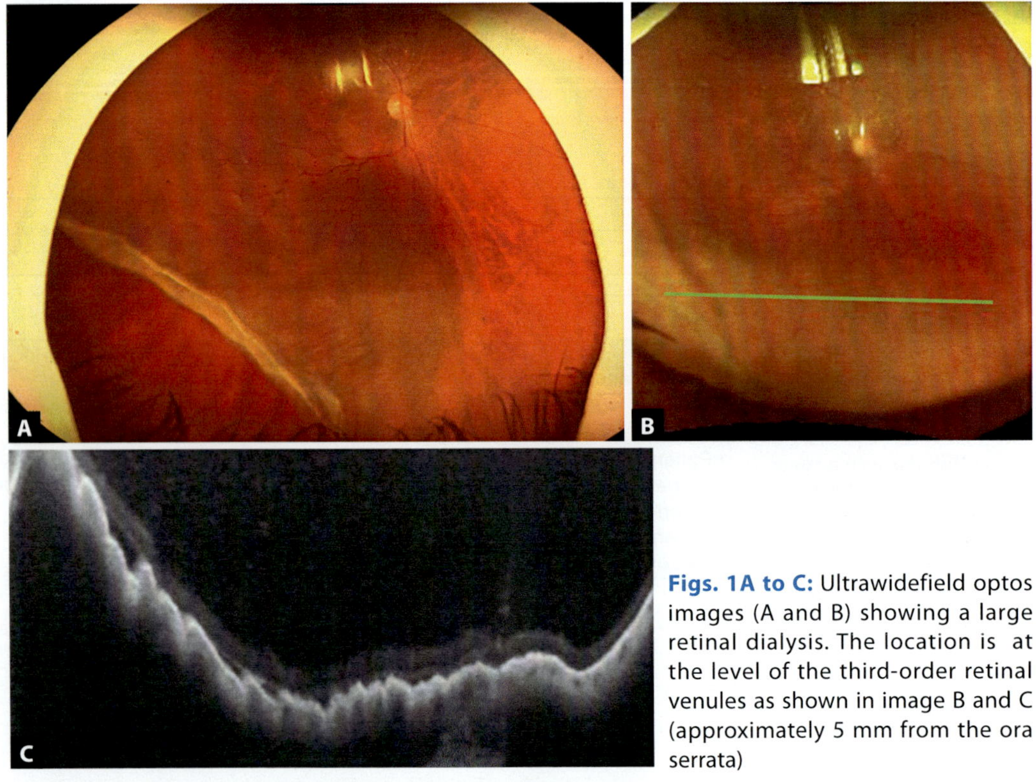

Figs. 1A to C: Ultrawidefield optos images (A and B) showing a large retinal dialysis. The location is at the level of the third-order retinal venules as shown in image B and C (approximately 5 mm from the ora serrata)

Treatment Plan

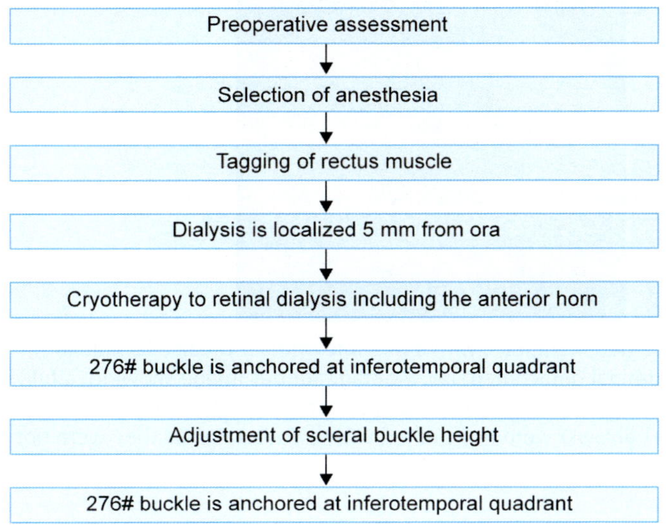

Thought Process

Decision	*Rationale*
Peripheral retinal breaks may appear more posterior on ultra-wide-field imaging due to image magnification	Hence, thorough examination with indirect ophthalmoscopy is essential for accurate localization and scleral buckle planning
Scleral buckle	Clear view, multiple peripheral breaks, and depressible breaks
Asymmetrical buckle	Provides greater indentation compared to symmetrical

OUTCOME SUMMARY

Postoperative fundus photograph and OCT show a fully attached retina following placement of a 276# buckle in the inferotemporal quadrant. The procedure was nondrainage.

Patient maintained a BCVA of 20/60 at the 4-month postoperative follow-up; the retina was attached, with the IOP of 10 mm Hg.

KEY POINTS

- A large retinal dialysis can be mistaken for a giant retinal tear; however, distinguishing features include a long history of symptoms (8 months), absence of posterior vitreous detachment on indirect ophthalmoscopy, and characteristic features of retinal dialysis.
- Other options, such as vitrectomy, are not recommended due to the high risk of recurrent RD.

FURTHER READING

1. Park SW, Kwon HJ, Byon IS, Lee JE, Oum BS. Impact of age on scleral buckling surgery for rhegmatogenous retinal detachment. Korean J Ophthalmol. 2017; 31:328-35.

CASE SCENARIO 2: MANAGEMENT OF SHALLOW RRD WITH HOLE WITHIN LATTICE

Case Summary

A 12-year-old male child presented with multiple lattice degenerations, with a possible primary break as a hole in the temporal lattice at 9:30 hours (arrow) associated with a shallow RD **(Fig. 2A)**. Preoperative fundus shows the lattice degeneration with a suspected hole.

Treatment Plan

Symmetrical scleral buckle is preferred in lattice degeneration and atrophic hole

↓

Non-drainage approach

Thought Process

Decision	*Rationale*
Immediate intervention	Macula-uninvolved retinal detachment
Concave scleral buckle	Provides an localized indentation without causing excessive distortion

OUTCOME SUMMARY

Patient maintained a best-corrected visual acuity (BCVA) of 20/40 at the 2-month postoperative follow-up; the retina was attached, with the intraocular pressure (IOP) of 13 mm Hg **(Fig. 2B)**.

KEY POINTS

- Multiple lattice degenerations are not a contraindication for SB.
- Accurate localization of the primary causative break using the Lincoff rule is critical for surgical planning.

FURTHER READING

1. Fallico M, Alosi P, Reibaldi M, Longo A, Bonfiglio V, Avitabile T, et al. Scleral Buckling: A Review of Clinical Aspects and Current Concepts. J Clin Med. 2022;11(2):314.

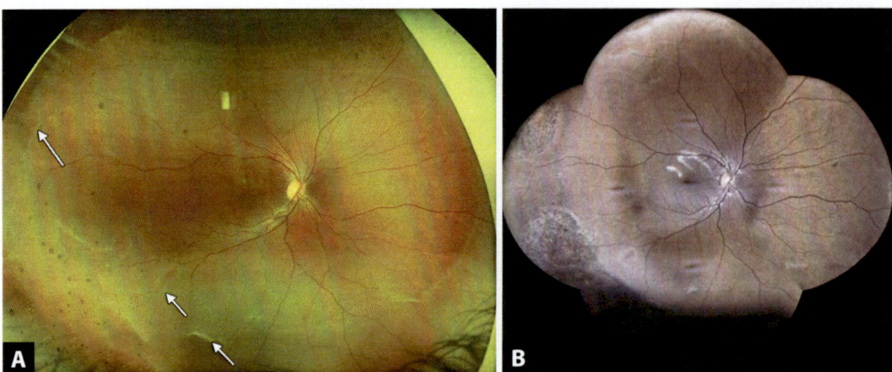

Figs. 2A and B: Ultrawide field fundus image showing multiple lattice degenerations, with a possible primary break as a hole in the temporal lattice at 9:30 hours (long arrow) associated with a shallow retinal detachment (A). Montage fundus image showing a fully attached retina is seen following placement of a 279# segmental buckle in the inferotemporal quadrant and a 360° encircling band (240#). The procedure was nondrainage. Two posterior lattices (short arrows) were not treated with cryotherapy, as they were not considered causative for the retinal detachment (B).

CASE SCENARIO 3: MANAGEMENT OF RRD WITH NO VISIBLE BREAK

Case Summary

A 27-year-old female presented with retinal detachment (RD). On examination, RD was present with cystoid changes noted in the macula **(Figs. 3A and B)**. No visible break was identified preoperatively. All suspicious areas were localized, and cryotherapy was done from 8 to 12 o'clock.

Treatment Plan

Nondrainage scleral buckling procedure.

The Lincoff rule may assist in localizing a suspicious or causative break

↓

An end-to-end buckle placed to cover the suspected area can effectively address the detachment

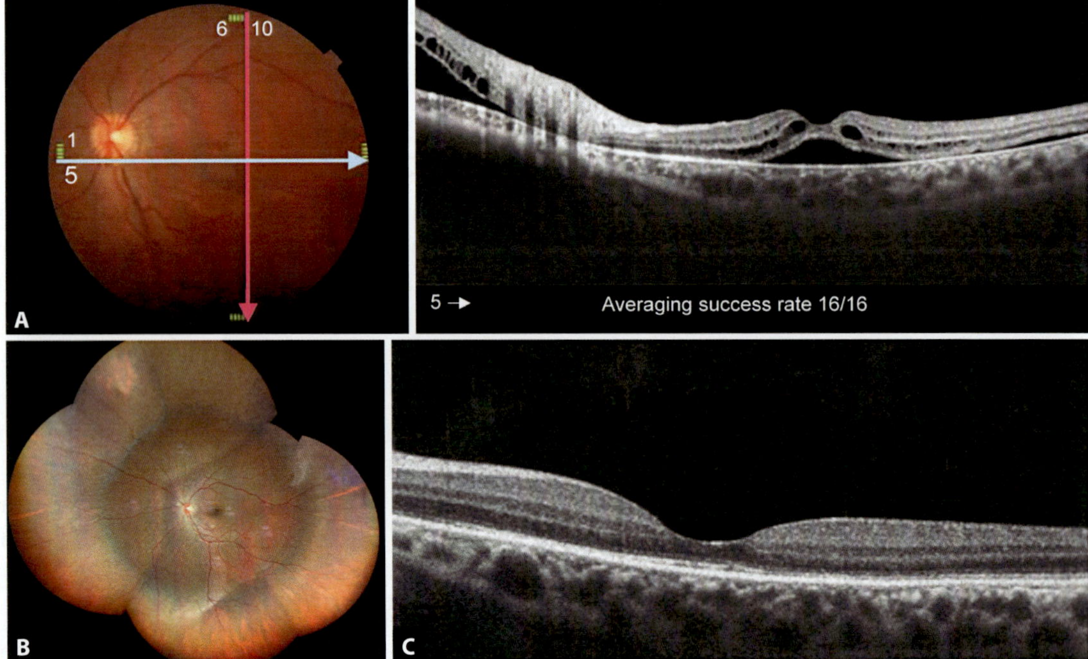

Figs. 3A to C: Color fundus and OCT images showing retinal detachment which was present with cystoid changes in the macula. (A) No visible break was identified preoperatively. All suspicious areas were localized, and cryotherapy was done from 8 to 12 o'clock. The patient underwent a nondrainage scleral buckling procedure. A fully reattached retina can be seen following placement of a 42# buckle (B and C).

Thought Process

Decision	Rationale
Absence of a visible break is not a contraindication for scleral buckling	360° encircling band can be used
Role of encerclage band	Supports the vitreous base, reduces chances of newer break formation

OUTCOME SUMMARY

Patient maintained a BCVA of 20/30 at the 3-year postoperative follow-up; the retina was attached, with the IOP of 15 mm Hg. A fully reattached retina can be seen following placement of a 42# buckle **(Figs. 3B and C)**.

KEY POINT

OCT can accurately delineate the extent of RD, particularly in cases with shallow subretinal fluid.

FURTHER READING

1. Sharma T, Challa JK, Ravishankar KV, Murugesan R. Scleral buckling for retinal detachment. Predictors for anatomic failure. Retina. 1994;14(4):338-43.

CASE SCENARIO 4: MANAGEMENT OF RRD WITH MULTIPLE LATTICES AND HOLES

Case Summary

A 42-year-old female with retinal detachment with lattice degeneration and a hole located 7 mm from the ora serrata, along with multiple lattices in the attached retina **(Fig. 4A)**.

Treatment Plan

279# buckle and a 240# encircling band were placed

↓

Subretinal fluid (SRF) drainage was performed

Thought Process

Decision	Rationale
SB with encircling band	Multiple lattices in the attached retina
# 279 buckle segment	Posterior edge of break at 7 mm from muscle insertion
SRF drainage	• To permit the apposition of the break to the buckle • *Chronic thick SRF:* It will take a longer time to get absorbed

OUTCOME SUMMARY

Patient maintained a BCVA of 20/60 at the 4-month postoperative follow-up; the retina was attached, with the IOP of 12 mm Hg **(Fig. 4B)**.

KEY POINTS

- When the break is localized beneath an extraocular muscle, one scleral suture should be placed on either side of the muscle.

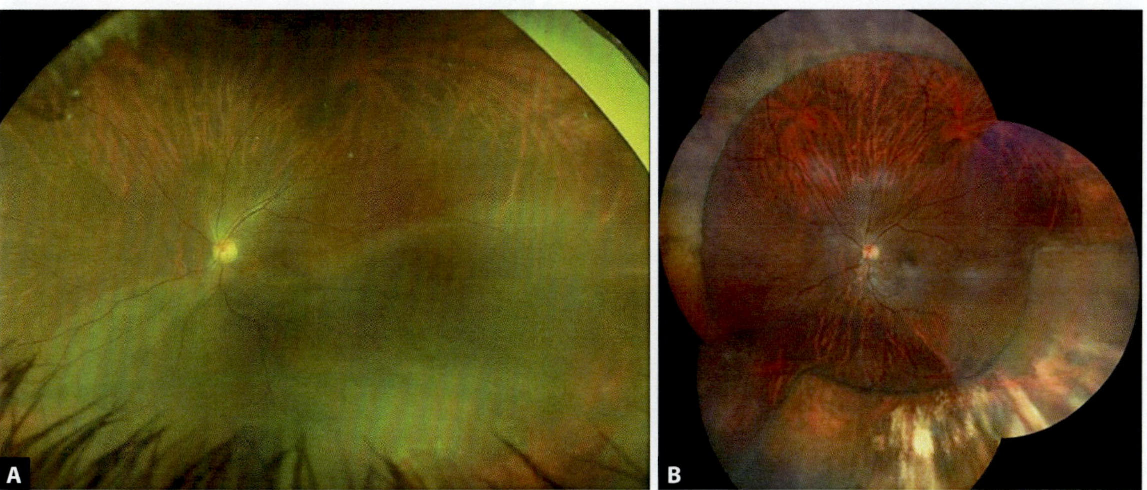

Figs. 4A and B: Ultrawide field optos image showing lattice degeneration and a hole located 7 mm from the ora serrata, along with multiple lattices in the attached retina. (A) Montage color fundus image shows attached retina with good buckle indent 4 months after 279# buckle and a 240# encircling band were placed, and subretinal fluid (SRF) drainage was performed (B).

- For a 7 mm-wide buckle (276#/277#/287#), the posterior scleral suture bite should be placed 9 mm from the ora serrata.
- For a 9 mm-wide buckle (289#/279#), the posterior scleral suture bite should be placed 11 mm from the ora serrata.
- For a 10 mm-wide buckle (280#), the posterior scleral suture bite should be placed 12 mm.

FURTHER READING

1. Roca JA, Maia M, da Cruz NFS, Polizelli MU, Chhablani J, Gangakhedkar S, et al. Non-contact wide-angled visualization with chandelier-assisted scleral buckling for primary uncomplicated rhegmatogenous retinal detachment. Graefes Arch Clin Exp Ophthalmol. 2020; 258(9):1857-61.

CASE SCENARIO 5: MANAGEMENT OF RRD WITH BREAKS IN MULTIPLE QUADRANT

Case Summary

A 43-year-old female presented with bilateral RRD with multiple breaks in multiple quadrant **(Figs. 5A and C)**.

Treatment Plan

287# buckle was placed in two quadrants in both eyes

↓

Cryotherapy was done to all lattices

↓

SRF was drained in the right eye

Thought Process

Decision	*Rationale*
Multiple breaks in multiple quadrants are not a contraindication for scleral buckle	Four quadrants and eight sutures are all required for a buckle suitable for RD!
SRF drainage within the buckle area	• In case of iatrogenic retinal damage in case of shallow fluid, it will be covered by the buckle indent • Careful localization of the drainage site to avoid draining the vitreous through the open break

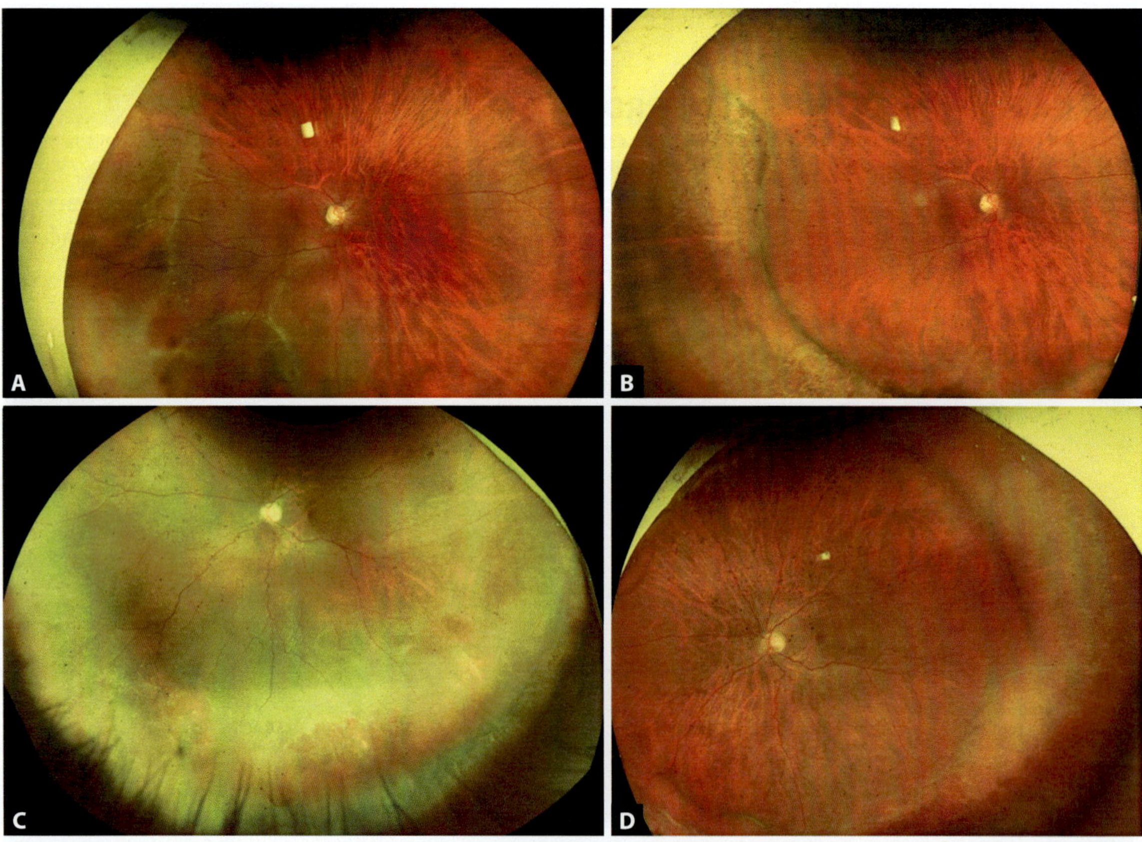

Figs. 5A to D: Ultrawide field fundus images showing bilateral retinal detachment (A and C). Postoperatively (B and D), a fully reattached retina is noted in both the eyes.

OUTCOME SUMMARY

Postoperatively **(Figs. 5B and D)**, a fully reattached retina is noted in both the eyes. Patient maintained a BCVA of 20/50 in the right eye and 20/30 in the left eye at the 5-month postoperative follow-up.

KEY POINTS

- Accurate indirect ophthalmoscopy of the retinal periphery is a must.
- Multiple breaks in multiple quadrants are not a contraindication.

FURTHER READING

1. Shanmugam PM, Ramanjulu R, Mishra KCD, Sagar P. Novel techniques in scleral buckling. Indian J Ophthalmol. 2018;66(7):909-15.

CASE SCENARIO 6: MANAGEMENT OF RRD WITH INFERIOR HORSESHOE TEAR (HST) IN YOUNG PATIENT

Case Summary

A 31-year-old male phakic presented with decreased vision in the left eye. A horseshoe tear was noted at 8 mm from the ora on the color fundus photo **(Fig. 6A)**.

Treatment Plan

Inferotemporal 280# buckle and nondrainage procedure

Thought Process

Decision	*Rationale*
280# scleral buckle	Asymmetrical buckle provides better anterior scleral indentation particularly useful in horseshoe tear

OUTCOME SUMMARY

Patient had improvement of BCVA from 20/400 to 20/320 at the 1-month postoperative follow-up; the retina was attached **(Fig. 6B)**, with the IOP of 14 mm Hg.

KEY POINTS

- The actual localization of the posterior margin of the break is crucial.
- *Morphology of RD:* Understanding posterior vitreous detachment status is important.
- Chronic shallow RD with subretinal PVR changes (demarcation lines/intraretinal cysts)—buckle is the choice.

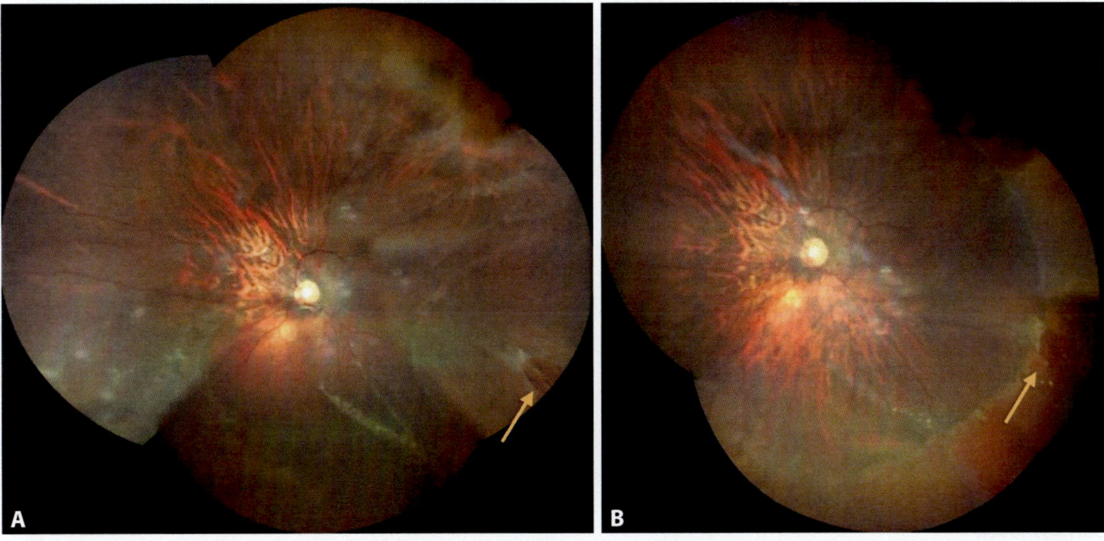

Figs. 6A and B: Montage color fundus image showing a horseshoe at 8 mm from the ora (A). Postoperative fundus photo showing a fully reattached retina, following an inferotemporal 280# buckle and nondrainage procedure (B).

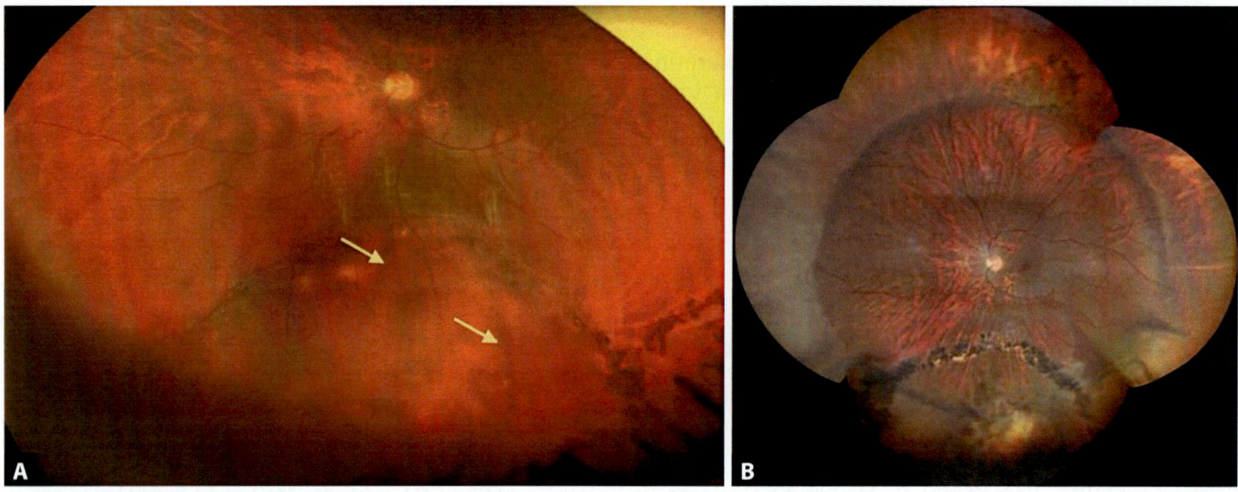

Figs. 7A and B: (A) Fundus image showing an inferior rhegmatogenous retinal detachment with visible laser marks (arrows); and (B) Postoperative image shows a fully reattached.

FURTHER READING

1. Fallico M, Alosi P, Reibaldi M, Longo A, Bonfiglio V, Avitabile T, et al. Scleral Buckling: A Review of Clinical Aspects and Current Concepts. J Clin Med. 2022;11(2):314.

CASE SCENARIO 7: MANAGEMENT OF RRD WITH BREAK WITHIN PRE-EXISTING LASER BARRAGE SCARS

Case Summary

A 24-year-old phakic male with only one seeing eye presented with decreased vision in the right eye. The patient had a prior history of barrage laser in the same eye. Fundus examination revealed an inferior RRD with visible laser marks **(Fig. 7A)**.

Treatment Plan

A convex buckle is preferred to relieve the tractional component adequately

↓

Symmetrical buckle like 287# can provide uniform indentation

Thought Process

Decision	*Rationale*
Confluent laser spots are needed in barrage laser.	To prevent migration of SRF
Closer follow-up is needed.	To rule out posterior migration of SRF till laser scars are formed.

OUTCOME SUMMARY

A fully reattached retina following placement of an inferior 287# buckle and a 360° encircling band (240#) **(Fig. 7B)**. Patient maintained a BCVA of 20/30 at the 3-year post-operative follow-up; the retina was attached, with the IOP of 15 mm Hg.

KEY POINTS

- Posterior barrage laser scars are not a contraindication for SB; however, they can represent areas of retinal thinning or weakness and may influence surgical planning.
- Subclinical RD is defined as a localized detachment extending up to two disk diameters. Considering that one disk diameter corresponds to approximately 1,500 µm and laser delimitation should be restricted to within two disk diameters from the margin of the detachment.

FURTHER READING

1. Wang A, Snead MP. Scleral buckling-a brief historical overview and current indications. Graefes Arch Clin Exp Ophthalmol. 2020;258(3):467-78.

CASE SCENARIO 8: MANAGEMENT OF CHRONIC SHALLOW RRD

Case Summary

A 24-year-old phakic female with lattice degeneration located at 12 o'clock, with shallow subretinal fluid approximately 7 mm from the ora serrata **(Figs. 8A and B)**.

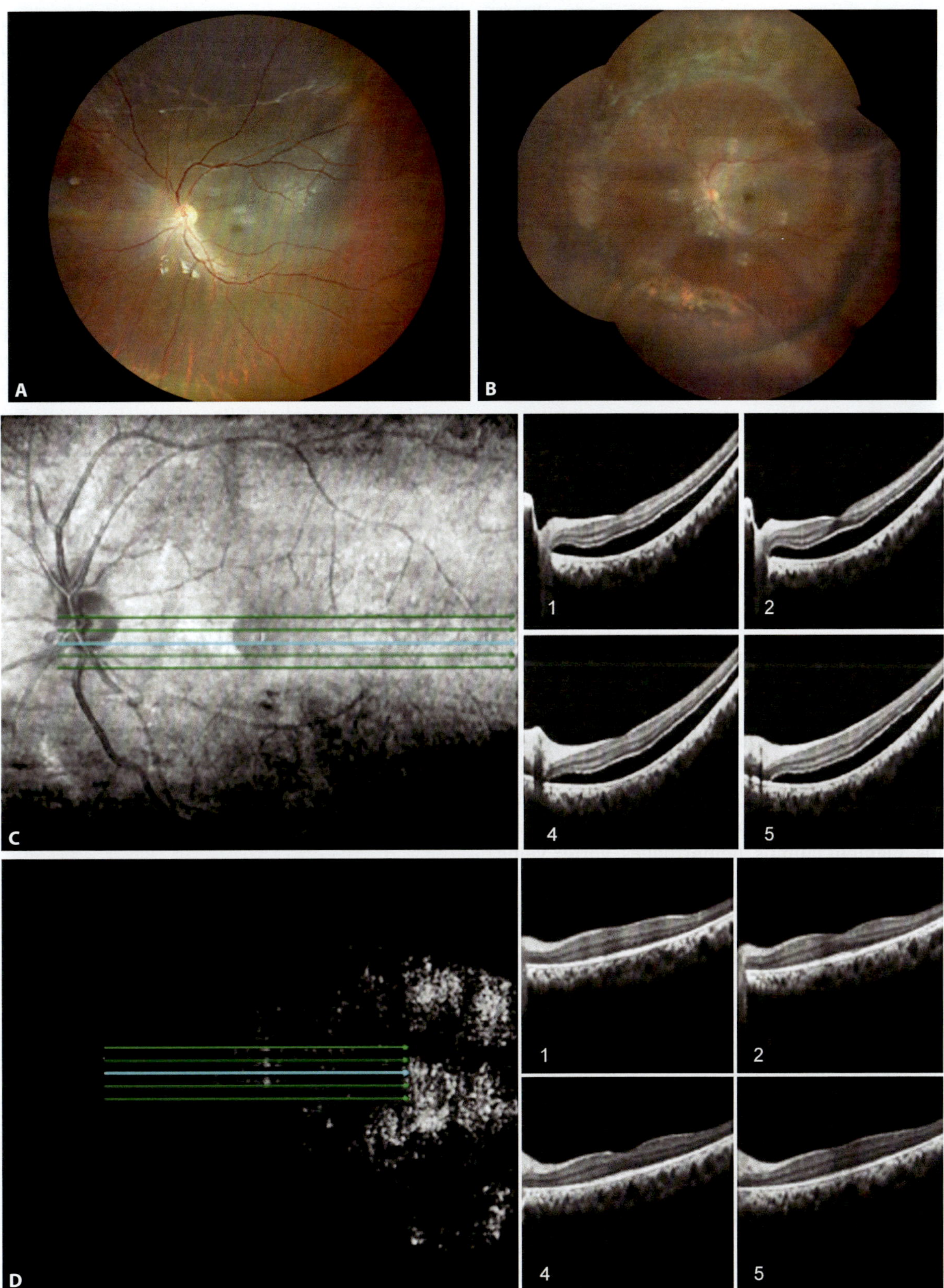

Figs. 8A to D: Color fundus image showing lattice degeneration located at 12 o'clock, approximately 7 mm from the ora serrata (A and B). Spontaneous absorption of subretinal fluid was noted over a 2-year follow-up period on optical coherence tomography (OCT) (C and D)

Treatment Plan

Nondrainage SB procedure using a 279# element, with the retina attached

↓

Chronic shallow subretinal fluid associated with lattice degeneration may resolve spontaneously following successful buckle placement

Thought Process

Decision	*Rationale*
279# scleral buckle	Symmetrical buckle provides uniform indentation

OUTCOME SUMMARY

The patient underwent a nondrainage SB procedure using a 279# element, with the retina attached. Patient maintained a BCVA of 20/25 at the 3-month postoperative follow-up; the retina was attached. Spontaneous absorption of subretinal fluid was noted over a 2-year follow-up period on OCT **(Figs. 8C and D)**.

KEY POINTS

- A detailed fundus drawing is essential to localize all retinal breaks and delineate the extent of RD. It helps to guide the surgical approach and serves as a valuable reference for postoperative monitoring and patient education. A well-prepared fundus drawing also helps to determine between SB and vitrectomy, ensuring the best possible surgical outcome. Key features such as folds, pigment clumps, hemorrhages, vortex veins, and retinal vessels can serve as important landmarks and provide indirect clues for break localization. As the saying goes, *"Breaks that are difficult to see are easy to close; those easily seen are often difficult to close."*
- Conjunctival peritomy can be either *limbal* or *perilimbal*, with a small frill of conjunctiva preserved.
- Adequate *relaxing incisions of 2–3 mm* should be made at *3 and 9 o'clock* positions to allow proper exposure and facilitate surgical manipulation. Using curved tenotomy scissors is recommended for optimal precision and efficiency.
- Muscle tagging is performed *beneath the insertion of each rectus muscle tendon* to facilitate controlled rotation and manipulation of the globe. While engaging the muscle hook, care must be taken *not to pass it posterior to the equator,* as this may injure the *vortex veins.*
- After muscle tagging, perform an *adequate quadrant inspection* to identify any *areas of scleral thinning* and to note the *location and course of vortex veins.* This step ensures safe placement of sutures and minimizes the risk of intraoperative complications.
- Localizing retinal breaks can be challenging, as they may appear more posterior than their true position. *Begin indentation anteriorly* in the suspected meridian for accurate localization. *Pigment clumps at the RPE* can serve as indirect clues to the break site. *Localization marks* should be made using a localizer held *perpendicular to the scleral surface,* and the corresponding points marked with a *scleral marker.* These marks are then *measured from the ora serrata,* using the *spiral of Tillaux* (muscle insertions) as the anatomical reference.
- Cryotherapy should be performed *before draining subretinal fluid.* The cryoprobe must be held *perpendicular to the scleral surface,* avoiding contact with the eyelids. *Freezing continues until a dull orange-gray "graying" is visible* around the retinal break, achieved by indenting with the *tip (not the shaft)* to prevent posterior burns. The goal is *light retinal whitening* with smooth, confluent, nonoverlapping spots and adequate anterior coverage. Avoid freezing the *center of the break,* bare RPE, or refreezing to reduce the risk of *PVR.*
- Ensure the probe is *fully thawed before moving* to another site, as premature removal may cause *new linear breaks or retinal hemorrhages.* The assistant should *wet the cornea first, then the probe* to prevent the formation of a large freeze ball and facilitate smooth thawing.
- The *configuration of the scleral buckle* depends on the *number, size, and location of retinal breaks,* as well as the *presence of vitreoretinal traction.* A *radial buckle* is suitable for a *single and localized break,* whereas *multiple or widely separated breaks* across different quadrants are best supported by a *wider and circumferential buckle.*
- The *buckle dimensions* should provide support extending approximately *2 mm anterior and posterior* to the localized retinal break. The *height of the buckle effect* is primarily achieved by *suture placement and adjustment,* rather than excessive tightening of the *encircling band.*
- Before performing *SRF drainage,* assess for *shifting SRF* and evaluate *IOP*—a *high IOP* increases the risk of *retinal incarceration,* while a *low IOP* may lead

to *inadequate drainage.* Carefully *recheck for large choroidal vessels* under *high magnification* to avoid inadvertent injury during drainage.

- Complications during *subretinal fluid drainage* can be minimized by carefully *selecting the drainage site*—preferably at the *area of maximum fluid,* close to the *horizontal meridians.* Avoid draining over regions with *subretinal fibrosis, fixed retinal folds, vascular choroid, or directly over a retinal break* to reduce the risk of intraoperative complications.
- In the event of *vitreous loss after SRF drainage,* management includes *excising the prolapsed vitreous, closing the sclerotomy,* and applying *cryotherapy to the drainage site.* If the site lies *outside the buckle bed,* provide *additional buckle support* to ensure adequate tamponade and retinal reattachment.
- Periodic *indirect ophthalmoscopy-assisted retinal examination* should be performed at key surgical steps—*during localization, cryotherapy, after buckle placement* (to assess the need and optimal site for drainage), and *during drainage* (if a dry tap or subretinal hemorrhage is encountered). At each stage, it is important to *evaluate optic nerve head perfusion—a pale disk with pulsations or absence of pulsations* indicates compromised perfusion and warrants *immediate anterior chamber paracentesis.*

NEWER MODIFICATIONS

- The *chandelier endoillumination system* enhances visualization during SB by providing *wide-angle, diffuse illumination* for clear identification, and precise cryotherapy of retinal breaks, including those in the far periphery. This reduces missed breaks—an important cause of recurrence—and enables the use of the *operating microscope with live video,* improving *teaching, demonstration, and supervision* for trainees.
- Care must be taken while using a *chandelier endoillumination system,* as its *intraocular placement can cause vitreous disturbance.* The *light source should be removed after retinopexy is completed* to avoid inadvertent *lens touch or intraocular injury.* Additionally, the intraocular entry of the chandelier may *increase the risk of epiretinal membrane formation* following SB.
- *Sutureless scleral buckle:* This technique employs a *silicone band (typically 2.5 mm wide)* anchored to the sclera through *partial-thickness scleral tunnels* in each quadrant. It eliminates the need for sutures, thereby *avoiding suture-related complications* and promoting faster healing.
- *Scleral buckle in combined RD:* Used as an adjuvant procedure in cases with extensive peripheral membranes where safe peripheral membrane dissection is not feasible, providing additional support to relieve traction and enhance retinal reattachment.
- *Suprachoroidal buckling:* This surgical technique is designed for selected cases of *RD with peripheral retinal tears, myopic macular holes, or myopic foveoschisis.* It can be performed *alone or combined with vitrectomy* and is particularly useful in patients with *thin or deformed sclera* or *posterior staphyloma.* The procedure involves *injecting a long-lasting filler, such as hyaluronic acid, into the suprachoroidal space* through a specially designed *catheter or cannula,* creating localized choroidal elevation to support the retina.

FURTHER READING

1. Rani PK, Narayanan R, Deshpande RS, Balakrishnan D, Ali MH. Scleral Buckling Versus Sutureless Pars plana Vitrectomy in the Management of Primary Rhegmatogenous Retinal Detachment. Cureus. 2020;12(11):e11579.

CHAPTER 7

Decision Making in Surgical Management of Pediatric Retinal Pathologies

Saumya Johri, Virangi Doshi, Sushma Ratna Jayanna

ALGORITHMIC APPROACH FOR MANAGEMENT OF PEDIATRIC RETINAL DETACHMENTS

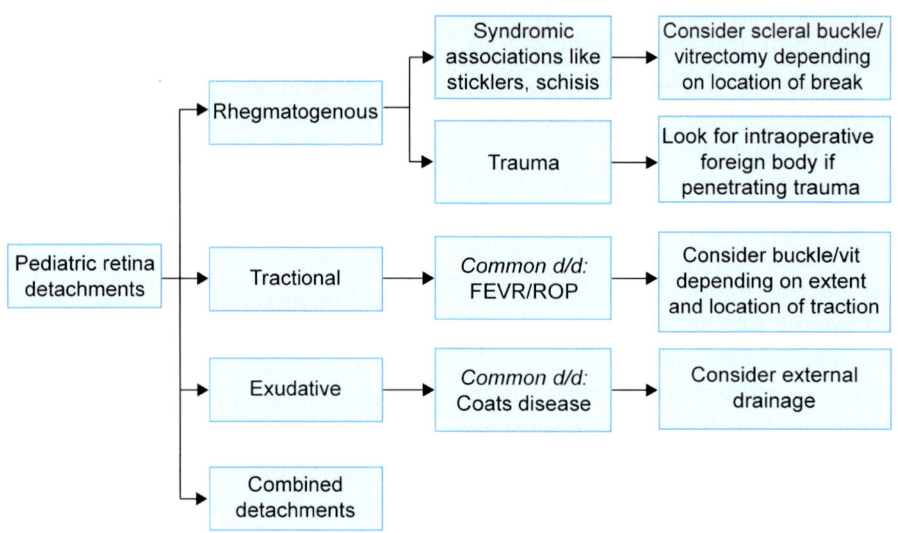

(FEVR: familial exudative vitreoretinopathy; ROP: retinopathy of prematurity sb/vit: scleral buckle/vitrectomy; d/d: differential diagnosis)

CASE SCENARIO 1: MANAGEMENT OF RETINAL DETACHMENT WITH SYNDROMIC ASSOCIATION

Case Summary

A 13-year-old male with a documented history of Axenfeld–Rieger syndrome characterized by corectopia and polycoria, bilateral open-angle glaucoma status post-trabeculectomy, and grade 1 subcapsular cataract presented with decreased visual acuity to counting fingers in the left eye. Examination revealed a rhegmatogenous retinal detachment, necessitating urgent surgical intervention **(Figs. 1A to C)**.

Treatment Plan

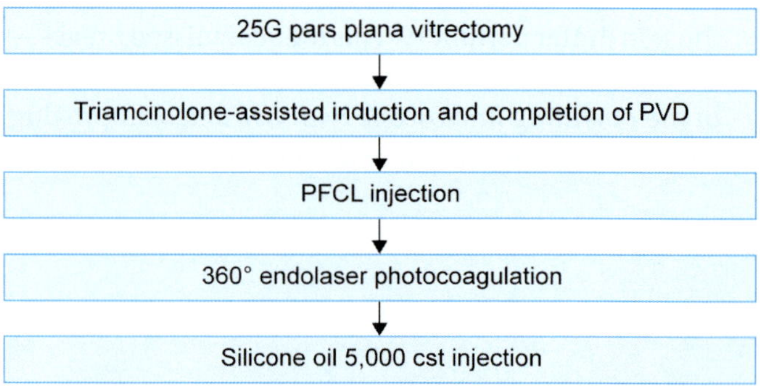

(PFCL: perfluorocarbon liquid; PVD: posterior vitreous detachment)

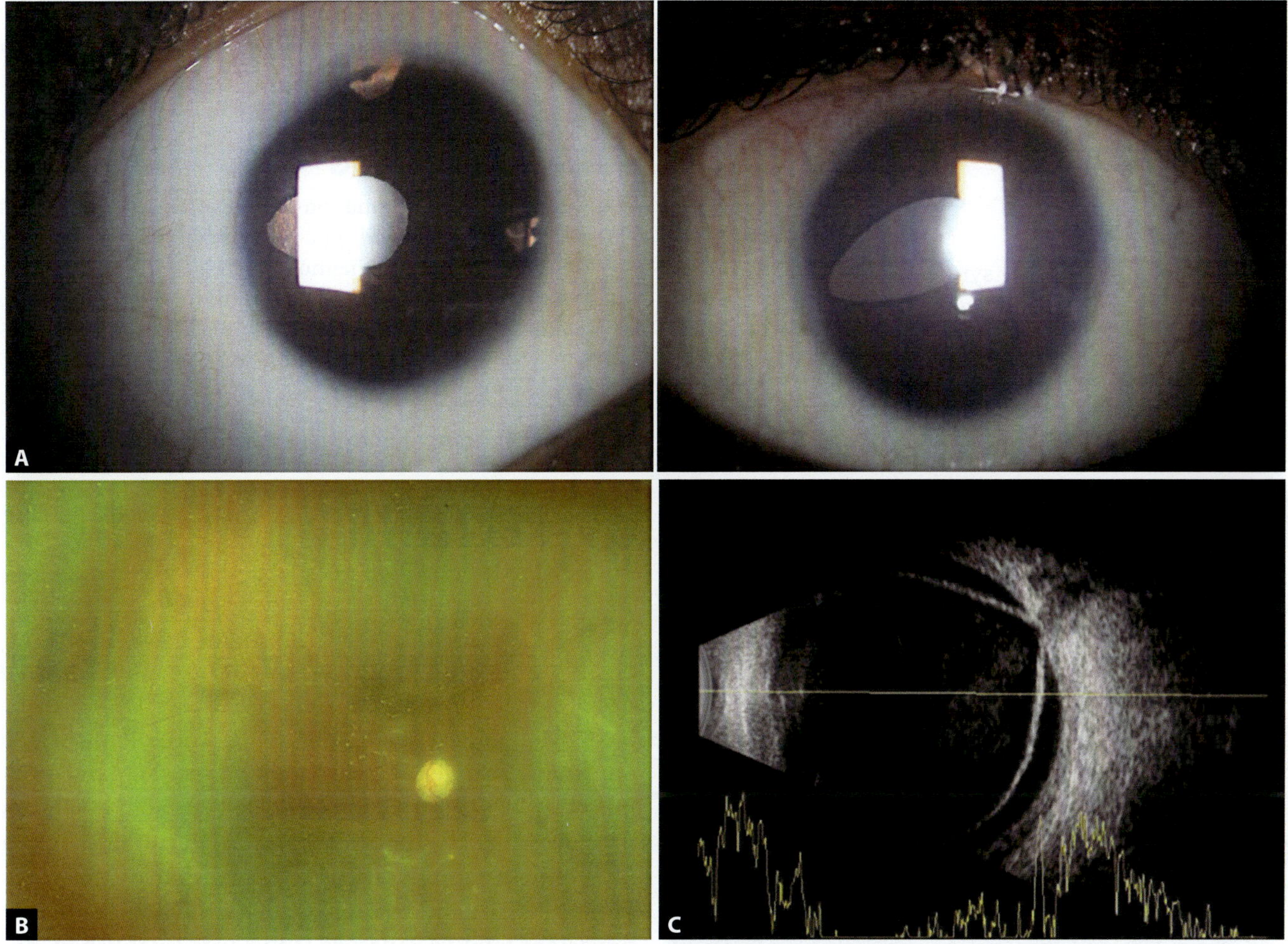

Figs. 1A to C: Depicts BE polycoria and corectopia on slit lamp examination (A). LE shallow retinal detachment seen in both color fundus photo and ultrasound B-scan (B and C).

Thought Process

Decision	*Rationale*
Avoid belt buckle	Glaucoma patient with trabeculectomy—avoid conjunctival scarring to preserve future surgical options
Avoid lensectomy	Lens clear enough to provide a good view for surgery
Avoid drainage retinotomy	To minimize potential PVR-related complications
Use PFCL to drain fluid	Chosen for its effectiveness in displacing subretinal fluid through an anteriorly located break
PFCL–air exchange	Performed to stabilize the retina and facilitate further surgical steps
360° laser photocoagulation	To make sure the unseen anterior microbreaks if any are covered
Usage of 5000 cst silicone oil	To prevent early emulsification and related complication like raised IOP

(IOP: intraocular pressure; PFCL: perfluorocarbon liquid; PVR: proliferative vitreoretinopathy)

OUTCOME SUMMARY

Postoperative vision improved to 6/36 with a well-attached retina under silicone oil. His intraocular pressure remained within normal limits, managed by anti-glaucoma medications **(Fig. 2)**.

KEY POINTS

- Retinal detachment in syndromic cases should be approached with a comprehensive multidisciplinary perspective.
- Sparing the conjunctiva and lens whenever feasible can help prevent future complications and facilitate further medical or surgical interventions.

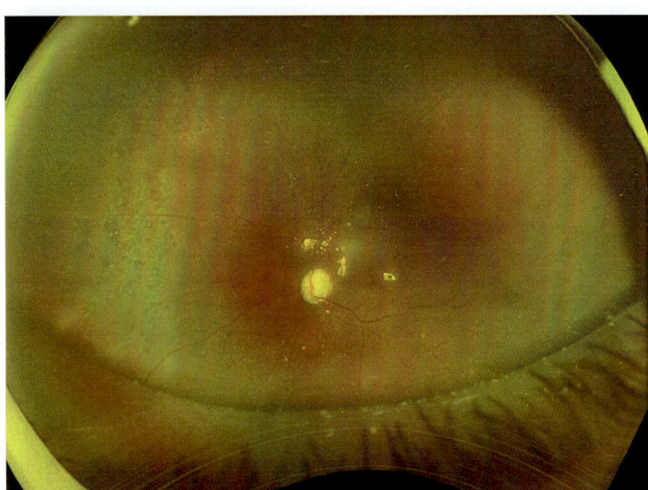

Fig. 2: Depicting attached retina under silicone oil with laser photocoagulations scars in periphery.

- Close follow-up is essential to monitor for recurrence, proliferative vitreoretinopathy (PVR) changes, and of the fellow eye.

FURTHER READING

1. Khandwala NS, Ramappa M, Edward DP, Mocan MC. Axenfeld–Rieger syndrome in the pediatric population: A review. Taiwan J Ophthalmol. 2023;13(4):417-24.
2. Spallone A. Retinal detachment in Axenfeld-Rieger syndrome. Br J Ophthalmol. 1989;73:559-62.

VIDEO LEGEND

Video 5: RRD in Axenfeld-Rieger Syndrome.

CASE SCENARIO 2: MANAGEMENT OF PERSISTENT FETAL VASCULATURE

Case Summary

A 11-month-old full-term infant presented with a unilateral white reflex observed by the parents since birth. Examination revealed a clear cornea of normal size and shape, a quiet anterior chamber, and a paracentral posterior lens opacity with a stalk attachment associated with optic disc drag and anterior peripheral retinal attachment to the stalk. The remainder of the retina appeared attached **(Fig. 3)**. A clinical diagnosis of persistent fetal vasculature (PFV) was established, and the patient was scheduled for a lens-sparing pars plana vitrectomy (LSV).

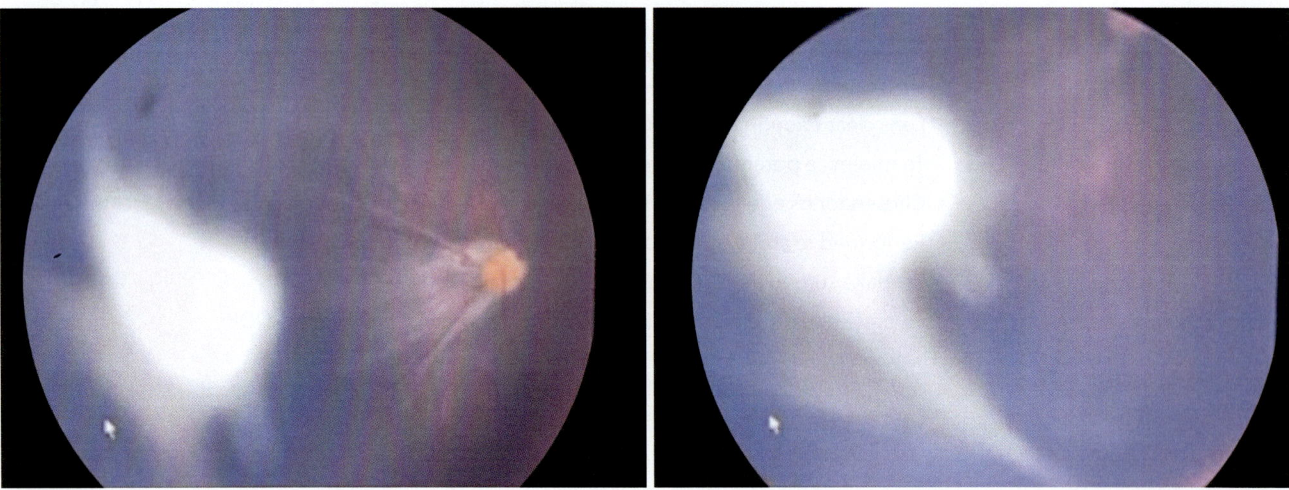

Fig. 3: Persistent fetal vasculature with attachment to peripheral anterior retina causing active anteroposterior traction.

Treatment Plan

25G 3 ports were made with nasal infusion placement

↓

Bridging membrane between the retinal fold and posterior lens capsule was carerfully released using microscissors without touching the lens

↓

Vitreous around the retinal fold was trimmed. Residual membrane attachment to pararcentral posterior lens capsule was trimmed

↓

Rest of the periphery checked for breaks or avascular retina, thin PFV stalk was trimmed

↓

Partial fluid air exchange was performed, ports were removed without any leak

(PFV: persistent fetal vasculature)

Thought Process

Decision	*Rationale*
Spare the lens	PFV-related aphakia can have long-term complications including glaucoma, hence preserve the lens whenever possible
Using microscissors instead of cutter	Scissors gives better navigation to approach localized membranes with good plane
Nasal infusion	Avoid temporal placement because of the retinal fold extending anteriorly
Meticulous periphery check	Posterior and combined PFVs can have tractional detachments and very thin retina
Trim the posterior stalk	Total removal of the PFV stalk is avoided as part of retinal fold can be integrated along with stalk hence trim and cauterize the tip if bleeds
Avoid induction of PVD	Extremely adherent vitreous and thin retina can induce breaks while induction hence prefer good trimming of vitreous around the fold and avoid iatrogenic breaks

(PFV: persistent fetal vasculature; PVD: posterior vitreous detachment)

OUTCOME SUMMARY

One month after surgery, a well-separated retinal fold was observed from the posterior lens capsule, with residual membrane attachment noted in the paracentral area of the posterior capsule. The remainder of the lens was clear, and the retina appeared attached with reduced disc drag **(Figs. 4A and B)**.

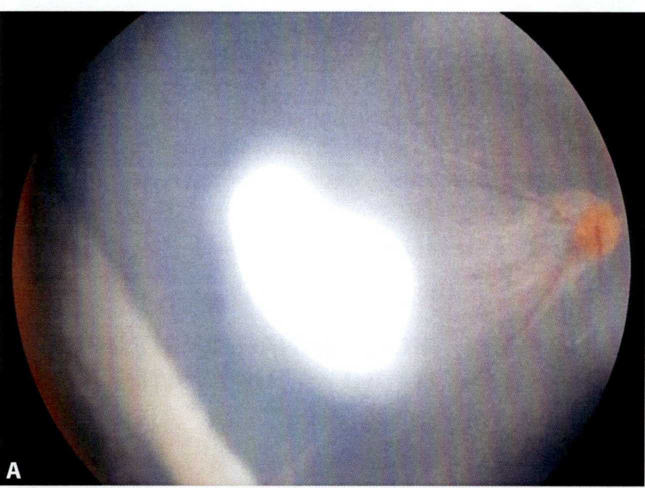

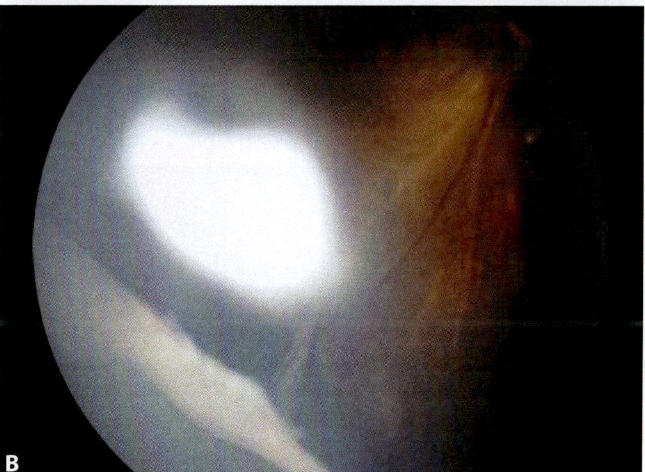

Figs. 4A and B: 1 month postoperative peripheral retinal fold appeared fallen back free from anterior traction with focal residual membrane in posterior lens capsule. Rest of the lens appeared clear.

KEY POINTS

- PFV with clear lens with paracentral focal attachment can be managed without sacrificing the lens.
- B-scan ultrasonography should be considered in cases of media opacity, and alternative causes of retinal fold—such as FEVR and ROP—should be excluded through thorough examination of the fellow eye.
- Aggressive induction of posterior vitreous detachment (PVD) should be avoided due to the presence of a thin retina and highly adherent vitreous.

FURTHER READING

1. AlGhazal F, Semidey VA, Rubio-Caso MJ, AlSulaiman SM, Sesma G. Surgical Parameters and Prognostic Factors in Persistent Fetal Vasculature: Insights from a Retrospective Cohort Study. Ophthalmol Ther. 2025;14(3):515-28.

2. Chen C, Xiao H, Ding X. Persistent Fetal Vasculature. Asia Pac J Ophthalmol (Phila). 2019;8(1):86-95.
3. Radder S, Radder N. Persistent Hyperplastic Primary Vitreous With Complete Retinal Detachment in an Infant: Imaging Characteristics and Clinical Management. Cureus. 2025;17(11):e96420.

VIDEO LEGEND

Video 6: Lens sparing vitrectomy in PFV.

CASE SCENARIO 3: MANAGEMENT OF TRAUMATIC MACULAR HOLE WITH CHOROIDAL RUPTURE

Case Summary

A 10-year-old boy with a history of cricket ball trauma 2 months prior presented with progressive right eye vision loss from 6/12 to 6/24. Fundus examination revealed a full-thickness macular hole and a radial juxtafoveal chorioretinal scar due to choroidal rupture and absence of PVD **(Figs. 5A and B)**. OCT confirmed a full-thickness foveal defect with cystic changes at the hole's edges, and a linear hyperreflective juxtafoveal choroidal scar. Given the vision decline and duration, surgical intervention was planned.

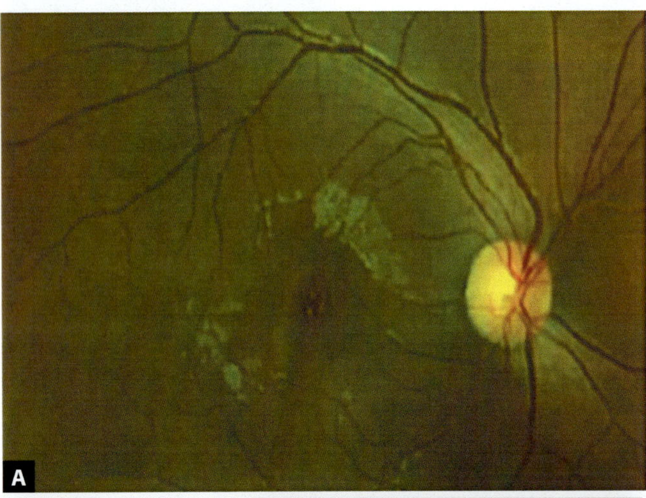

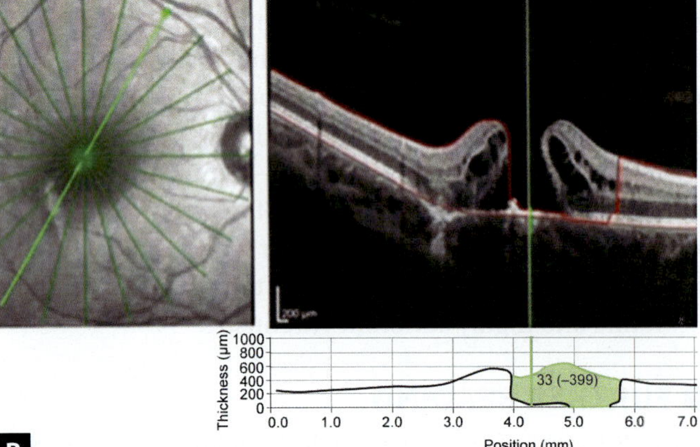

Figs. 5A and B: (A) Traumatic macular hole and juxtafoveal scarring probably due to choroidal rupture; (B) RE OCT showing full thickness macular hole along with a hyperreflective linear choroidal scar.

Treatment Plan

25G 3 ports valved cannula placement 4 mm from limbus in superotemporal, superonasal and inferotemporal (infusion) quadrant

↓

After minimal core vitrectomy, PVD was intiated with minimal traction over fovea and the choroidal scar and was completed with assistance of triamcinolone acetate (4%)

↓

Periphery was meticulously checked for breaks, ILM staining was done using brilliant blue dye under air

↓

ILM peeling was initiated under fluid, ILM flap was created and placed over the macular hole gently using ILM peeling forceps, avoiding intiation over the scar. Residual overlying posteior hyaloid was also peeled along with ILM nasal to fovea

↓

Fluid air exchange was perfomed with cutter mouth away from the flap to prevent dislodgment, c3f8 12% gas tamponade was injected at the end. Strict prone positioning was advised for 3–4 weeks

(PVD: posterior vitreous detachment)

Thought Process

Decision	*Rationale*
Surgical intervention	Reducing vision with duration of hole
Triamcinolone assisted PVD	Vitreous in children is extremely adherent, needs dye assistance for PVD induction, completion and confirmation
Avoid active pull over fovea and choroidal scar	Active vitreous pull over fovea may enlarge the hole and active pull over the scar might induce iatrogenic retinal breaks due to abnormal strong adhesion of vitreous along the scar
ILM stain under air	Under air, ILM staining for 60–90 seconds helps in efficient and longer hold of the dye by the tissue
Flap over the hole	Traumatic etiology and size of the hole

(PVD: posterior vitreous detachment)

OUTCOME SUMMARY

At 4 weeks postoperatively, the patient's vision improved to 6/9, with closure of the macular hole confirmed both

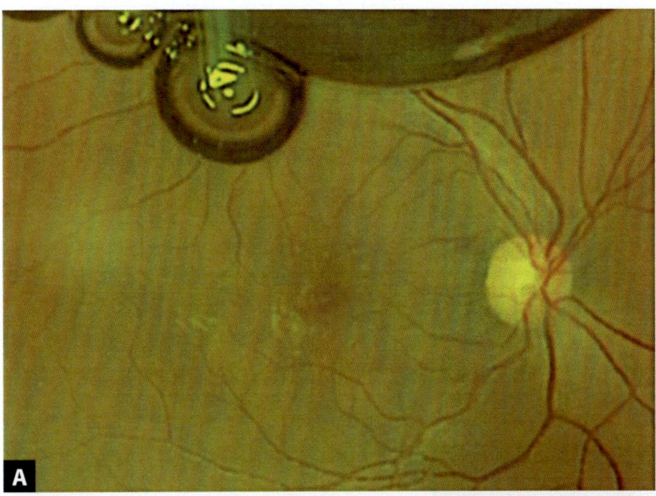

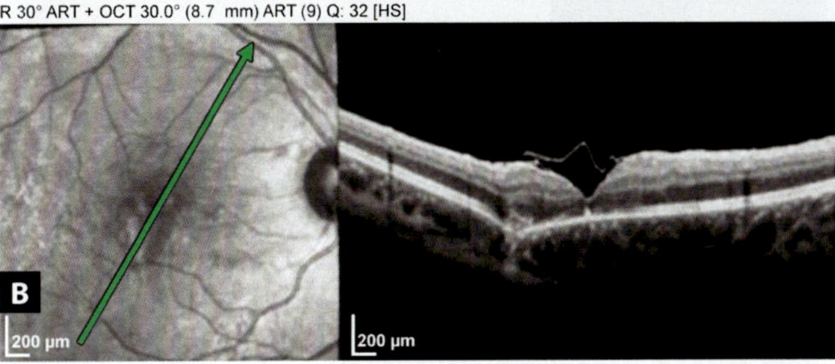

Figs. 6A and B: (A) 4 weeks postoperative macular hole closed with vision improvement to 6/9; (B) On OCT, a residual bridging ILM over the closed hole can be seen.

clinically and on OCT. Intraocular pressure remained well controlled. OCT imaging demonstrated a hyperreflective internal limiting membrane (ILM) flap bridging the closed hole **(Figs. 6A and B)**.

KEY POINTS

- Spontaneous closure of a traumatic macular hole in children is possible, so observation is recommended unless there is progressive vision loss or an increase in the size of the hole.
- In cases of traumatic macular hole, always check for additional intraocular trauma with a thorough eye examination, including gonioscopy for angles and inspection of the peripheral and posterior retina for other lesions.

FURTHER READING

1. Cui Y, Wang G, Shi X. Characteristics and surgical outcomes of pediatric traumatic macular holes. BMC Ophthalmol. 2025;25(1):291.
2. Liu W, Grzybowski A. Current Management of Traumatic Macular Holes. J Ophthalmol. 2017;2017:1748135.

VIDEO LEGEND

Video 7: Traumatic macular hole.

CASE SCENARIO 4: MANAGEMENT OF RETINOSCHISIS

Case Summary

A 7-year-old boy referred with suspected retinal detachment in both eyes. His best-corrected visual acuity in RE was 6/60 and in left eye was 6/36. On clinical examination, BE had good red glow with bullous schitic cavities with inner and outer retinal breaks **(Fig. 7A)**. Ultrasound B-scan showed low to medium spike corresponding to the schitic inner layers. There were no signs of retinal detachment on B-scan **(Fig. 7B)**. BE OCT showed schitic cavities with foveal involvement **(Fig. 7C)**.

Treatment Plan

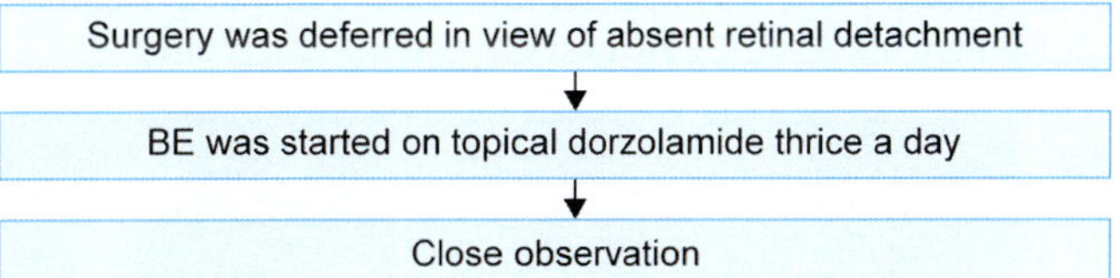

Thought Process

Decision	*Rationale*
Surgical intervention	Bullous retinoschisis that blocks the visual field or involves the fovea may indicate the need for surgery. However, conservative management can be attempted to allow the schisis fluid to resolve spontaneously, which occasionally occurs
Topical dorzolamide	Topical dorzolamide is known to reduce the cystic fluid macula in x-linked juvenile schisis
Imaging	Careful imaging with OCT and B-scan is recommended

OUTCOME SUMMARY

At the 3-month follow-up, a marked decrease in schisis fluid was observed clinically, as well as confirmed by B-scan and OCT imaging **(Figs. 8A to C)**.

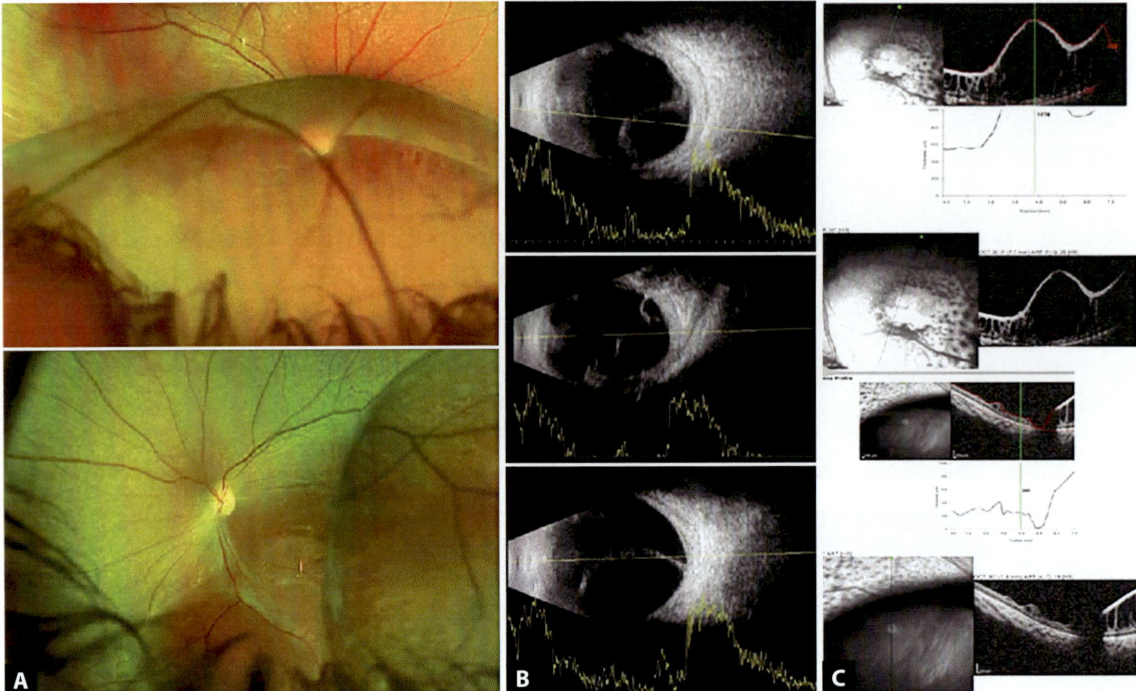

Figs. 7A to C: (A) A 7-year-old boy was referred with suspected retinal detachment in both eyes. BE fundus had good red glow with bullous schitic cavities with inner retina breaks; (B) Ultrasound b-scan both eyes showed low to medium spike corresponding to inner schitic layer. It did not show any signs of retinal detachment; (C) Both eyes OCT showed bullous schitic cavities with foveal area involvement (RE > LE). (BCVA: best-corrected visual acuity)

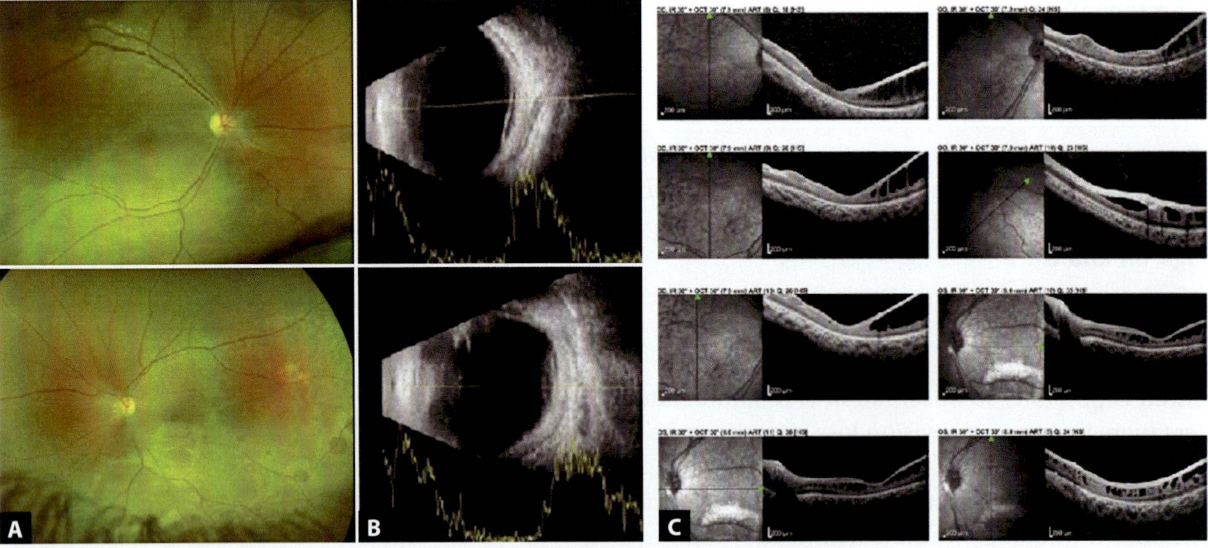

Figs. 8A to C: Both eyes show a marked decrease in schisis fluid was observed clinically, as well as confirmed by B-scan and OCT imaging.

KEY POINTS

- Vitreous hemorrhage, retinal detachment, and macular edema are potential complications of retinoschisis.
- Laser photocoagulation helps distinguish schisis (visible laser marks) from retinal detachment (no laser spots).
- Surgery may involve draining schisis fluid (externally or internally), trimming the inner retinal layer, and treating the schisis area if the retina is attached.
- In cases of schisis with retinal detachment, carefully examine the peripheral retina for breaks and address outer retinal holes in the schisis area.

FURTHER READING

1. Jeroudi AM, Shah V, Blinder KJ, Shah GK. Management of Degenerative Retinoschisis-Associated Retinal Detachment. Ophthalmol Retina. 2017;1(4):266-71.
2. Swaminathan S, Starr MR. Clinical and surgical approach to retinoschisis. Curr Opin Ophthalmol. 2026. Epub ahead of print.

CASE SCENARIO 5: MANAGEMENT OF VITREOUS HEMORRHAGE SECONDARY TO TERSON SYNDROME IN PRETERM

Case Summary

A 2-month-old preterm infant (34 weeks gestational age, 40 weeks postmenstrual age) presented with clear lens in both eyes and bilateral vitreous hemorrhage. The left eye had no fundus view due to dense hemorrhage and showed low to medium membranous echoes on B-scan **(Fig. 9)**. The infant was diagnosed with intraventricular hemorrhage by the pediatrician. Clinical diagnosis of bilateral vitreous hemorrhage secondary to Terson syndrome was made. LSV was planned for the left eye due to persistent dense hemorrhage, while the right eye was managed conservatively as the hemorrhage was clearing sufficiently to allow retinal visualization.

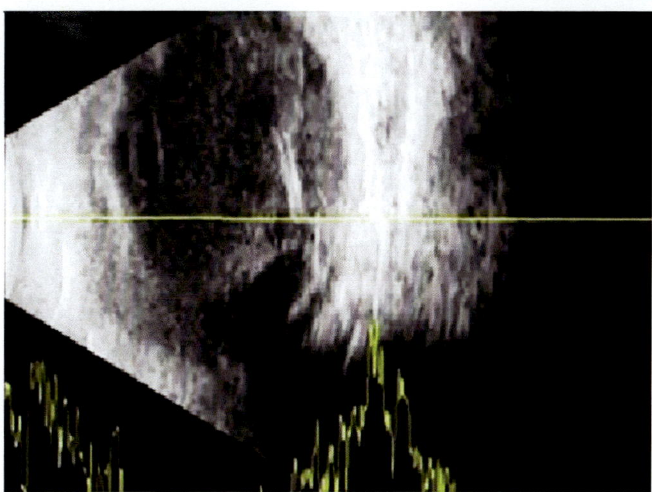

Fig. 9: LE B-scan showing low to medium reflective spikes s/o vitreous hemorrhage.

Treatment Plan

25G 3 valved cannula was placed 1.5 mm from the limbus

↓

All instrumentation were made sure to be vertically held to prevent lens touch

↓

Infusion cannula was placed in inferior qudrant carefully and position was verified before switching on the infusion

↓

Core vitrectomy was initiated with vacuum of 300–350 on constellation machine with cut rate of 10,000

↓

Midvitreous blood was cleared initially until the disc and posterior pole retina were visible and found to be attached

↓

Peripehral vitreous was trimmed with care to prevent inadvertent traction over immature retina and periphery was examined for any breaks

↓

Residual adherent posterior hyaloid over surface of the retina was trimmed, followed by partial fluid air exchange

Thought Process

Decision	*Rationale*
Early surgical intervention	As baby was premature, status of ROP could not be assessed which was crucial
Placement of infusion instead of AC maintainer	Prior to placing the trocar, a thorough examination was conducted to ensure the region was clear for trocar placement. This decision was made to achieve additional goal of preserving the lens. If the view of the infusion tip had not been clear, an AC maintainer would have been considered, as it can also be safely inserted without touching the intact lens
Defer induction of PVD	The strong vitreous adhesion in children and the fragile, immature retina in preterm infants require minimizing traction to prevent iatrogenic retinal breaks
Vertical placement of instruments.	To avoid touching the lens—which is larger relative to the globe in preterm infants—instruments should not be placed obliquely as they are placed in adults; doing so increases the risk of lens contact. Additionally, we try not to cross instruments beyond the vertical meridian for the same reason. However, it is safe to cross over beyond the lens if the instruments are kept sufficiently vertical

(PVD: posterior vitreous detachment; ROP: retinopathy of prematurity)

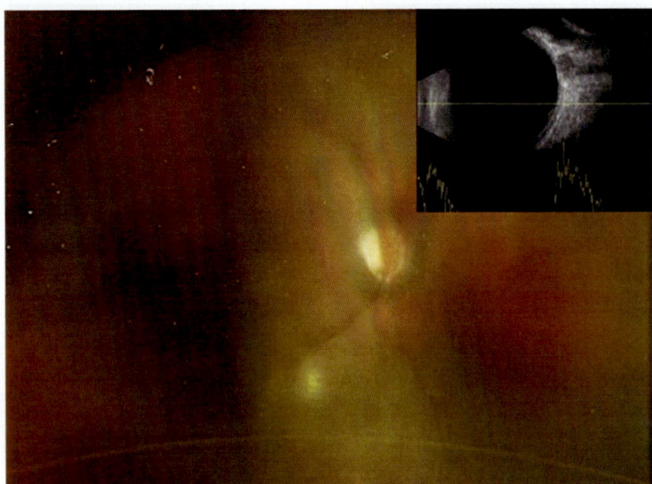

Fig. 10: Fundus image and B-scan (inset) showing postoperative attached retina with no new hemorrhage.

OUTCOME SUMMARY

At the 1-month follow-up, the media and lens were clear, and the retina was well attached with no new hemorrhage. The baby was scheduled for ongoing ROP follow-ups **(Fig. 10)**.

KEY POINTS

- Not all vitreous hemorrhage in preterm infants is attributable to ROP; it is important to also consider alternative causes of vitreous hemorrhage in newborns. Early surgical intervention should be considered in such cases, as ongoing monitoring for ROP remains essential.
- Proper infusion placement is a critical aspect of management. If the posterior segment view is compromised, we can consider using an AC maintainer as preserving the retina is of utmost importance. LSV is feasible with careful placement of the anterior chamber maintainer.

FURTHER READING

1. Alobaid MM, Alhaidari AI, Adhi MI, Nabeel Refka M. Terson Syndrome in Two Infants: Case Report and Literature Review. Cureus. 2024;16(12):e75102.
2. Hayreh SS. Pathogenesis of Terson syndrome. Indian j ophthalmol. 2022;70(12):4130-7.

VIDEO LEGEND

Video 8: VH secondary to Terson's syndrome.

CASE SCENARIO 6: MANAGEMENT OF PRESUMED PRE-PHTHISICAL EYE

Case Summary

A 4-year-old girl came for review who was diagnosed with pre-phthisical left eye after undergoing corneal tear repair 1 year prior elsewhere. She had no light perception, with corneal sutures present in the paracentral area, 360° posterior synechiae, a cataractous lens, and an obscured view of the fundus. The eye felt soft upon digital examination. B-scan ultrasonography revealed a clear vitreous cavity, an axial length of 18 millimeters, and an attached retina **(Fig. 11)**. Surgical intervention including pars plana lensectomy combined with vitrectomy was planned before definitively labeling the eye as phthisical.

Treatment Plan

Anterior chamber maintainer was placed in the inferotemporal quadrant, 25G ports were placed in superior quadrants

↓

Posterior synechiae was released, pars plana lensectomy was completed

↓

Posterior capsule was meticulously removed with help of micro forceps without causing retinal dialysis or ciliary body damage

↓

Posterior pole appeared clear with attached retina with mild chorioretinal folds and blurring of disc margins secondary to chronic hypotony

↓

Peripheral retina was meticulously examined, silicon oil was injected in view of hypotony

Thought Process

Decision	*Rationale*
A thorough examination under anesthesia followed by the necessary surgical intervention	Evidence for surgical intervention was provided by the axial length and the presence of a clear vitreous cavity on B scan
Meticulous removal of posterior capsule	Residual posterior capsule may contract and worsen existing hypotony
Silicone oil injection	Helps in preventing hypotony

OUTCOME SUMMARY

One week after surgery, the retina was attached with clear media and intact corneal sutures. Retinal folds and blurred disc margins resolved during follow-ups. The child

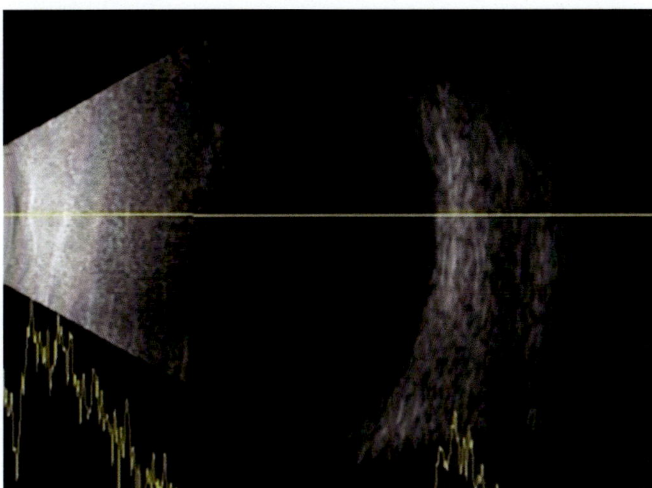

Fig. 11: B-scan ultrasonography revealed a clear vitreous cavity, an axial length of 18 millimeters, and an attached retina.

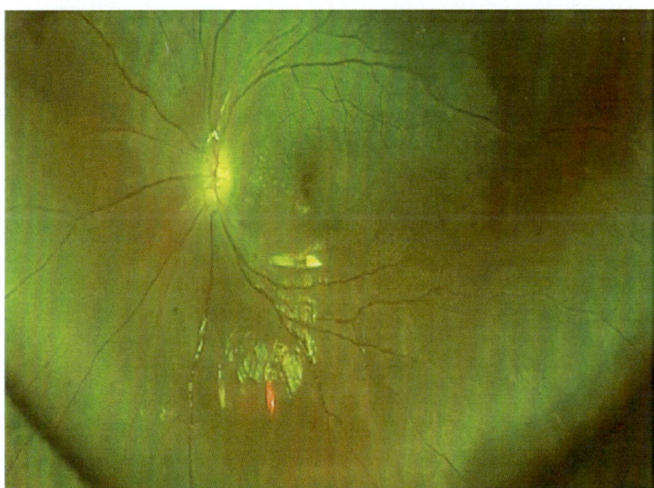

Fig. 12: Postoperatively retina was well attached and there was resolution of blurry disc margins and chorioretinal folds. Child has good light perception and follows light.

perceived and followed light, and was treated with an aphakic contact lens and patching therapy **(Fig. 12)**.

KEY POINTS

- A thorough surgical assessment should be conducted prior to designating any eye as "best left untreated."
- Visual rehabilitation is equally vital as surgical intervention in achieving optimal functional outcomes.

FURTHER READING

1. Puodžiuvienė E, Jokūbauskienė G, Vieversytė M, Asselineau K. A five-year retrospective study of the epidemiological characteristics and visual outcomes of pediatric ocular trauma. BMC Ophthalmol. 2018;18(1):10.
2. Scott IU, Flynn HW Jr, Azen SP, Lai MY, Schwartz S, Trese MT. Silicone oil in the repair of pediatric complex retinal detachments: a prospective, observational, multicenter study. Ophthalmology. 1999;106(7):1399-407; discussion 1407-8.

VIDEO LEGEND

Video 9: Presumed pre-phthisical eye.

CASE SCENARIO 7: MANAGEMENT OF TRD IN FAMILIAL EXUDATIVE VITREORETINOPATHY

Case Summary

A 6-month-old full-term infant presented with leukocoria in both eyes. The birth history was unremarkable, with no reports of fever or sepsis. There was no parental consanguinity, and this was the couple's first child. Fundus examinations for both parents revealed complete vascularization. On examination, both lenses were clear; with no view of posterior segment, B-scan ultrasonography identified closed funnel retinal detachments in both eyes **(Figs. 13A and B)**. Clinically, a diagnosis of stage 5 familial exudative vitreoretinopathy was made. The parents were recommended to seek genetic evaluation, and surgical intervention was planned.

Treatment Plan

25G translimbal infusion cannula was placed, 2 corneal side ports were created using 25G MVR blade

↓

PPL was performed. Posterior capsule was removed using micro forceps

↓

With BIOM assisted visualization and transiris approach, posterior vitrectomy was initiated

↓

Careful trimming and releasing of vitreous strands and membranes anteriorly and posteriorly, around the nasal fold was performed

↓

Nasal anterior attachment was trimmed without much manipulation in view of extremely thin retina with adherent membranes

↓

Partial fluid air exchange was performed. Anterior chamber was formed using viscoelastic substance
Side ports were hydrated
Infusion was safely removed
No sutures were placed as there was no wound leak

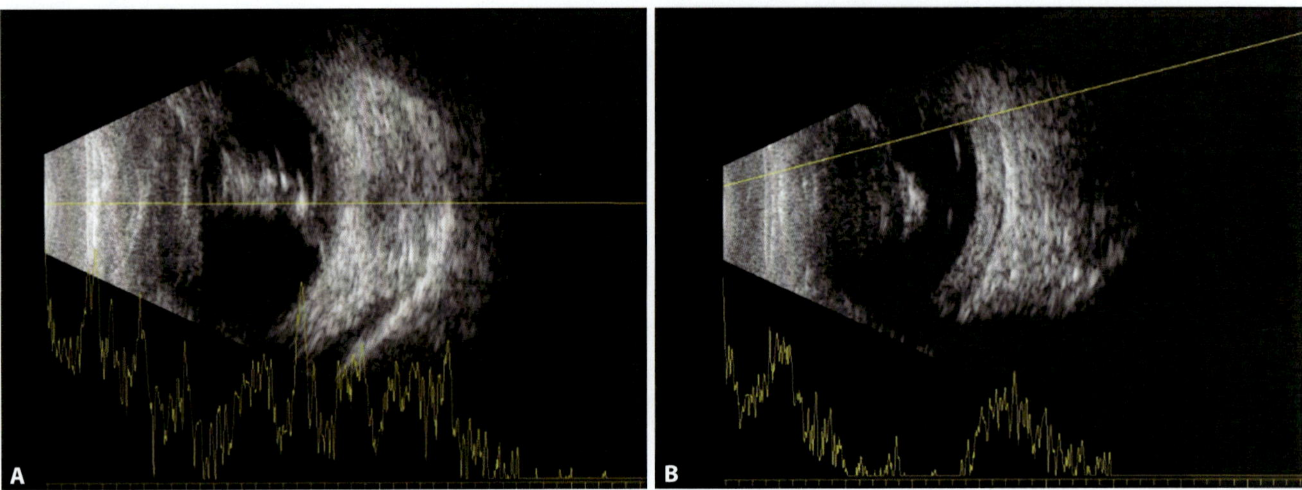

Figs. 13A and B: B-scan ultrasonography showing closed funnel retinal detachments in both eyes (A) Right eye and (B) Left eye.

Thought Process

Decision	*Rationale*
Translimbal infusion instead of AC maintainer	AC maintainer can frequently slip during membrane dissection
Trans-iris approach instead of complete iridectomy	If, following limited iridectomy, the membranes are both accessible and visible, trans-iris manipulation can be carried out
Trimming of membranes instead of complete dissection	Since iatrogenic breaks may lead to significant complications, it is advisable to avoid disturbing membranes once active traction has been addressed. Rather than attempting further dissection, simply trim any loose membrane
Sutureless surgery	With the development of smaller gauge instruments, pediatric retinal surgeries often do not require port suturing if the wound is secure and leak-free. Likewise, when using 23,25-gauge MVR blades, corneal side ports typically do not need suturing; adequate hydration of these ports usually keeps them sealed

(MVR: micro vitreoretinal)

OUTCOME SUMMARY

Eight weeks post-surgery, an open retinal funnel with relaxed folds and no ongoing traction was observed. Surgery on the other eye was planned, and rehabilitation therapy was initiated **(Fig. 14)**.

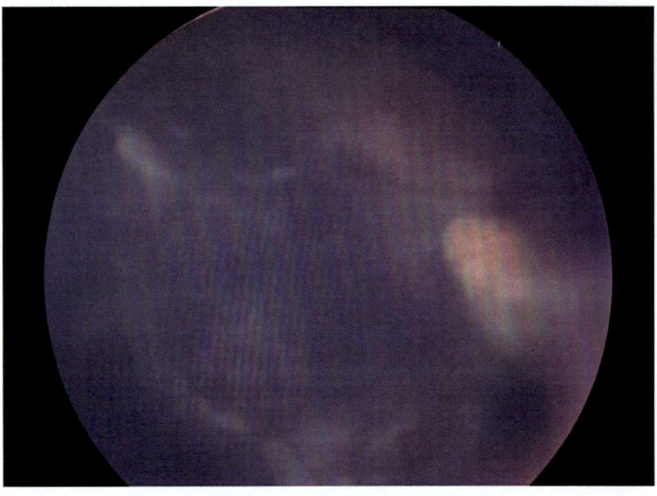

Fig. 14: 8 weeks postsurgery, open funnel with relaxed retinal fold with no active traction were noted.

KEY POINTS

- Familial exudative vitreoretinopathy (FEVR) presenting at stage 5 at birth is associated with a poor surgical prognosis; however, it does not constitute an absolute contraindication for surgical intervention.
- Intraoperatively, membranes in stage 5 FEVR are typically more adherent to and integrated with the retinal tissue compared to those observed in retinopathy of prematurity (ROP). The presence of subretinal crystals detected by B-scan may further suggest an unfavorable prognosis.

- Suturing should be performed if a wound leak is suspected, but routine suturing in all pediatric retinal surgeries is unnecessary due to smaller gauge instruments and reduced side port sizes.

FURTHER READING

1. Oga T, Mano F, Kuniyoshi K, Iwahashi C, Kondo H, Kusaka S. Fluorescein Angiography May Predict Surgical Outcomes of Tractional Retinal Detachment in Familial Exudative Vitreoretinopathy. Ophthalmol Retina. 2025;9(8):739-46.
2. Tauqeer Z, Yonekawa Y. Familial Exudative Vitreoretinopathy: Pathophysiology, Diagnosis, and Management. Asia Pac J Ophthalmol (Phila). 2018;7(3):176-82.
3. Xia F, Lyu J, Fei P, Zhao P. Diagnosis of complicated FEVR preoperatively and intra-/post-operatively: characteristics and risk factors for diagnostic timing. BMC Ophthalmol. 2019;19(1):126.

VIDEO LEGEND

Video 10: TRD in familial exudative vitreoretinopathy.

CHAPTER 8

Decision Making in Surgical Management of Retinopathy of Prematurity

Shreeya Jain, Sushma Ratna Jayanna, Subhadra Jalali

MANAGEMENT ALGORITHM FOR RETINAL DETACHMENT IN RETINOPATHY OF PREMATURITY

"ROP retinal detachments are the most difficult surgeries that a retinal surgeon does."

—Dr Tatsuo Hirose, Boston, USA

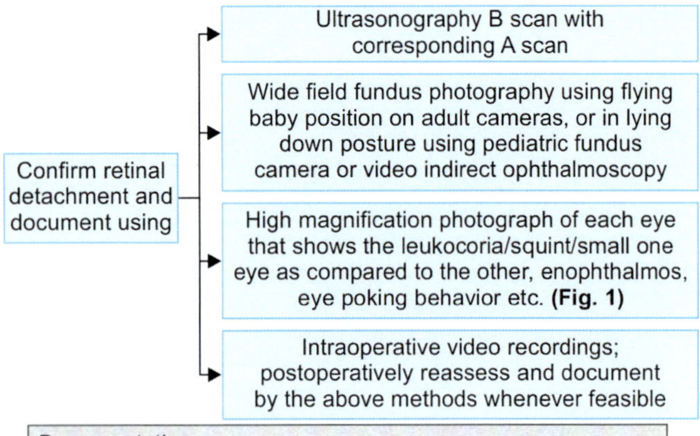

Documentation:
- Many times, the child may be asymptomatic or with minimal symptoms while the underlying pathology may be quite advanced or aggressive.
- It helps in educating parents, teaching students, following up the condition using objective tools.
- Self-learning
- Using as evidence in any medicolegal or mis-understanding situation with the caregivers

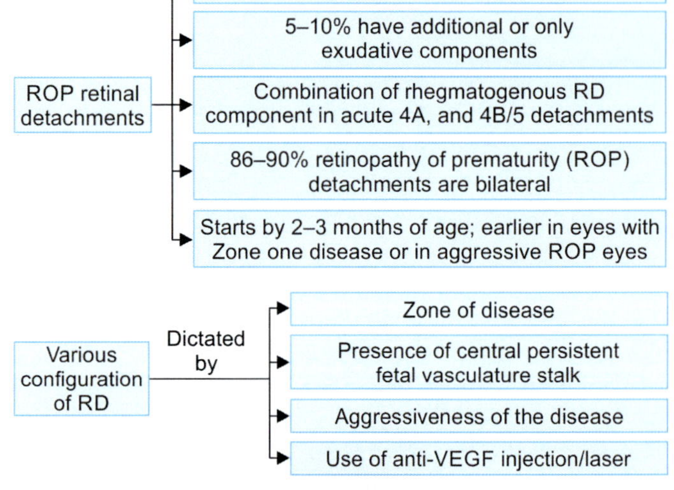

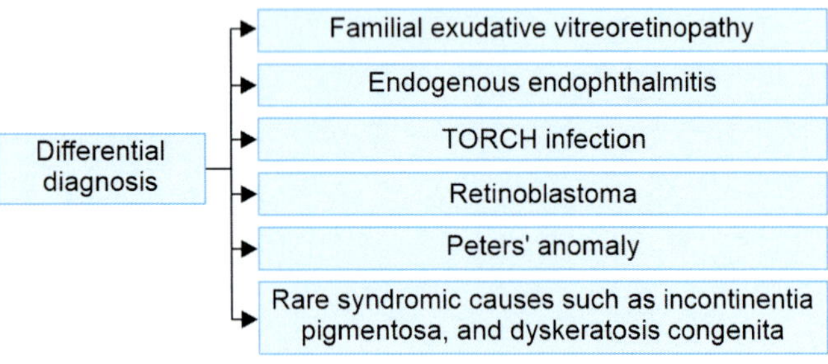

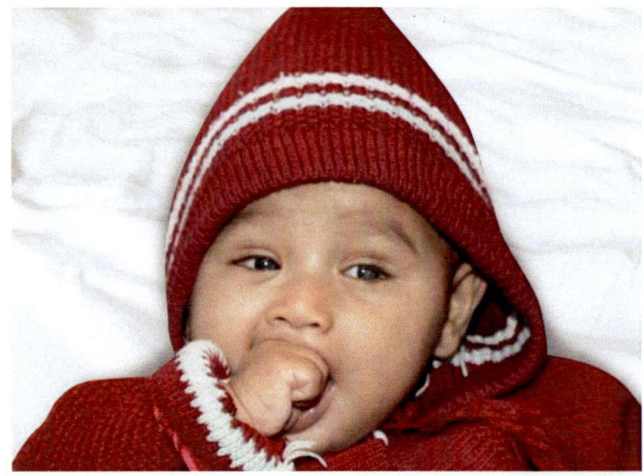

Fig. 1: Face photograph documenting bilateral leukocoria and early enophthalmos, from advanced stage 5 retinal detachment.

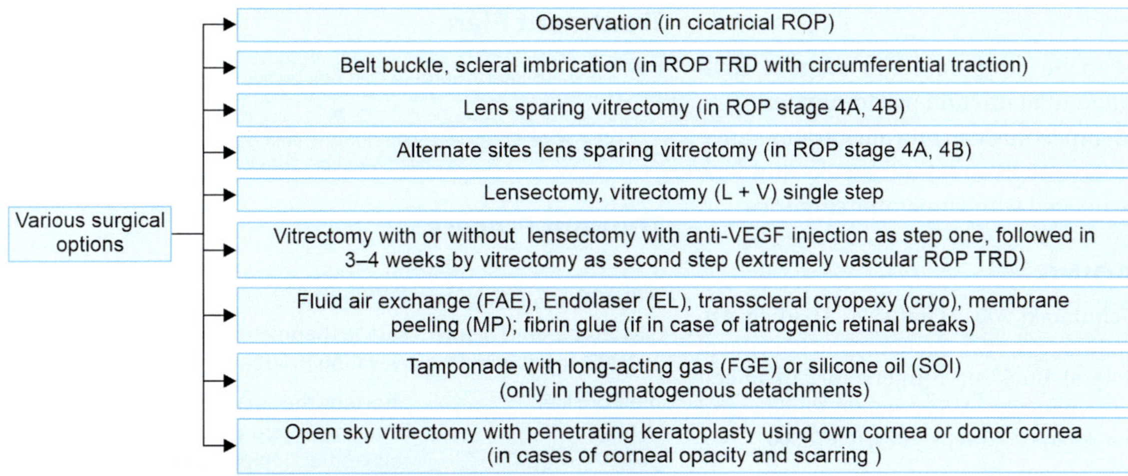

MANAGEMENT ALGORITHM FOR ATYPICAL BLEB-LIKE RETINAL DETACHMENT IN ROP

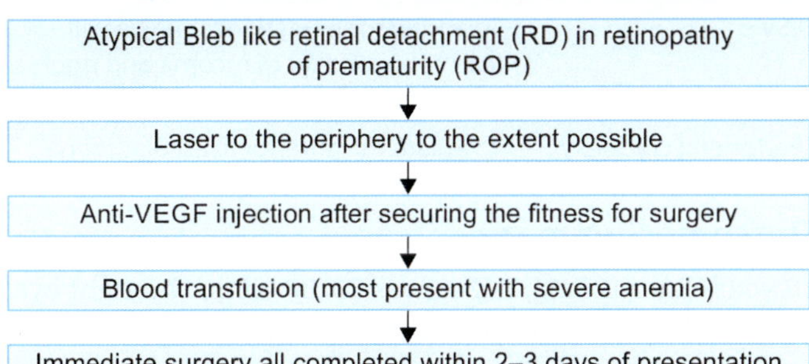

CASE SCENARIO 1: MANAGEMENT OF ROP STAGE 4A PLUS IN THE RIGHT EYE AND NEOVASCULAR GLAUCOMA WITH TOTAL RETINAL DETACHMENT STAGE 5 PLUS IN THE LEFT EYE (YEAR 1998)

Case Summary

A baby born at 28-week gestational age and 800 g birth weight presented at 6 weeks with retinal detachment, stage 4A plus in the right eye and neovascular glaucoma with total retinal detachment stage 5 plus disease in the left eye. The left eye was not salvageable. The zone 2 retina and the ridge showed tractional elevation temporally in a circumferential configuration. There was no persistent fetal vasculature (PFV) stalk, so macular dragging was flat.

Treatment Plan

Belt buckle in right eye

Thought Process

Decision	*Rationale*
Belt buckle	To support and counter the circumferential elevation during the active acute phase of the disease
Low vision aids	To give best vision to the child—help maximize the remaining vision

Outcome Summary

Photograph **(Fig. 2)** taken 1 year later shows stable retina. Even after release (not removal) of the belt buckle condition has remained stable till date (2025). Current visual acuity is 20/125, N8 improving with telescope and magnifying visual aids to 20/50, N6. Child pursuing PhD in biological sciences now.

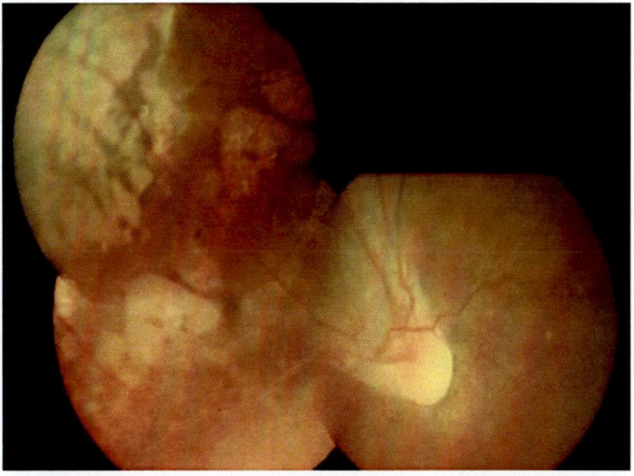

Fig. 2: Fundus photo of the right eye showing attached retina with disk drag and peripheral laser scars.

KEY POINTS

- Scleral buckle can be considered in stage 4 ROP whenever circumferential traction predominates.
- Scleral buckle (SB) procedure can prevent intraoperative dreaded complication such as retinal breaks and lens touch which is associated with vitrectomy surgeries.

FURTHER READING

1. Kottaridou E, Seliniotaki AK, Mataftsi A, Haidich AB, Lithoxopoulou M, Koutra A, et al. Anatomic and Functional Outcomes of Scleral Buckling Surgery for Advanced Retinopathy of Prematurity: A Systematic Review and Proportional Meta-Analysis. Cureus. 2024;16:e76000

CASE SCENARIO 2: MANAGEMENT OF ROP STAGE 4B TRACTIONAL RETINAL DETACHMENT (TRD) IN THE RIGHT EYE AND COMBINED RHEGMATOGENOUS AND TRD WITH MACULAR HOLE IN THE LEFT EYE (2013)

Case Summary

At 28 weeks, 800 g baby was brought at 9 months of age with a squint noted recently.

On examination under anesthesia, there was stage 4B TRD in the right eye and combined rhegmatogenous and TRD with macular hole in the left eye **(Figs. 3A and B)**. No PFV (persistent fetal vasculature) stalk was seen. Refraction before surgery: Right eye -4.25 D sphere/ -2.25 Dcyl at 180°; left eye: +5.00/-2.50 at 180°.

Treatment Plan

Bilateral surgery with belt buckle in right eye

↓

Left eye-belt buckle + vitrectomy + fluid gas exchange (FGE) + peripheral cryopexy

Thought Process

Finding	*Rationale*
Hyperopic shift nearly +9.00D in left eye	Due to rhegmatogenous retinal elevation in left eye
Belt buckle	Shortens the circumference thereby reducing antero-posterior traction, relaxes traction on macula and even posterior pole
Macular hole in retinopathy of prematurity (ROP)	Is tractional, need to address the A-P and tangential traction; ILM peeling not required
LSV	To address the traction; aphakia will lead to secondary glaucoma and poor visual rehabilitation
Peripheral cryopexy	To ablate the anterior avascular retina

Outcome Summary

10 years later (2023), BCVA was 20/80 N8 in the right eye and 20/500 in the left eye. Right eye improved to 20/40 with a telescope lens. Both retinas remain attached. Refraction after 10 years of surgery: Right eye 5.00/-2.00 at 115°; left eye -2.00D sphere/-5.00 Dcyl at 180°.

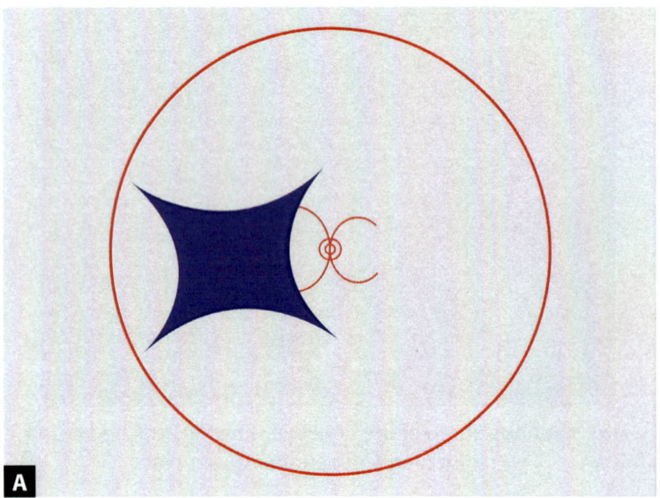

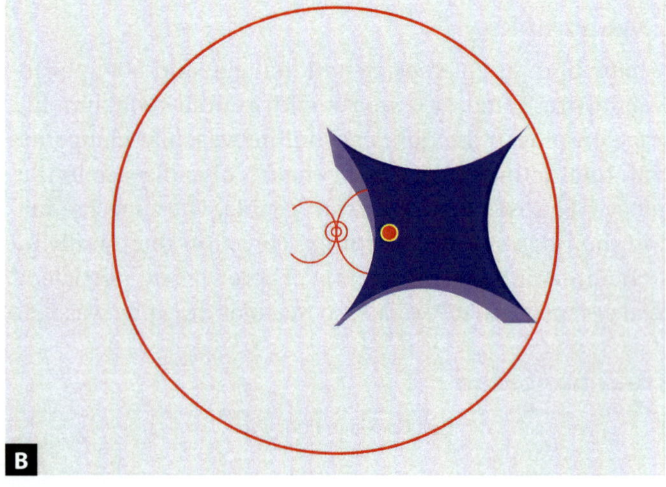

Figs. 3A and B: Digital fundus diagram of right eye showing stage 4B tractional retinal detachment and left eye showing combined retinal detachment with macular hole.

Current axial length at 11 years of age: right eye 21.47 mm and left eye 19.41 mm.

KEY POINTS

Belt buckle alone in stage 4B ROP detachments moves the vitreous base anteriorly, relieves the A-P traction (anterio posterior traction), and avoids the risk of lens touch, iatrogenic retinal break, and development of proliferative vitreoretinopathy changes.

Retinopathy of prematurity detachments is usually tractional. In this case, in left eye component of rhegmatogenous retinal detachment was also seen due to the development of a macular hole due to traction. ILMP here is not required, and focus should be on addressing the traction in ROP.

FURTHER READING

1. Patel A, Padhy SK, Saoji K, Saldna M, Multani PK, Khalsa A, et al. Bleb-like posterior combined retinal detachment in severe retinopathy of prematurity: clinical characteristics, management challenges, and outcome. Eye (Lond). 2021; 35(11):3152-5.

CASE SCENARIO 3: MANAGEMENT OF TRACTIONAL RETINAL DETACHMENT 4A ROP WITH PRERETINAL HEMORRHAGE (2013)

Case Summary

A baby born at 28-week gestational age and 750 g birth weight presented with tractional retinal detachment 4A ROP in both eyes with pre-retinal hemorrhage **(Figs. 4A and B)**.

Treatment Plan

Laser indirect ophthalmoscopy both the eyes
↓
Belt buckle in both the eyes

Thought Process

Decision	*Rationale*
Laser indirect ophthalmoscopy	Ablates peripheral avascular retina and decreases metabolic demand, reduces VEGF load
Belt buckle	Shortens the circumference thereby reducing antero-posterior traction, relaxes traction on macula and even posterior pole

Outcome Summary

A scan check and suggest 11 years of age in the right eye was 23.78 mm, and the left eye was 25.18 mm. Lens thickness in the right and left eye was 4.23 mm and 3.66 mm, respectively.

Av K readings were 50.47D and 48.49D in the right and left eye, respectively.

Refraction was -15.50D sph in the year 2023, which was increased as compared to -12.00D sph in 2021. Hence, buckle release was indicated **(Figs. 5A and B)**.

KEY POINTS

Postoperative complications may include refractive errors due to changes in the contour of the globe, infection, extrusion or intrusion of the buckle, ischemia of the anterior or posterior segment, secondary strabismus, and resulting diplopia.

The encircling bands are typically cut or removed after 6–9 months to permit normal ocular growth and to minimize the development of myopic shift.

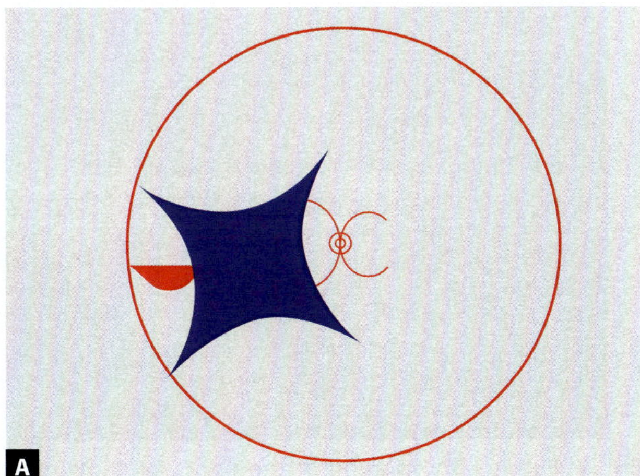

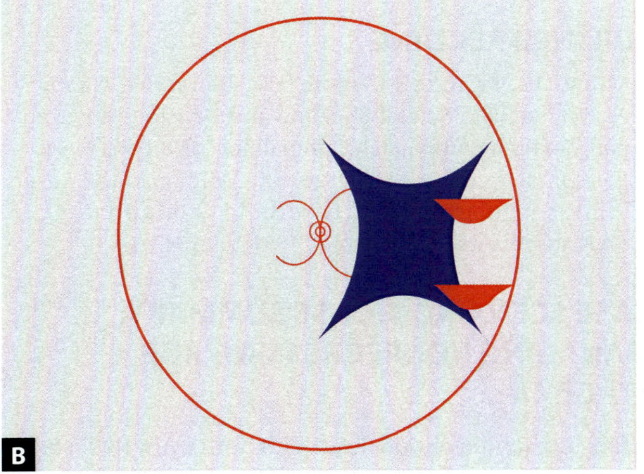

Figs. 4A and B: Digital fundus diagram of the right and left eye showing stage 4B tractional retinal detachment with pre-retinal hemorrhage.

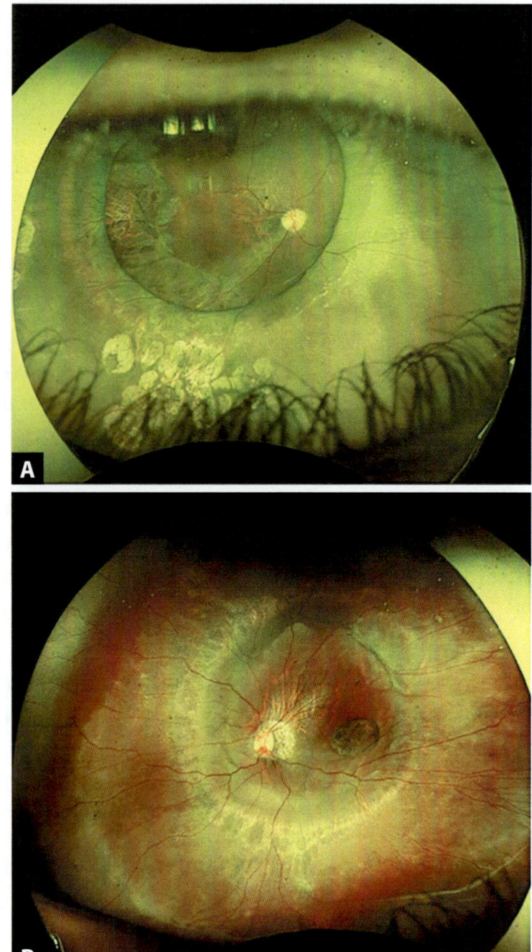

Figs. 5A and B: Wide-field fundus photograph of the right and left eye showing attached retina with tilted disk and retinal pigment epithelium (RPE) atrophic patch seen adjacent to fovea. Prominent posterior buckle effect seen.

FURTHER READING

1. Chow DR, Ferrone PJ, Trese MT. Refractive Changes Associated with Scleral Buckling and Division in Retinopathy of Prematurity. Arch Ophthalmol. 1998;116:1446-8.
2. Iverson DA, Trese MT, Orgel IK, Williams GA. Laser Photocoagulation for Threshold Retinopathy of Prematurity. Arch Ophthalmol. 1991;109:1342-3.

CASE SCENARIO 4: CASE SUMMARY: MANAGING NONREGRESSING ROP STAGE 4A

The baby presented to our clinic with both eyes, ROP stage 4A, and tractional retinal detachment in the right eye **(Figs. 6 to 9)**.

Treatment Plan

Laser indirect ophthalmoscopy in the right eye

↓

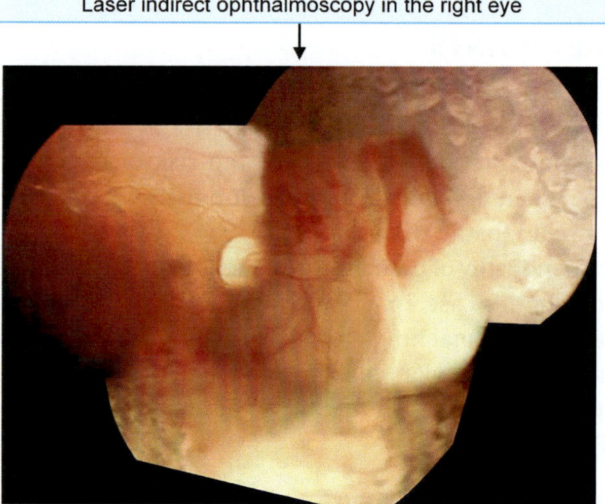

Fig. 6: Fundus photograph of the right eye showing attached retina, extensive laser scars showing "only laser traction".

↓

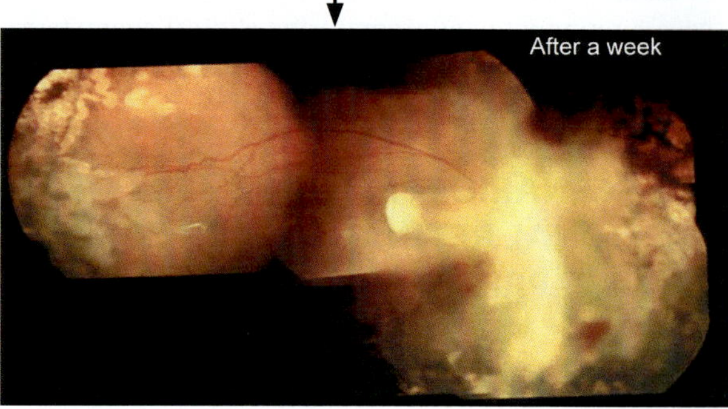

Fig. 7: Fundus photograph of the right eye showing the reduced plus and hemorrhages. There is an increase in nasal disk drag, and the contraction of members was slightly elevated and more consolidated than before.

↓ Review after 5 days

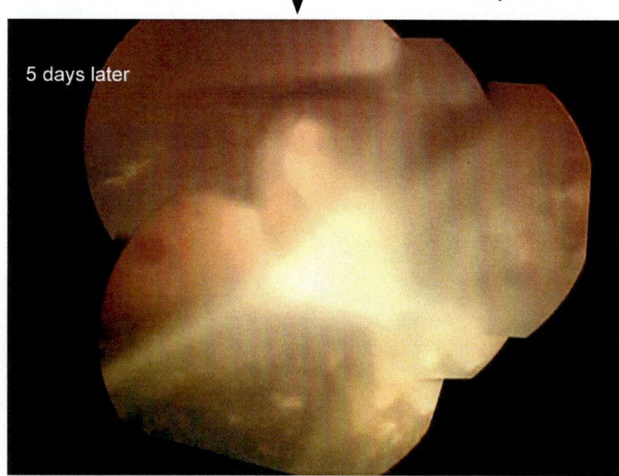

Fig. 8: Fundus photograph of the right eye showing rapid progression to stage 4B, the elevated ridge now threatening to reach the lens.

Immediate lens sparing vitrectomy planned

↓

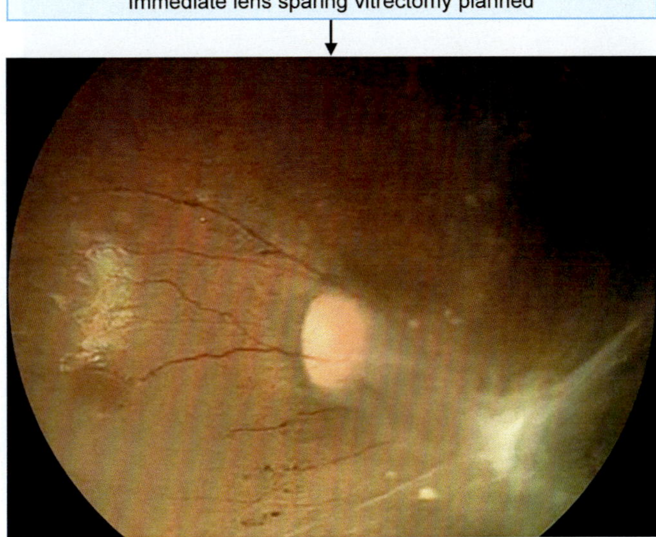

Fig. 9: Fundus photograph of the right eye showing attached retina, fibrous membranes nasally with peripheral laser scars.

Thought Process

Decision	*Rationale*
Laser indirect ophthalmoscopy	Ablates peripheral avascular retina and decreases metabolic demand, reduces VEGF load
Observation	After extensive laser, only laser traction so observed closely
Lens sparing vitrectomy	As there was rapid progression to stage 4B

KEY POINTS

Stage 4A TRD in the acute phase is rapidly progressive and can worsen within a day. After extensive laser, there was "only laser traction", so the child was reviewed after a week. There was a deceptive stability of ROP. However, the nasal disk drag had increased and on close follow-up, had converted into stage 4B, the elevated ridge now threatening to reach the lens. Immediate lens-sparing vitrectomy salvaged the situation. In hindsight, better macular and overall anatomical and functional outcomes could have been achieved by surgery at presentation or within a week.

FURTHER READING

1. Hubbard GB 3rd, Cherwick DH, Burian G. Lens-sparing vitrectomy for stage 4 retinopathy of prematurity. Ophthalmology. 2004;111:2274-7.

CASE SCENARIO 5: EARLY LENS-SPARING VITRECTOMY IN ROP

Case Summary

A preterm baby with post-lasered right eye stage 3 plus ROP, the ridge showed significant elevation in zone 2 with persistent plus disease **(Figs. 10A and B)**.

Treatment Plan

Immediate lens sparing vitrectomy

Thought Process

Decision	*Rationale*
Immediate lens sparing vitrectomy	Any ridge or retinal elevation >3 clock hours in acute phase ROP can progress rapidly either to stage 4B or to an adhesion between the lens and the ridge leading to a higher risk of need for lens removal/lens touch/cataract.

Outcome Summary

Immediate lens-sparing vitrectomy gave very good anatomical and visual outcomes, especially a pristine posterior pole. Cut edge of vitreous is seen in the posterior pole photo. A myopia of -7.00 D sphere developed by 9 months postoperatively, and glasses were prescribed and monitored every 6 months to improve visual acuity. At 10 years of age child has BCVA of 20/50 **(Fig. 11)**.

KEY POINTS

- Any ridge or retinal elevation >3 clock hours in the acute phase of ROP can progress rapidly either to stage 4B or to an adhesion between the lens and the ridge, leading to a higher risk of need for lens removal/lens touch/cataract.
- Doing the challenging lens-sparing vitrectomy under high-risk neonatal anesthesia, at this stage, gives excellent outcomes and faster recovery with intact, clear phakic status.
- Better visual outcomes and a low level of long-term complications (for example, glaucoma) of phakic eyes are hugely superior to aphakic eyes in these tiny children, making the challenge worth taking.

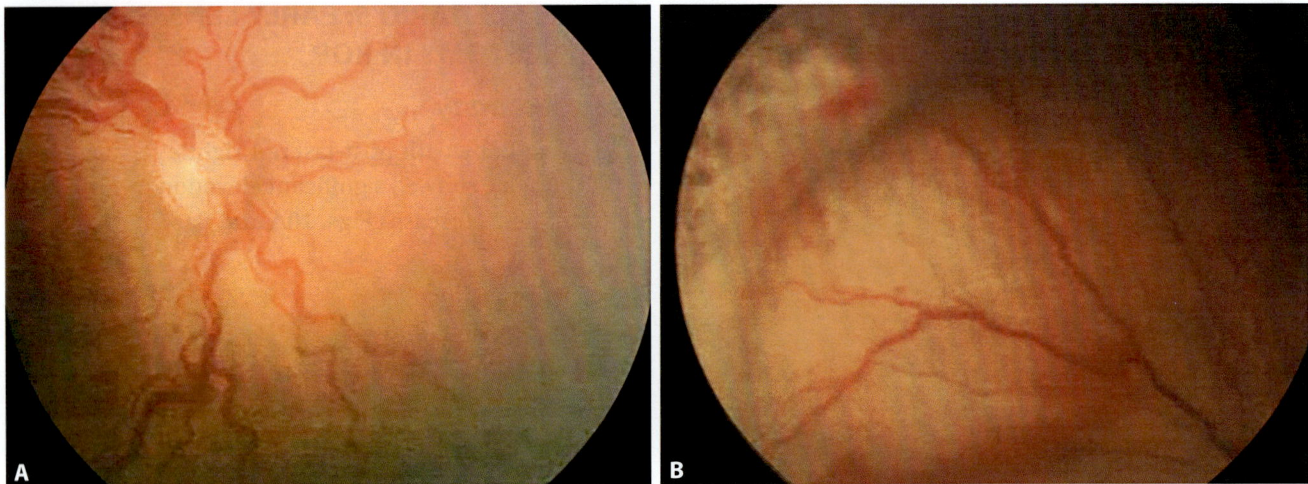

Figs. 10A and B: Fundus photograph of the right eye showing plus disease with laser scars and an elevated ridge in zone 2.

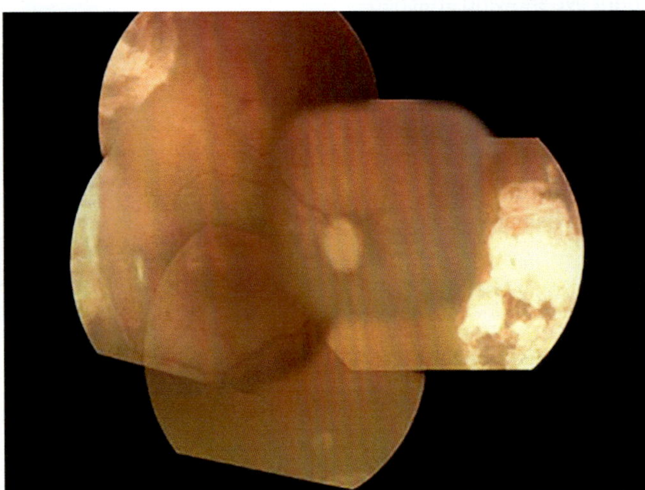

Fig. 11: Fundus photograph of the right eye showing reduced plus disease with attached retina and laser scars.

- In the post-anti-VEGF era, these detachments progress within a few days and should be operated as an emergency and not kept under 1–2 weekly observations.
- Any media haze in the vitreous is also a sign of ongoing smoldering activity and should be directed to urgent surgery.

FURTHER READING

1. Macor S, Pignatto S, Capone A Jr, Piermarocchi S, Lanzetta P. Lens-sparing vitrectomy for stage 4A retinopathy of prematurity in infants with aggressive-posterior ROP: Anatomic and functional results. Eur J Ophthalmol. 2021;31:2020-6.

CASE SCENARIO 6: MANAGEMENT OF STAGE 5 ROP

Case Summary

A baby hailing from a far-off place (1,200 miles away), born at 28-week gestational age, and 1,100 g birth weight, presented at 7 months of age with bilateral leukocoria. In the year 2021, the B scan of the both eyes shows tractional retinal detachment and multiple folds **(Figs. 12A and B)**. The child was evaluated in a child rehabilitation center preoperatively and noted to perceive light in all directions in both eyes, had early eye poking behavior and delayed motor milestones. Parents were advised to discourage eye poking by keeping their hands busy with some harmless

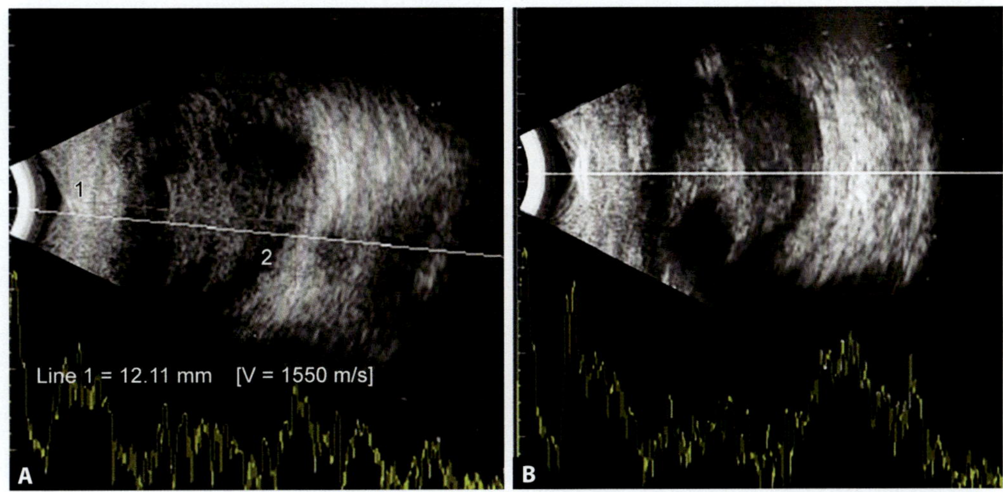

Figs. 12A and B: B-scan of the both eyes showing closed funnel retinal detachment (RD).

sticky material and toys. The vision exercises that need to be done postoperatively were demonstrated by a vision therapist, and an evaluation by a physiotherapist demonstrated physiotherapy to improve motor development. Neonatologist, pediatric anesthesiologist, and nurses trained in postoperative neonatal care teamed up well to facilitate the 3-hour simultaneous surgery of two eyes.

Treatment Plan

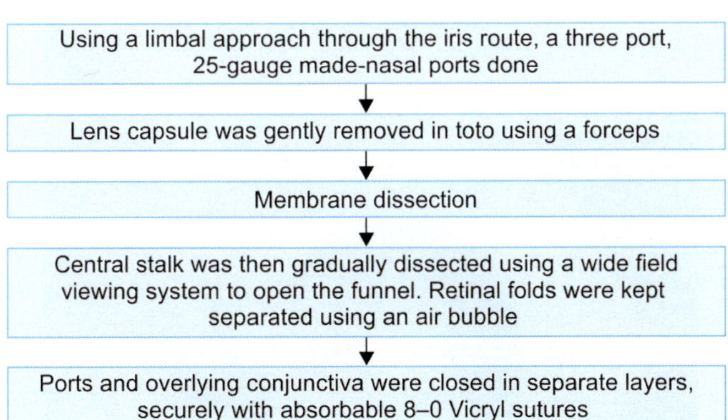

Thought Process

Decision	*Rationale*
Visual rehabilitation preoperatively	The presence of PL suggests that the optic nerve and visual pathways retain basic functional integrity. In contrast, absence of PL points toward severe retinal dysplasia, optic nerve involvement, or prolonged retinal ischemia—no benefit from surgery
Avoiding eye poking behavior	In children with retinal disease or low vision, eye poking can further compromise already limited visual potential. Causes progressive structural damage
Limbal approach for vitrectomy	As retina is too close to the lens, making the ports away can cause iatrogenic retinal tears
Lensectomy	The lens is frequently incorporated into or lies in close proximity to the retrolental fibrovascular tissue. Removing the lens facilitates release of traction on the ciliary body and retina and helps minimize additional tractional injury during membrane dissection
Membrane dissection	Membrane dissection done carefully at its attachment all around to the ciliary processes, taking utmost care not to put any stress on the peripheral vitreous base and ora that are very close to the dissection site

Contd...

Contd...

Outcome Summary

The child was prescribed aphakic glasses on postoperative day 1 and started visual rehabilitation training at home on postoperative day 3. Regular follow-up for IOP and refraction was done through video teleconsultations after local consultation from the referring doctor, and a yearly visit to our center. The right eye did not do well. (As the child grows and the eyeball enlarges over the next 3–4 years, the retinal folds gradually open up, leading to reduced hypermetropia and improved visual function.)

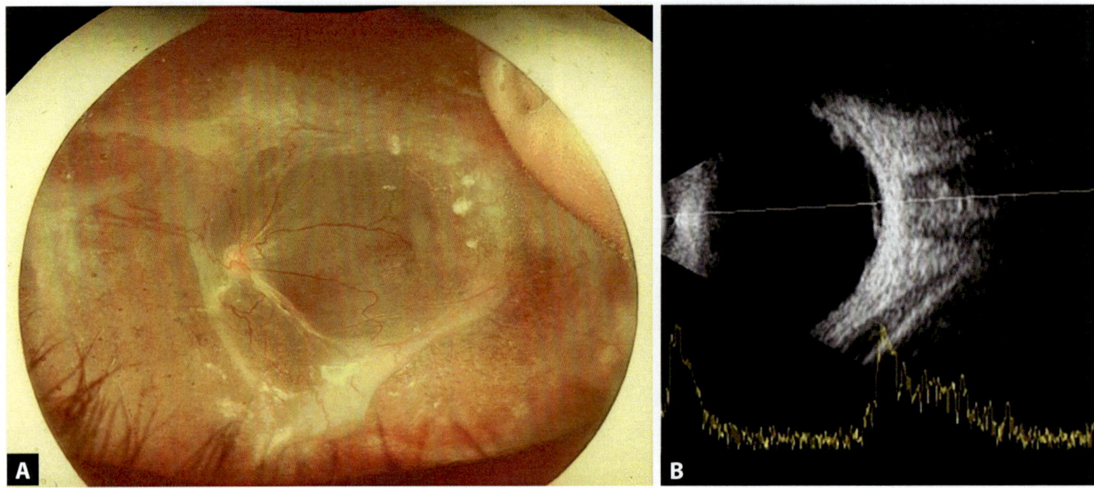

Figs. 13A and B: Wide-field fundus photograph and B-scan of the left eye showing attached retina with few membranes.

The left eye retina reattached well with most of the tractional retinal folds opened, a normal optic disk and not much subretinal cholesterol or retinal pigment epithelium (RPE) degeneration. Fundus photograph in 2025 shows a well-attached retina, and the anatomic restoration of the posterior segment is very well seen on the corresponding B scan **(Figs. 13A and B)**. Child now at 4 years of age has a visual acuity of 20/600, is independently mobile, can recognize her family members and colors and is advised bifocal aphakic glasses of +18.00 D-sphere with an add of +3.00 D-sphere now. Monitoring of intraocular pressure and avoiding falls/trauma, along with continued vision training, has been counselled to the family. The child has no developmental delay now.

KEY POINTS

Bilateral simultaneous ROP surgery is feasible in patients travelling from far away or where there is a high risk of repeated general anesthesia. Surgery for stage 5 retinal detachment is hugely rewarding, though the results are seen only in 3–4 years, unlike other eye surgeries, where 6 weeks is a routine time to assess surgical outcomes. It requires not only surgical skill, but a team of skilled anesthetists, pediatrician/neonatologist, trained neonatal nurses, opticians and vision therapists, along with multidisciplinary therapists and onboarding of local ophthalmologists who play a crucial role in monitoring complications, especially glaucoma. Outcomes of surgery are measured not only in the functional vision outcomes but also in the developmental milestones that are affected due to vision loss in these babies **(Figs. 14A and B)**.

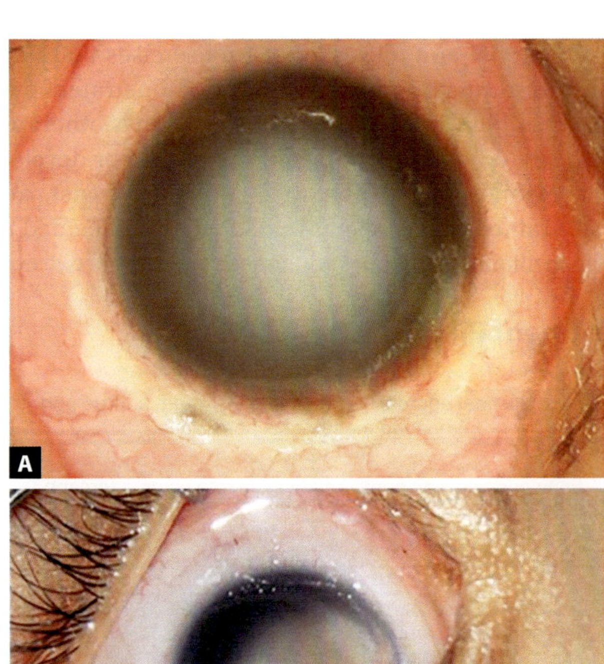

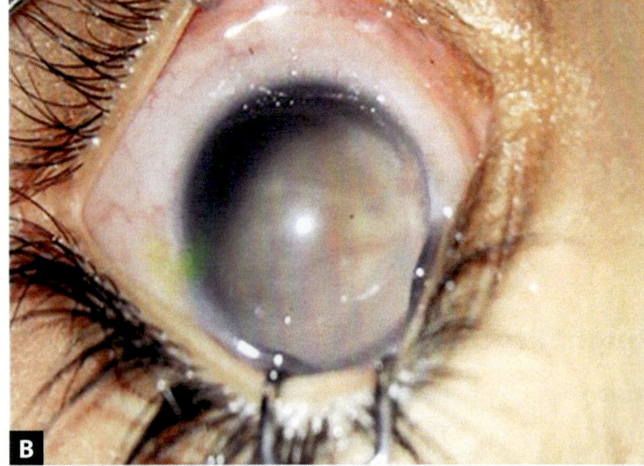

Figs. 14A and B: The right figure shows an unoperated stage 5 retinopathy of prematurity (ROP) with secondary glaucoma and a painful blind eye being treated with trans-scleral photocoagulation; (A) The left side figure shows an operated stage 5 eye with a clear cornea, opened funnel and some visual potential. Surgery in these eyes is rewarding in different ways (B).

FURTHER READING

1. Gopal L, Sharma T, Shanmugam M, Badrinath SS, Sharma A, Agraharam SG, et al. Surgery for stage 5 retinopathy of prematurity: the learning curve and evolving technique. Indian J Ophthalmol. 2000;48:101-6.

CASE SCENARIO 7: SURGERY IN EYES WITH STAGE 5C ROP

Case Summary

Premature baby diagnosed with stage 5 ROP referred with denied surgical intervention in view of extreme guarded prognosis **(Figs. 15A and B)**.

Treatment Plan

The right eye with stage 5C was operated on in two steps.

↓

The left eye in a single step

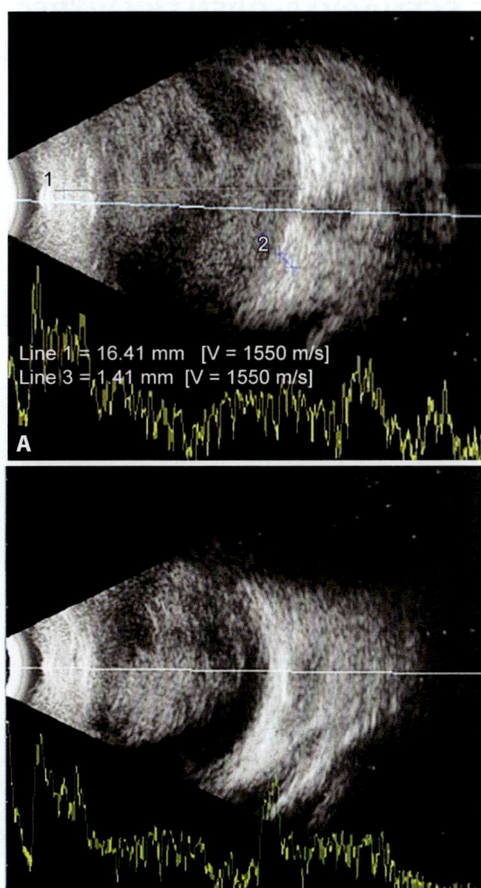

Figs. 15A and B: Preoperative B scan of the right eye and left eye shows advanced stage 5 retinopathy of prematurity (ROP) pathology that may discourage surgery.

Thought Process

Finding	*Rationale*
Corneal edema in ROP	Corneolenticular adhesions cause corneal edema and later scarring, in untreated stage 5 ROP
Single step procedure in stage 5 ROP	Eyes with mild corneal scarring can undergo a single-step procedure if the scar is central and mild
Two-step procedure in stage 5 ROP	Two-step procedure where initially only lens and capsule removal is done, followed after 4–5 weeks with the rest of the surgery as the corneal edema and scarring reduce substantially during this period
Glaucoma	Often due to angle damage from the flat anterior chamber and needs long term, life-long treatment

Outcome Summary

Except for a small residual corneal scar in the right eye, the right eye gained some vision and good retinal reattachment. The left eye had a much better retinal reattachment but developed secondary glaucoma, intercalary staphyloma at surgical sites and disk cupping. The child has very good ambulatory vision and is able to identify book pictures and colors at 3 years of age **(Figs. 16 and 17)**.

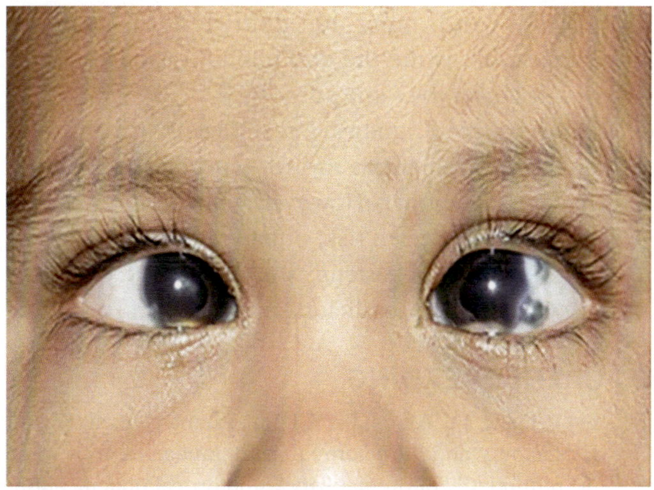

Fig. 16: Diffuse image of the right and left eye showing a corneal scar in the right eye and intercalary staphyloma in the left eye.

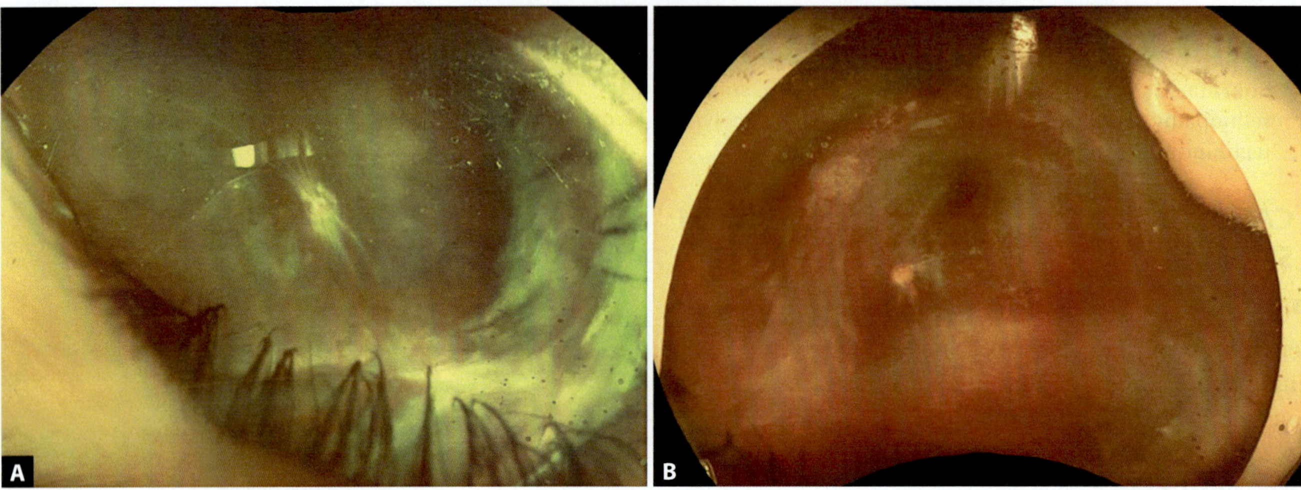

Figs. 17A and B: Wide-field fundus photograph of the right and left eye showing attached retina with tilted disk and minimal drag with few membranes.

KEY POINTS

- In untreated stage 5 ROP, corneolenticular adhesions lead to corneal edema, which later progresses to scarring. Eyes with minimal corneal scarring may be managed with a single-stage surgery if the scar is mild and centrally located.
- Alternatively, a two-stage approach can be adopted, where the first stage involves removal of the lens and capsule alone, followed 4–5 weeks later by completion of the remaining surgery. During this interval, corneal edema and scarring often decrease significantly.
- Intraoperatively, corneal epithelial edema commonly develops and must be debrided to improve visualization, while the endothelium is coated with viscoelastic for the same purpose.
- Postoperatively, many eyes demonstrate some visual improvement as the cornea frequently shows substantial recovery. However, glaucoma remains a significant long-term risk, often resulting from angle damage due to a persistently shallow anterior chamber, and typically requires lifelong management.

FURTHER READING

1. Fei P, Liang TY, Peng J, Xu Y, Luo J, Zhang Q, et al. Staged lensectomy and vitrectomy in the management of stage 5C retinopathy of prematurity with corneal opacification: long-term follow up. Int J Ophthalmol. 2022;15:1437-43.

CASE SCENARIO 8: OPEN SKY VITRECTOMY FOR STAGE 5 ROP WITH SUBSTANTIAL CORNEAL SCARRING

Case Summary

An 8-month aged preterm born baby was presented with substantial corneal scarring, a flat anterior chamber and corneolenticular adhesion from stage 5 ROP. B scan showed funnel retinal detachment with no subretinal echoes. IOP and corneal diameter were normal **(Figs. 18 to 22)**.

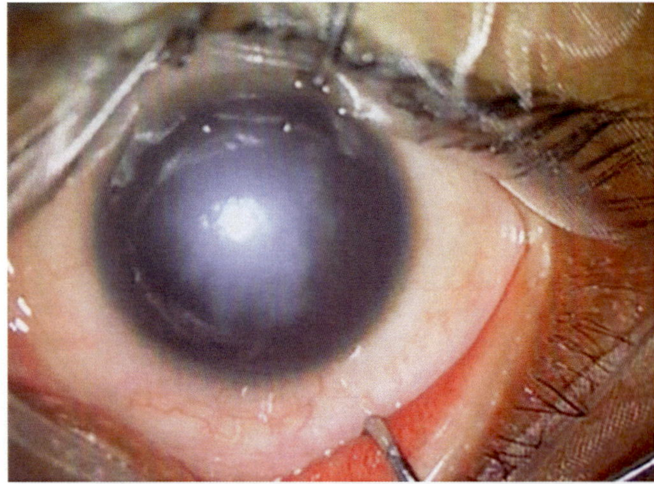

Fig. 18: Diffuse illumination of the eye showing retinopathy of prematurity (ROP) stage 5 with corneal opacity, corneolenticular touch and flat AC.

Treatment Plan

Along with a corneal surgeon, an open sky approach was planned

↓

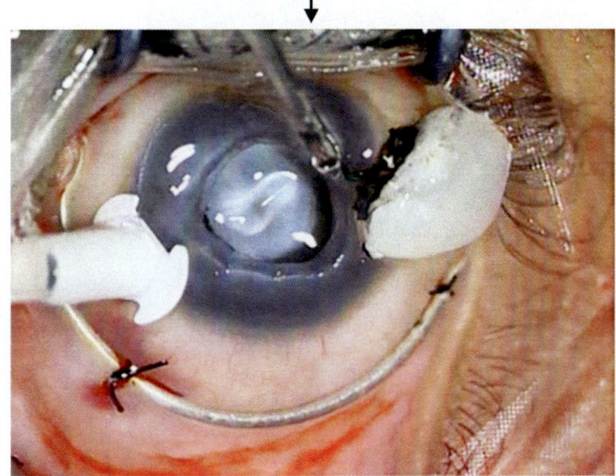

Fig. 19: Corneal button is trephined after securing the infusion cannula and Flieringa ring. Dense cataract is removed, exposing the underlying retrolenticular fibrous membrane.

↓

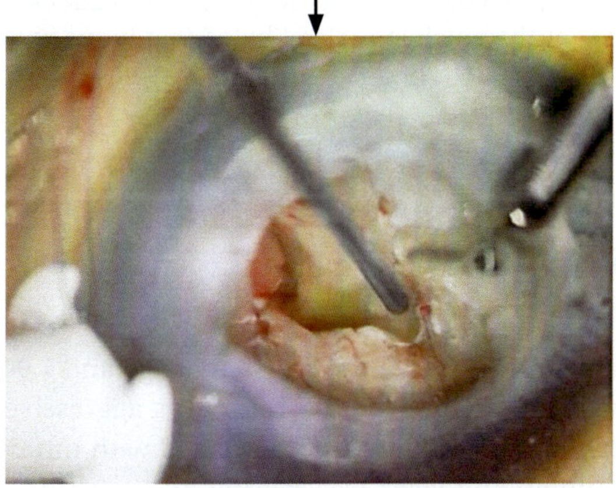

Fig. 20: Using a viscoelastic, sterile small coverslip, forceps, scissors, and the special Trese's spatula (instrument to the right) to dissect membranes, the folds are opened up, and the macula (yellow spot) is visualized.

↓

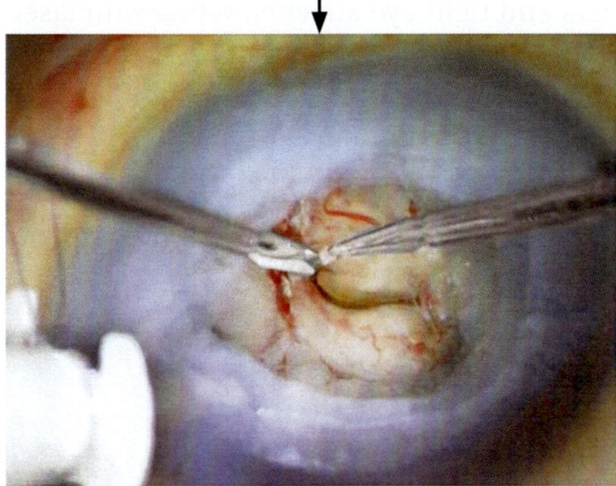

Fig. 21: The stalk is finally reached and cut gently after separating it from the peripapillary and perifoveal adhesions using scissors, forceps, viscoelastic and direct visualization using a microscope and a cover slip on the open globe.

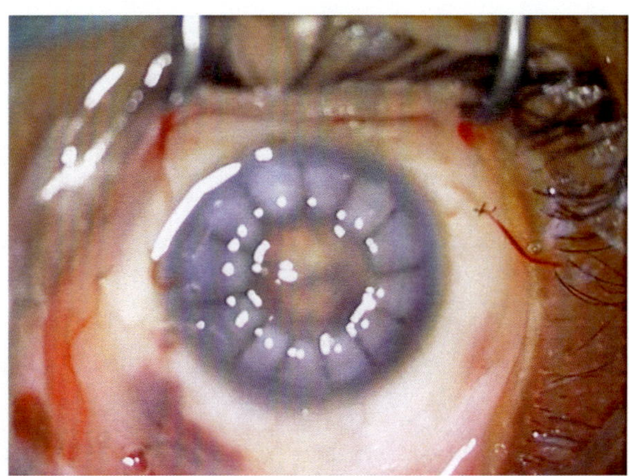

Fig. 22: The wound is closed with a corneal graft.

Thought Process

Decision	*Rationale*
Open sky approach	The underlying retina behind the corneal scar is viable, has no macular ischemia or PVR changes, has visual gain
Use of Flieringa ring	To avoid globe collapse during surgery
Use of trimmed small cover slip (used in pathology slides)	Is placed on the open globe and gives a clear view up to the base of the stalk, which is carefully removed from the disk and foveal adhesions
Use of viscoelastics	Aids in membrane dissection

KEY POINTS

The underlying retina behind the corneal scar is viable, has no macular ischemia or PVR changes. Left alone, the eye will go into phthisis or secondary glaucoma. Surgery offers a chance for vision and anatomic recovery, albeit small. In case of a non-dense scar, the child's own corneal button can also be sutured back in place.

FURTHER READING

1. Hirose T, Katsumi O, Mehta MC, Schepens CL. Vision in Stage 5 ROP after open-sky vitrectomy. JAMA Ophthalmol.

CASE SCENARIO 9: SCLERAL IMBRICATION ALONE OR WITH ADDITIONAL BUCKLE FOR COMBINED RETINAL DETACHMENTS OR EVOLVING TRACTIONAL RETINAL DETACHMENTS

Case Summary

A baby was presented with combined detachment with temporal retinal fold secondary to stage 4 ROP along with rhegmatogenous configuration of the detachment with no obvious location of break **(Figs. 23 and 24)**.

Treatment Plan

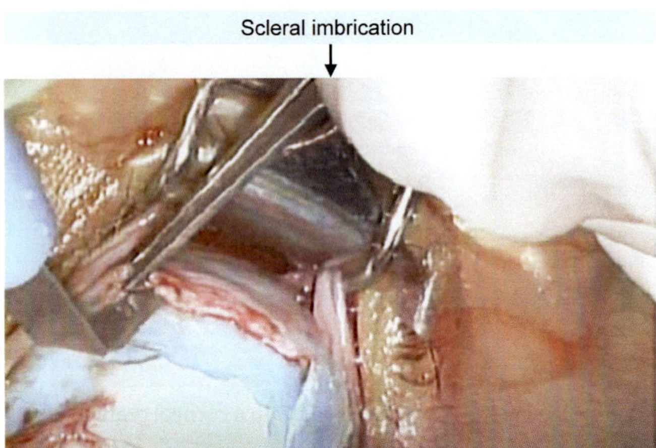

Fig. 23: Shows scleral flap dissection placed on either side of the equator.

Thought Process

Decision	*Rationale*
Scleral imbrication	Helps to shorten the globe and acts like a posterior buckle. It also allows the bottom of the globe to flatten, changing the vector forces that keep the retina detached to forces that allow retinal reattachment.

KEY POINTS

- S Jalali's modified technique of square flaps and adding a buckle increases the success of this procedure in eyes with combined rhegmatogenous and tractional retinal detachments, especially in neonatal and pediatric onset retinal diseases, where a retinal fold and traction often hamper reattachment using normal scleral buckling procedures.
- No additional instrumentation or material is needed from what one uses in routine scleral buckling, and only the additional step of quadrant-wise scleral flaps and imbrication using tight non-absorbable sutures is needed.
- Cryopexy/laser/ SRF drainage can be done as in routine buckling. Long-term, transiently elevated intraocular pressure and myopic shift in refraction need to be managed.

FURTHER READING

1. Belenje A, Jalali S. Combined rhegmatogenous and tractional retinal detachment in a child with incontinentia pigmenti managed by scleral imbrication with scleral buckle. BMJ Case Rep. 2023;16:e253738.

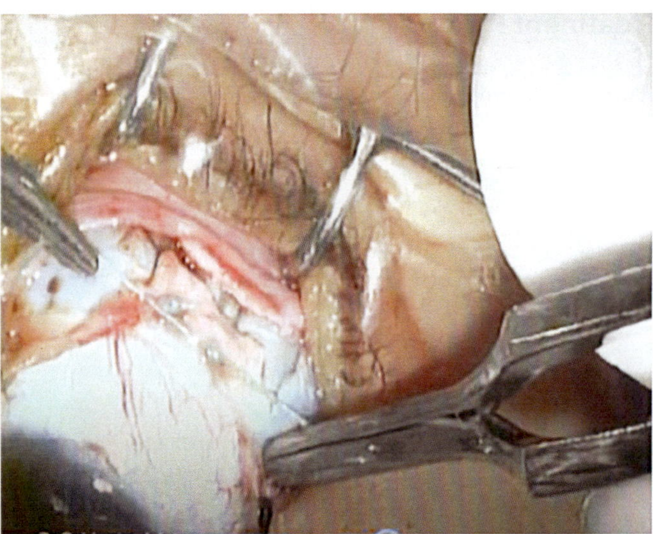

Fig. 24: Imbrication by tightening the flaps using 5–0 Dacron/ Ethibond sutures after external SRF drainage or paracentesis to soften the globe. Buckle element, usually circumferential. The tire is then placed over this to provide additional buckle indent, especially at the adjoining scleral bulge that forms under the muscles.

CASE SCENARIO 10: STAGE 4B—NASAL APPROACH

Case Summary

The baby born at 28 weeks, gestational age and 1,000 gm birth weight, diagnosed with both eyes aggressive retinopathy of prematurity (AROP), treated with intravitreal bevacizumab and laser, was referred to our clinic for LE zone 2 ROP stage 4B on subsequent follow-ups. The baby currently weighed 3.2 kg and was 3 months of age. Baby had left eye zone 2, stage 4B, temporal lifted retina with laser scars and right eye attached retina with laser scars and tortuous vessels **(Figs. 25A and B)**.

Treatment Plan

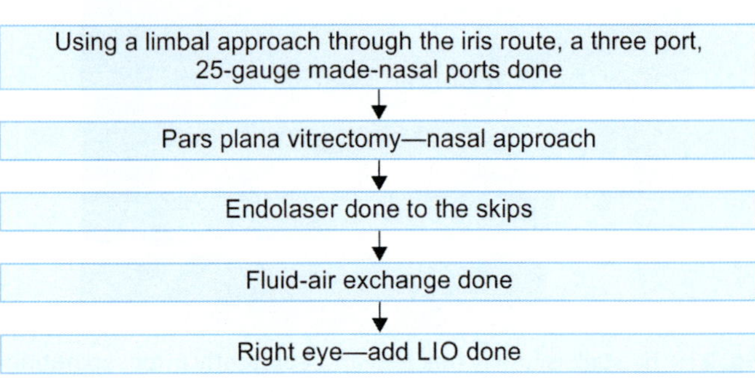

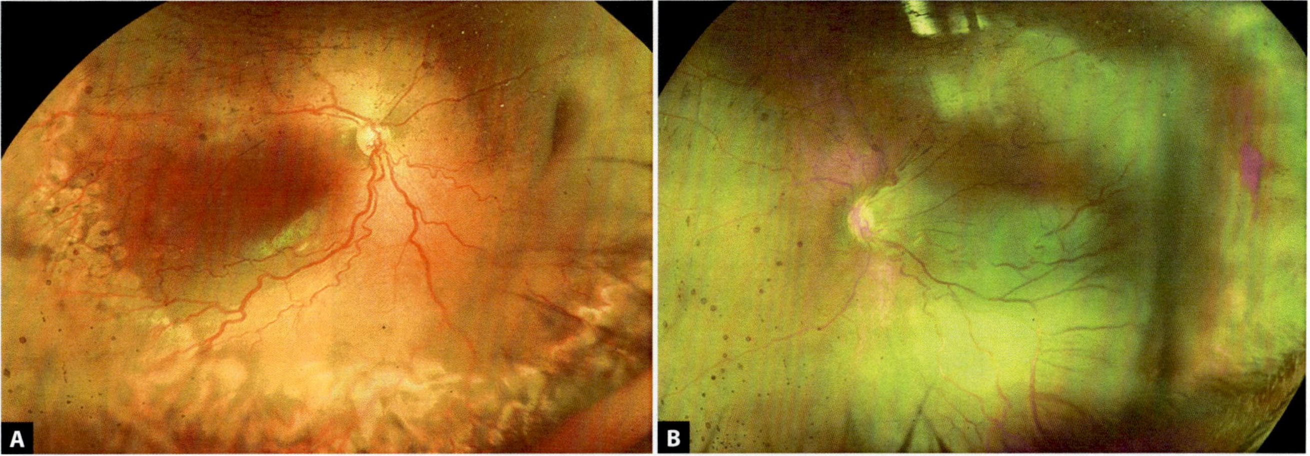

Figs. 25A and B: Wide-field fundus photography of the right eye showing attached retina with tortuous vessels, healthy disk, and macula and with laser scars, left eye showing zone 2P, stage 4B temporally lifted retina, with peripheral laser scars.

Thought Process

Decision	*Rationale*
Nasal approach in ROP	The main tractional forces are temporal; entering nasally offers safer access to the tractional membranes, facilitates lens-sparing surgery, and minimizes the risk of damage to the retina and crystalline lens

Outcome Summary

Postoperatively baby had a vitreous hemorrhage in the left eye with attached retina, right eye retina attached with laser scars and fresh laser marks.

KEY POINTS

In stage 4B ROP, traction is frequently greatest on the temporal side, causing anterior elevation of the retina and increasing the risk associated with temporal sclerotomy placement. An all-nasal approach offers a safer entry into the vitreous cavity, minimizing the risk of injury to both the lens and the retina.

FURTHER READING

1. Dogra MR, Singh SR, Katoch D, Dogra M, Moharana B, Jain S, et al. "All-Nasal" Approach for 25-Gauge Lens Sparing Vitrectomy in stage 4B Retinopathy of Prematurity. Retina. 2022;42:1619-22.

OBSERVATION/NO SURGERY

Scenario 1

See **Figure 26**.

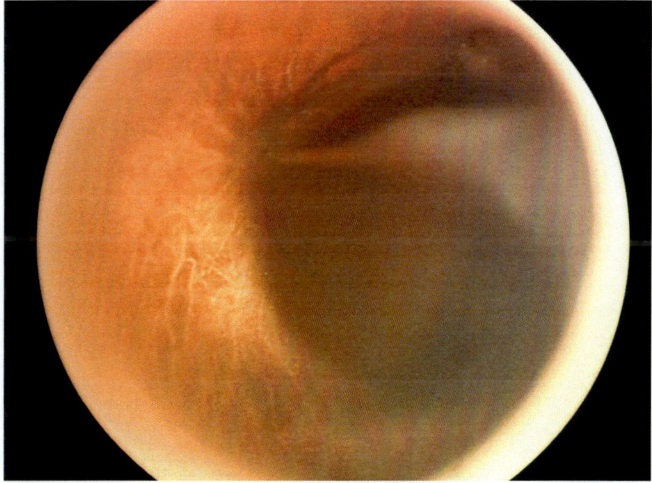

Fig. 26: Fundus photo of the left eye showing complete retinal dysplasia with total retinal detachment (RD) and optic nerve aplasia/hypoplasia/no vessels seen. Likely to have no PL.

Scenario 2 (Fig. 27)

They are generally stable, minimum vision, a cicatricial ROP retinal fold, and a dragged disk.

Scenario 3

See **Figure 28**.

Conditions wherein no Surgery is Advised in Retinopathy of Prematurity

- Stable, cicatricial stage 4B/stage 5 ROP eyes. Discourage eye poking, provide and monitor vision therapy and vision and other milestone development. Monitor IOP.

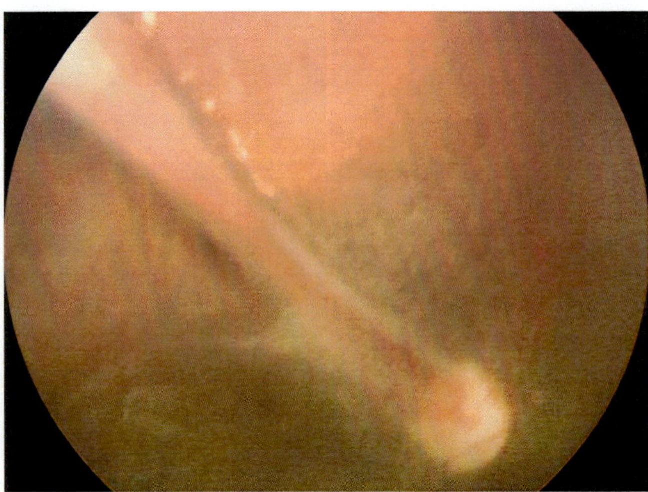

Fig. 27: Fundus photo of the right eye showing stage 4B ROP—diffuse retinal pigment epithelium (RPE) degeneration, poor vascularity. Do not operate.

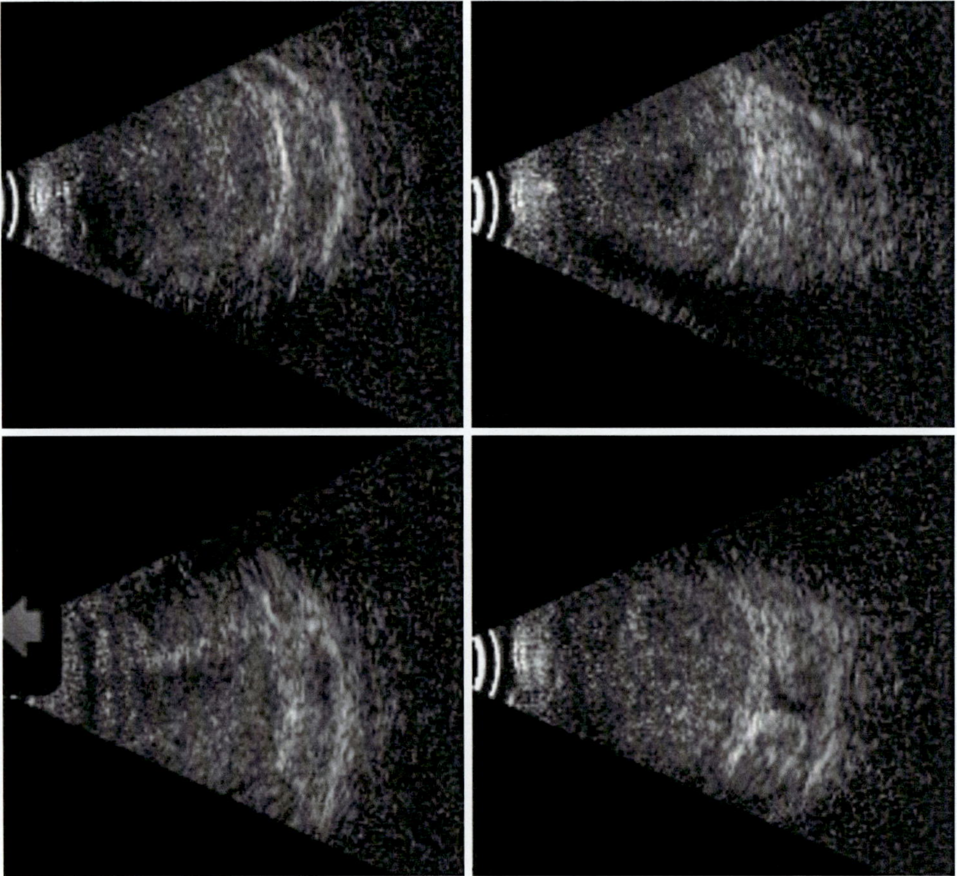

Fig. 28: B scan showing severe hyperechoic subretinal echoes suggestive of cholesterol crystals, old massive subretinal hemorrhage, funnel retinal detachment, and calcification of ocular coats. Surgery in such eyes will not be helpful and cause more misery to the baby by developing irritable, blind eyes.

- Age beyond 2 years (relative) since eyeball growth after this age is very minimal and so the folds will not open.
- Unilateral stage 5 ROP (relative contraindication)—surgery is offered depending on age of child, extent of stage 5 pathology, condition of other eye, motivation of parents etc.
- Eyes with buphthalmos following stage 5 ROP, as this is usually due to extensive intraocular hemorrhage.
- Extensive subretinal echoes (relative contraindication) as this denotes cholesterol deposition and RPE atrophy so even with anatomical reattachment, functional vision is quite poor.
- Documented optic atrophy (example from severe untreated hydrocephalus) or calcified coats of eyeball on USG (eyeball cannot expand)

CHAPTER 9

Decision Making in Surgical Management of Myopic Tractional Maculopathy

Pradeep Susvar, Divya Balakrishnan

MYOPIC TRACTION MACULOPATHY

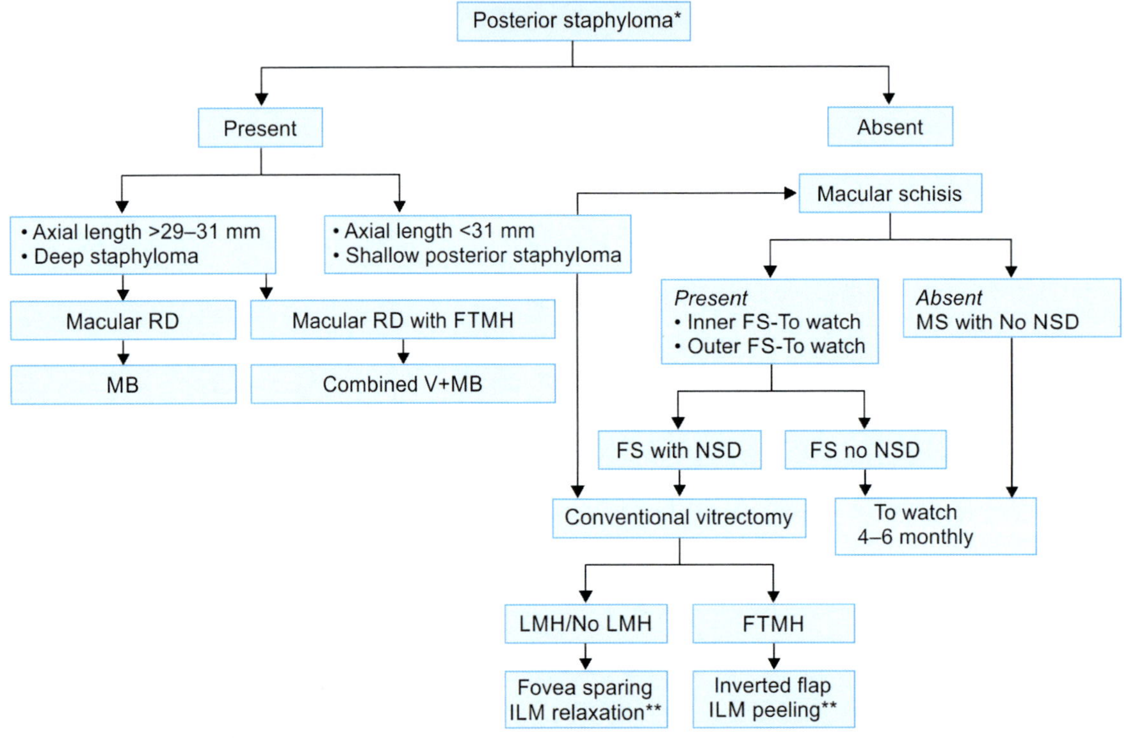

*With Symptomatic presentation/Recent progression

**Gas/ SOI situation based

(FS: foveoschisis; FTMH: full-thickness macular hole; ILM: internal limiting membrane; LMH: lamellar macular hole; MS: maculoschisis; NSD: neurosensory detachment; RD: retinal detachment)

Effective surgical decision making in myopic traction maculopathy (MTM) requires recognizing how evolving posterior pole changes arise from the dynamic balance between perpendicular and tangential tractional forces. The parolini myopic traction maculopathy staging system (MSS), comprising four retinal and three foveal stage offers a structured, morphology-based approach for selecting appropriate interventions according to the dominant tractional mechanism.

Factors to be considered:

- Visual acuity
- Duration of onset of symptoms
- Axial length
- Degree of staphyloma
- Status of vitreomacular interface changes:
  - Degree of retinoschisis
  - Foveal involvement
  - Presence of macular hole
  - Presence of macular detachment
- Rate of progression on serial OCT

CASE SCENARIO 1: DEEP POSTERIOR STAPHYLOMA WITH FULL THICKNESS MACULAR HOLE AND MACULAR DETACHMENT

A 60-year-old male presented with sudden decrease in vision in his right eye (RE). His best corrected visual acuity (BCVA) was 20/320 and 20/200 in RE and left eye (LE) respectively. Fundus examination showed deep posterior staphyloma (PS) with patchy choroidal atrophy in both eyes. LE showed myopic traction maculopathy (MTM) changes, full thickness macular hole (FTMH) and macular detachment (MD) **(Figs. 1A and B)**. Axial length (AL) was 34.8 mm in RE and 32.5 mm in LE. Optical coherence tomography (OCT) showed thin retinal layers, foveal schisis (FS), FTMH, and MD **(Figs. 2A and B)**.

Treatment Plan

Macular buckle (Morin-Devin T-shaped buckle) in RE.

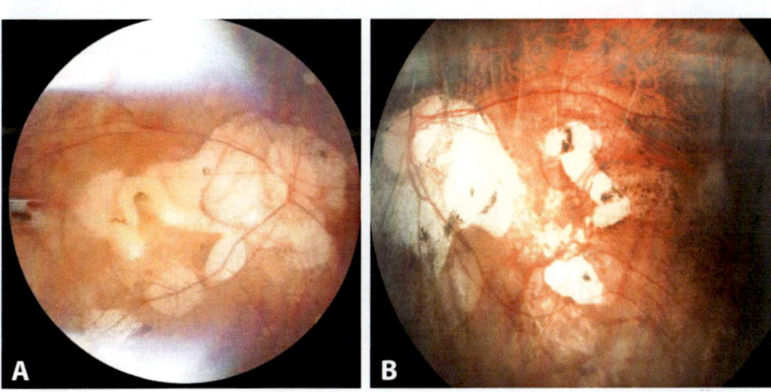

Figs. 1A and B: Fundus images showing PS with patchy chorioretinal atrophy in both eyes (A and B) with MD in RE (A).

Conjunctival peritomy performed with isolation and tagging of the four rectus and two obliques muscles

↓

Morin-Devin macular buckle assembly prepared by threading the Morin band into the Devin wedge

↓

Both ends of the Devin band passed from the temporal side beneath the oblique and rectus muscles and positioned superior and inferior to the medial rectus muscle

↓

Macular buckle positioned and indentation titrated under direct visualization using a 25-G Chandelier illumination system

↓

Plate end secured with sutures under the lateral rectus muscle on either side to stabilize the buckle position

↓

Nasal ends of the band marked on sclera, sutured securely, and free edges trimmed

↓

Paracentesis done

↓

Conjunctiva mobilized and sutured in two layers

Thought Process

Decision	*Rationale*
Macular buckle	In eyes with deep staphyloma, macular indentation by MB reduces the axial length and apposes the retinal layers thereby addressing the primary cause
Chandelier light	Provides widefield illumination to position and adjust the buckle under direct visualization

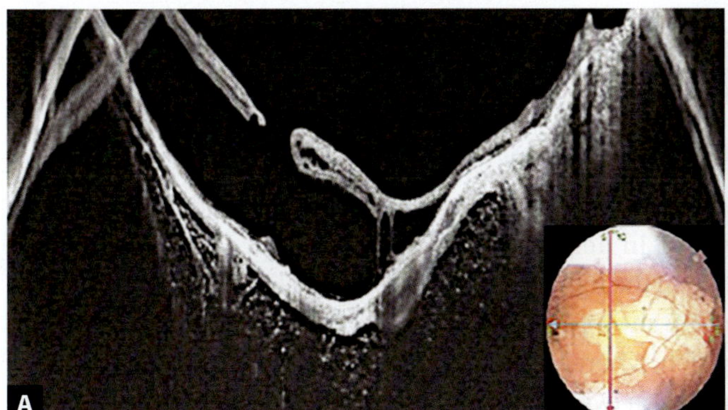

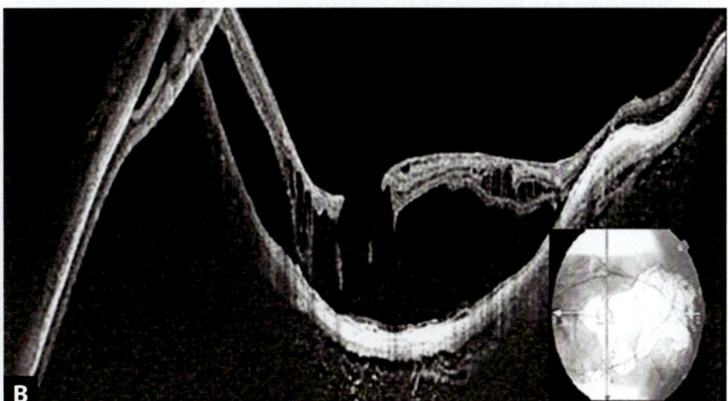

Figs. 2A and B: Widefield optical coherence tomography (OCT) showing posterior staphyloma, foveoschisis (FS), full-thickness macular hole (FTMH) with MD.

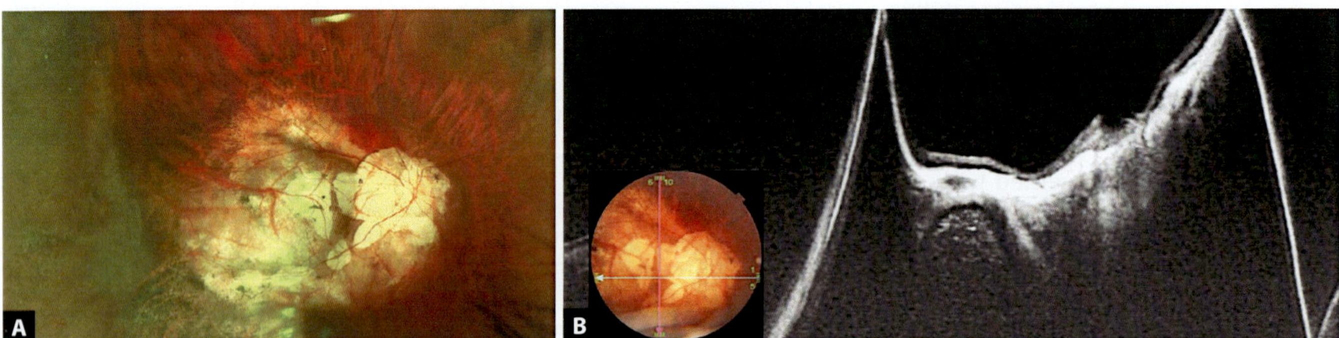

Figs. 3A and B: Postoperative widefield image illustrating attached macula with indentation of macular buckle (A). Postoperative OCT showing reduced axial length with MB resulting in attached macula with closed macular hole (B).

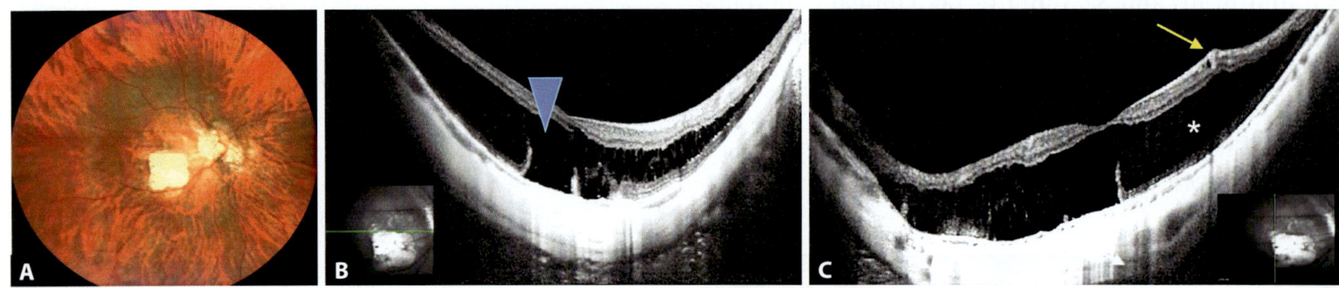

Figs. 4A to C: Fundus image showing PS with patchy choroidal atrophy (A). Widefield OCT showing posterior staphyloma, (blue arrow) O-LMH, (*) MS, (yellow arrow) retinal microfold (B and C).

OUTCOME SUMMARY

Macular buckle effectively shortened the posterior staphyloma resulting in closure of FTMH and resolution of the MD **(Figs. 3A and B)**. BCVA improved to 20/200.

KEY POINTS

- Macular buckle reduces the risk of intraoperative complications of vitrectomy in these eyes with foveal schisis and thin atrophic retina.
- Preoperative widefield OCT is essential to localize the breaks in high myopic eyes with choroidal atrophy and poor fundus contrast.
- Chandelier illumination eliminates the need for repeated use of indirect ophthalmoscopy intraoperatively.

FURTHER READING

1. Serhan HA, Ahmed A, Chaudhry M, Nadeem ZA, Ahmed F, Kamal UH, et al. Macular buckling for myopic traction maculopathy: a comprehensive systematic review and meta-analysis. Am J Ophthalmol. 2025;270:25-34.
2. Susvar P, Sood G. Current concepts of macular buckle in myopic traction maculopathy. Indian J Ophthalmol. 2018;66(12):1772-84.
3. Zhao X, Li Y, Ma W, Lian P, Yu X, Chen S, et al. Macular buckling versus vitrectomy on macular hole associated macular detachment in eyes with high myopia: a randomised trial. Br J Ophthalmol. 2022;106(4):582-6.

VIDEO LEGEND

Video 11: Macular buckle surgery (Morin-Devin T-shaped Buckle)

CASE SCENARIO 2: MACULOSCHISIS WITH OUTER LAMELLAR MACULAR HOLE

Case Summary

A 50-year-old female presented with a sudden decrease in vision in her anisometropic amblyopic RE, BCVA was CF 3 m in the right eye and 20/20 in the LE. Fundus examination of RE showed a myopic fundus with chorioretinal atrophic patch, whereas the LE fundus was normal. AL was 29 mm in the right eye and 24 mm in the left eye. OCT of the right eye revealed maculoschisis (MS), an outer lamellar macular hole (O-LMH), and associated neurosensory detachment (NSD) **(Figs. 4A to C)**.

Treatment Plan

Pars plana vitrectomy (PPV) with foveal sparing internal limiting membrane (ILM) peel with C_3F_8 injection.

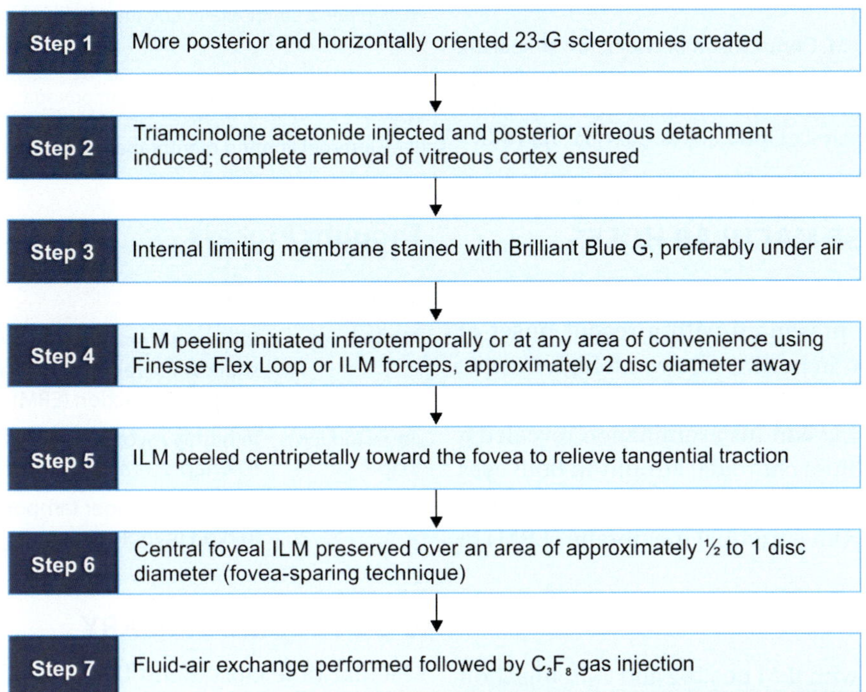

Thought Process

Decision	*Rationale*
Vitrectomy	Due to shallow posterior staphyloma with tangential traction more than vertical traction
23-G vitrectomy	23-G instruments are rigid and longer
PVD induction	Repeated attempts of PVD induction are often required to ensure complete vitreous removal
Brilliant blue G (BBG) dye	Stains the ILM which facilitates ILM peeling in myopic eyes with poor contrast. Often needs repeated staining
Scraper or Finesse flex loop	More controlled and reduces risk of iatrogenic breaks in thin retina in high myopic eyes

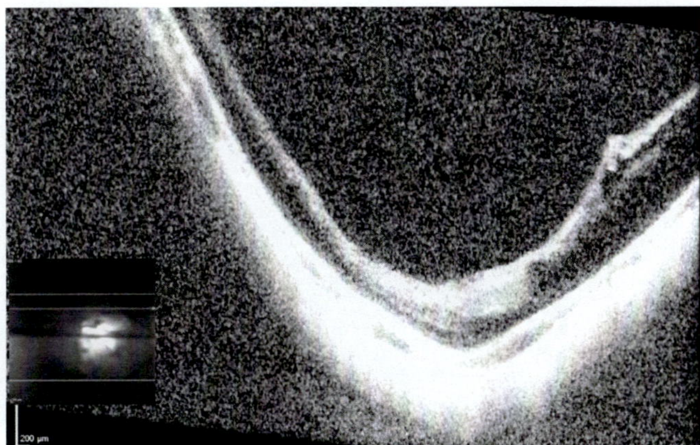

Fig. 5: Postoperative OCT showing attached macula with closure of O-LMH.

OUTCOME SUMMARY

MS resolved with closure of O-LMH. Her vision was maintained at 6 months of follow-up **(Fig. 5)**.

KEY POINTS

- Use of longer instruments, along with more posterior and horizontally aligned sclerotomy placement, enhances accessibility to the posterior pole in eyes with extreme axial elongation.
- Foveal sparing ILM peeling reduces the risk of iatrogenic macular hole formation in these eyes with thin retina.

FURTHER READING

1. Quiroz-Reyes MA, Quiroz-Gonzalez EA, Quiroz-Gonzalez MA, Lima-Gomez V. Novel surgical approaches for treating myopic traction maculopathy: a meta-analysis. BMC Ophthalmol. 2024;24(1):105.

2. Shimada N, Sugamoto Y, Ogawa M, Takase H, Ohno-Matsui K. Fovea-sparing internal limiting membrane peeling for myopic traction maculopathy. Am J Ophthalmol. 2012;154(4):693-701.
3. Zeng Q, Yao Y, Zhao M. Comparison between fovea-sparing and complete internal limiting membrane peeling for the treatment of myopic traction maculopathy: a systemic review and meta-analysis. Ophthal Res. 2021;64(6):916-27.

CASE SCENARIO 3: HIGH MYOPIA WITH FULL-THICKNESS MACULAR HOLES

Case Scenario

A 53-year-old female presented with a recent onset of difficulty in near vision in her LE. She was a high myope. BCVA was 20/100 with -21.00 DS in the RE and 20/200 with -20.00 DS in the LE. Fundus examination revealed a myopic fundus with diffuse choroidal atrophy in both eyes and full-thickness macular hole (FTMH) in the LE. OCT confirmed the FTMH with epiretinal membrane (ERM) in the LE **(Fig. 6)**.

Treatment Plan

Pars plana vitrectomy with ILM peeling and C_3F_8 injection in the LE.

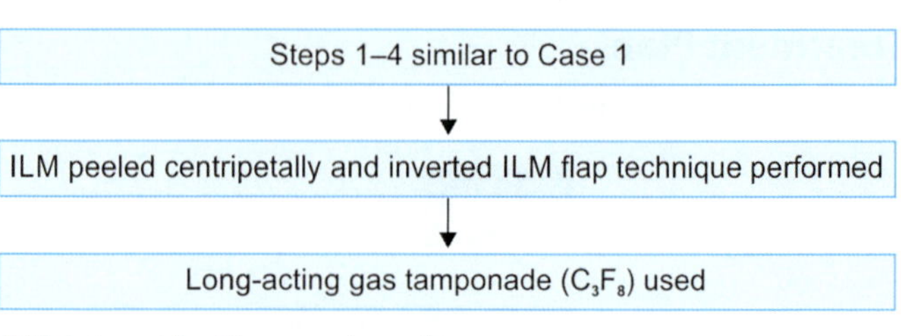

(ILM: internal limiting membrane)

Thought Process

Decision	*Rationale*
Vitrectomy	Recent decrease in vision with FTMH and shallow PS, relieves both anteroposterior and tangential traction (ERM)
Inverted ILM flap	In highly myopic eyes with large MH, inverted ILM flap acts a scaffold for hole closure
C_3F_8	It provides longer tamponade which is required in high myopic eyes

OUTCOME SUMMARY

Macular hole closed and BCVA improved to 20/60 p and patient is on regular follow-up **(Fig. 7)**.

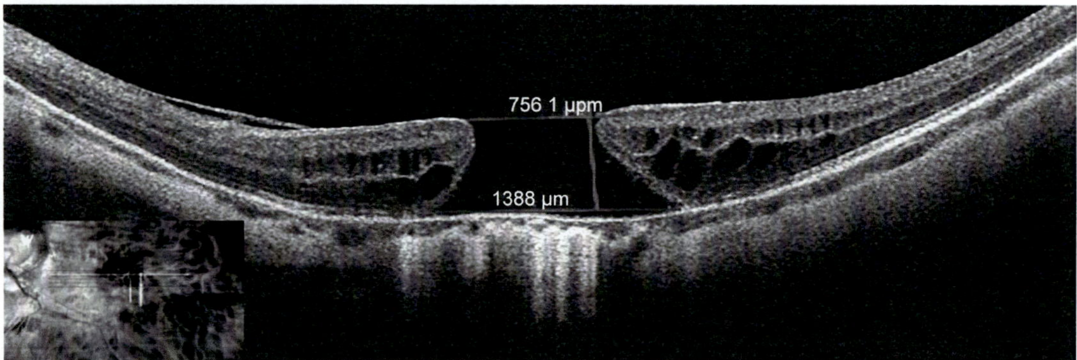

Fig. 6: OCT of LE showing FTMH, epiretinal membrane (ERM) and FS.

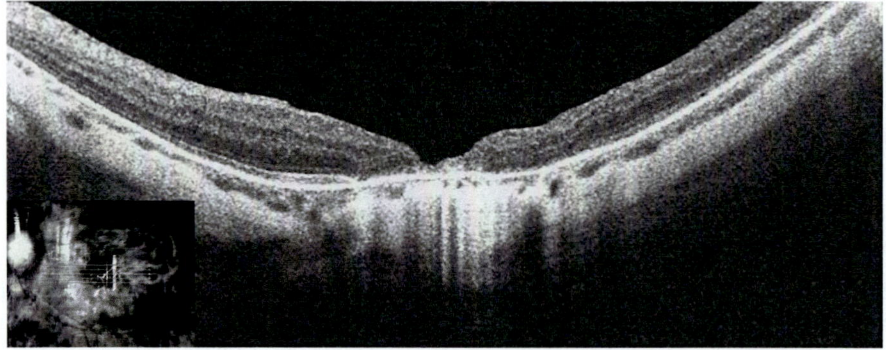

Fig. 7: Postoperative OCT showing closed MH.

KEY POINTS

- Highly myopic eyes with FTMH and ERM, when not associated with deep PS or MD, can be successfully managed with vitrectomy.
- Inverted ILM flap technique enhances the closure rate in these eyes.

FURTHER READING

1. Nakano H, Terashima H, Hasebe H, Fukuchi T. Inverted internal limiting membrane flap technique for macular hole retinal detachment in high myopia compared to internal limiting membrane peeling. Sci Rep. 2025;15:21537.
2. Shroff D, Gupta P, Atri N, Gupta C, Shroff C. Inverted internal limiting membrane (ILM) flap technique for macular hole closure: patient selection and special considerations. Clin Ophthalmol. 2019;13:671-8.

CASE SCENARIO 4: POSTERIOR STAPHYLOMA WITH MACULAR DETACHMENT

Case Summary

A 53-year-old female, high myope (–17.00/–1.50 D) presented with a 3-week history of gradual, painless visual decline in the RE, associated with intermittent photopsias. The LE was a painful blind eye following vitreoretinal surgery for retinal detachment 12 years earlier. She had previously been diagnosed with *myopic tractional maculopathy (MTM) with MD* in the RE and advised surgical intervention. Her BCVA was 20/80 in RE and NPL in LE. Fundus examination showed PS with patchy choroidal atrophy and MD in RE **(Fig. 8A)**. OCT showed PS with MD and FTMH in RE **(Figs. 8B and C)**.

Treatment Plan

- Plan A: MB
- Plan B: Vitrectomy with ILM relaxation with C3F8 under local anesthesia
- Barrage laser to HST present superiorly

The surgical steps were similar to those described in Case 2

Thought Process

Decision	*Rationale*
Vitrectomy and not macular buckle	Suspected rhegma at staphylomatous area one-eyed status of patient, and borderline IOP
Sclerotomy	In extremely long eyes, temporary removal of canula facilitates access to posterior pole
Gas and not silicone oil (SO)	In deep staphyloma gas conforms to staphyloma better than SO
Barrage laser	To superior retinal break

OUTCOME SUMMARY

MD resolved with type 2 MH closure and BCVA was stabilized on follow-up **(Figs. 9A to C)**.

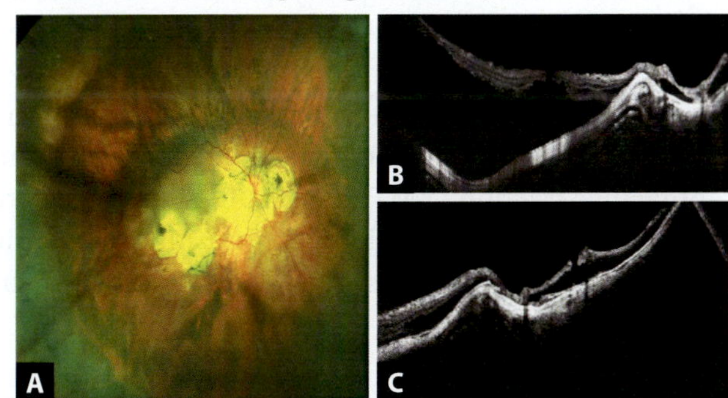

Figs. 8A to C: (A) Fundus image of RE showing PS with patchy choroidal atrophy with MD; (B) OCT showing PS with MD; (C) Macular hole.

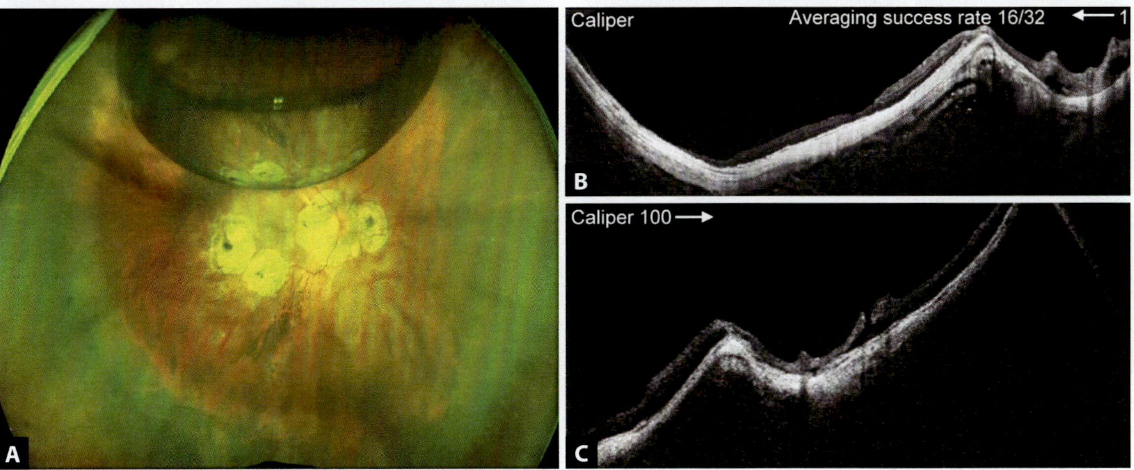

Figs. 9A to C: Postoperative (A) fundus optos image showing attached macula with small gas bubble; (B) OCT showing attached macula; (C) Type 2 closure of hole.

KEY POINTS

- The choice of surgical technique should be individualized considering various factors including one-eyed status, staphyloma depth, and coexisting glaucomatous changes.
- MB can be reserved as a second-stage procedure in cases of failed PPV.

FURTHER READING

1. Alkabes M, Mateo C. Macular buckle technique in myopic traction maculopathy: a 16-year review of the literature and a comparison with vitreous surgery. Graefes Arch Clin Exp Ophthalmol. 2018;256(5):863-77.
2. Parolini B, Matello V, Rosales-Padrón JF. Combined surgical approach for repair of refractory macular hole in myopic traction maculopathy. J Vitreoretin Dis. 2024;9(2):219-23.

CASE SCENARIO 5: MACULAR DETACHMENT WITH LAMELLAR MACULAR HOLE AND VMT

A 68-year-old female with high myopia (RE -9.00 DS, LE -11.50 DS) presented with a 1-month history of decreased vision in the RE. Examination revealed an axial length of 29 mm with a shallow PS **(Figs. 10A and B)**. OCT of the RE showed features of MTM with associated LMH and vitreomacular traction (VMT) **(Fig. 10C)**. Findings were consistent with tractional changes in a highly myopic eye, indicating risk of progression and potential need for surgical intervention.

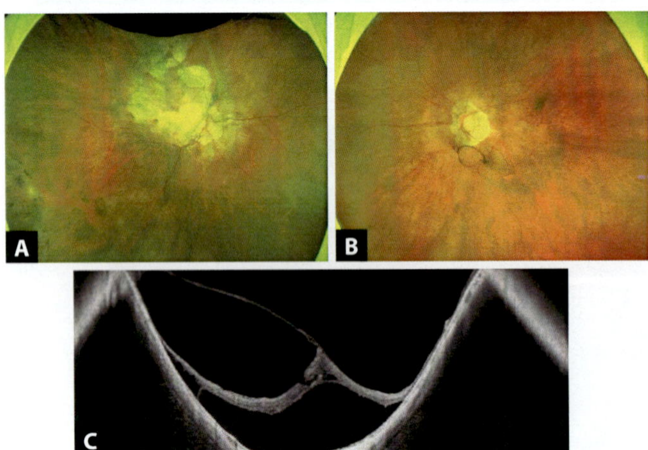

Figs. 10A to C: Optos wide field fundus image of (A) RE showing PS with patchy choroidal atrophy and MTM; (B) LE showing peripapillary atrophy and type 3 PS; (C) RE OCT showing shallow PS with MD with LMH and vitreomacular traction (VMT).

Treatment Plan

RE phacoemulsification with intraocular lens along with PPV. ILM peeling and gas injection.

The surgical steps were similar to those described in Case 2

Thought Process

Decision	*Rationale*
Vitrectomy	As AL was 29 mm with shallow PS, LMH, and vitreomacular traction, vitrectomy release the preretinal anteroposterior traction
ILM peeling	Release the tangential traction

(ILM: internal limiting membrane)

OUTCOME SUMMARY

MD resolved with stabilization of her BCVA at 2/60 in RE on follow-up **(Figs. 11 A and B)**.

KEY POINT

In cases with more of anteroposterior traction, vitrectomy can be preferred over macular buckle.

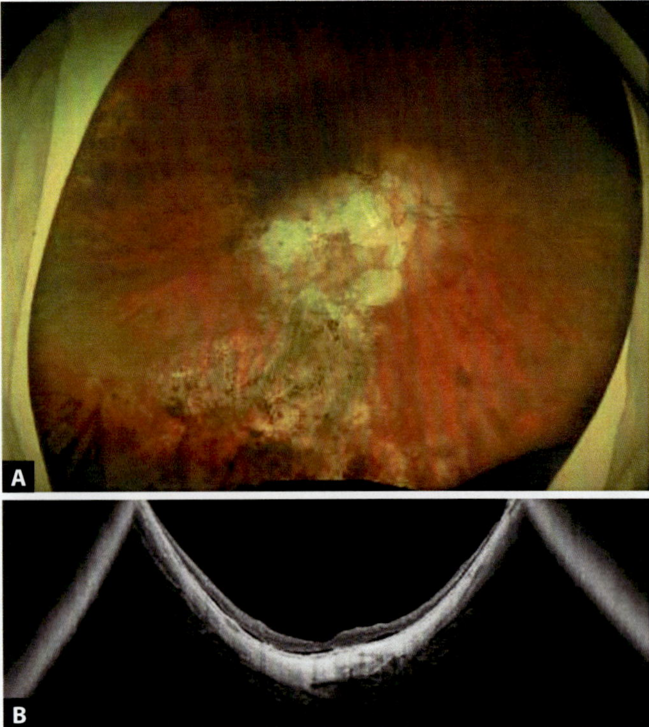

Figs. 11A and B: Postoperative (A) Optos image showing attached macula; (B) OCT showing settled MD and LMH.

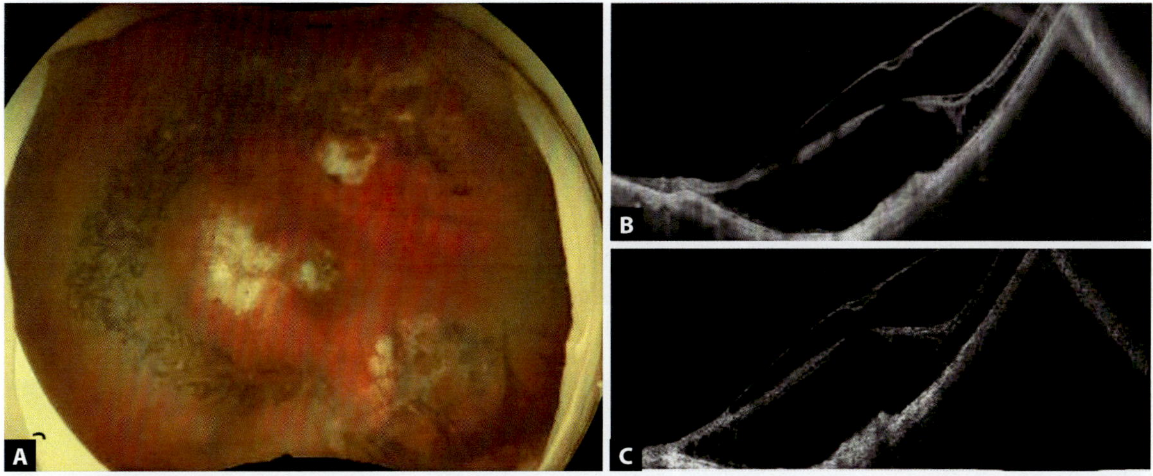

Figs. 12A to C: (A) Optos image of LE showing PS with patchy atrophy; (B and C) Follow-up OCT scan showing stable FS with stable vision.

FURTHER READING

1. Frisina R, Gius I, Palmieri M, Finzi A, Tozzi L, Parolini B. Myopic traction maculopathy: diagnostic and management strategies. Clin Ophthalmol. 2020;14:3699-708.
2. Parolini B, Palmieri M, Finzi A, Besozzi G, Frisina R. Myopic traction maculopathy: a new perspective on classification and management. Asia Pac J Ophthalmol (Phila). 2021;10(1):49-59.

CASE SCENARIO 6: MYOPIC TRACTIONAL MACULOPATHY WITH FOVEAL SCHISIS (CHRONIC)

Case Summary

A 67-year-old one-eyed female with chronic symptoms in her seeing left eye. Her BCVA was RE NPL, LE 2/60. Fundus examination revealed myopic fundus with PS and patchy choroidal atrophy **(Fig. 12A)**.

OCT revealed FS with incomplete PVD **(Figs. 12B and C)**.

Treatment Plan

To observe as one-eyed and vision and OCT remained stable over follow-up.

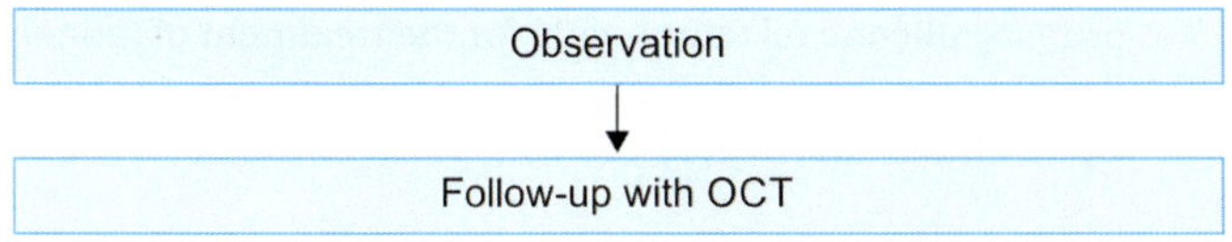

Thought Process

Decision	*Rationale*
Observe	One-eyed patient with chronic symptoms and no recent progression of symptoms or OCT features
OCT	Sequential OCT showed minimal or insignificant progression of schisis changes

KEY POINT

Thin and atrophic retina with chronic schitic changes may not benefit surgically for any visual improvement, in such cases prefer conservative approach.

FURTHER READING

1. Parolini B, Palmieri M, Finzi A, Besozzi G, Frisina R. Myopic traction maculopathy: a new perspective on classification and management. Asia Pac J Ophthalmol (Phila). 2021;10(1):49-59.

CASE SCENARIO 7: DEEP POSTERIOR STAPHYLOMA WITH MACULAR DETACHMENT AND FTMH

Case Summary

A 68-year-old man with sudden decrease in vision in RE of 20 days duration. His BCVA was 3/60 with –22.0 DS and 1/60 with –20.0 DS in RE and LE, respectively. Fundus examination showed PS in both eyes with MD in RE. B scan confirmed the PS and MD **(Fig. 13A)**. OCT showed deep PS with ERM and FTMH **(Fig. 13B)**.

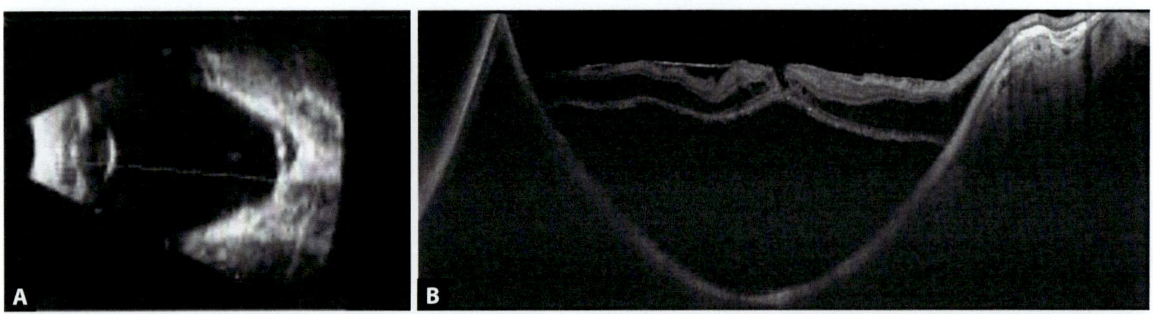

Figs. 13A and B: (A) B-scan of RE showing PS with MD; (B) OCT showing MD with ERM and LMH and PS.

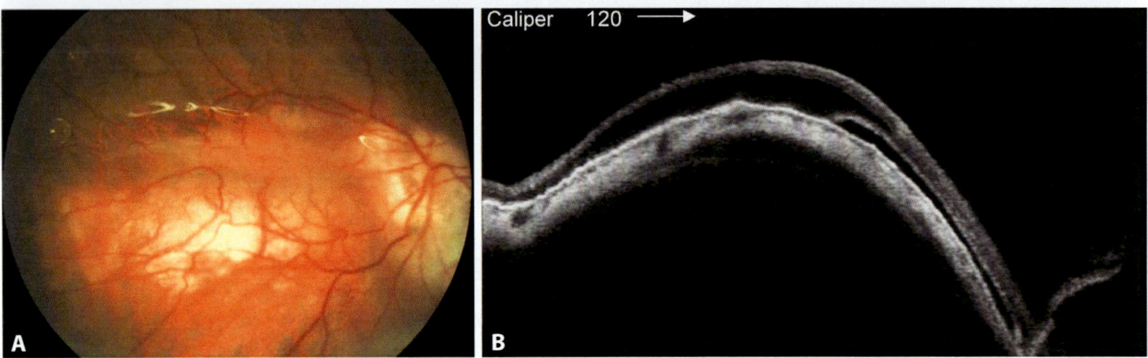

Figs. 14A and B: (A) RE fundus image showing attached macula with macular buckle indentation; (B) OCT showing attached macula with buckle indentation.

Treatment Plan

Combined macular buckle (MB), vitrectomy, ILM peel and silicone oil tamponade.

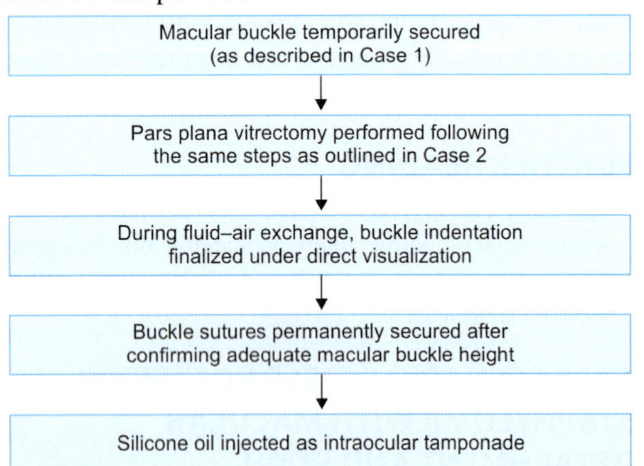

Thought Process

Decision	*Rationale*
Combined approach	Deep PS with MD and macular hole—needs to address both centrifugal and tangential traction
Macular buckle	Reduce centrifugal traction
Vitrectomy with ILM peel	Release tangential traction

OUTCOME SUMMARY

MD settled with closure of MH. Patients subsequently underwent silicone oil removal along with cataract surgery. Retina remained attached on follow-up with stable vision **(Figs. 14 A and B)**.

KEY POINTS

- Buckle is always placed first and then vitrectomy is performed.
- Buckle height titration to be done during FAE
- IOP control is crucial throughout surgery.

FURTHER READING

1. Ge JY, Jun Teo AW, Tsai ASH, Wei Tan GS, Lee SY, Cheung N, et al. Macular buckle, vitrectomy, or combined approach for the management of macular hole retinal detachment: a systematic review and network meta-analysis. Ophthalmol Retina. 2025:S2468-6530(25)00395-1.
2. Nishimura A, Kimura M, Saito Y, Sugiyama K. Efficacy of primary silicone oil tamponade for the treatment of retinal detachment caused by macular hole in high myopia. Am J Ophthalmol. 2011;151(1):148-55.

CHAPTER 10

Decision Making in Surgical Management of Macular Pathologies

CK Nagesha, Gaurav Malwe, Priya BV

ALGORITHMIC APPROACH FOR SURGICAL MANAGEMENT OF EPIRETINAL MEMBRANE

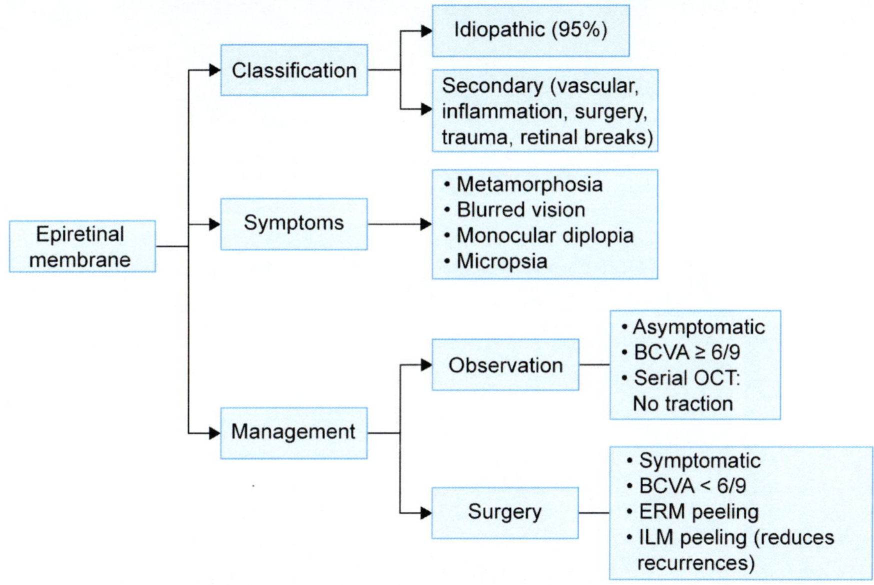

(BCVA: best-corrected visual acuity; ERM: epiretinal membrane; ILM: internal limiting membrane; OCT: optical coherence tomography)

CASE SCENARIO 1: MANAGEMENT OF ASYMPTOMATIC EPIRETINAL MEMBRANE

Case Summary

A 70-year-old male came for regular checkup. On examination, fundus RE showed ERM with RPE alterations in fovea with multiple retinal holes inferiorly **(Fig. 1)**. Left eye showed glaucomatous optic atrophy.

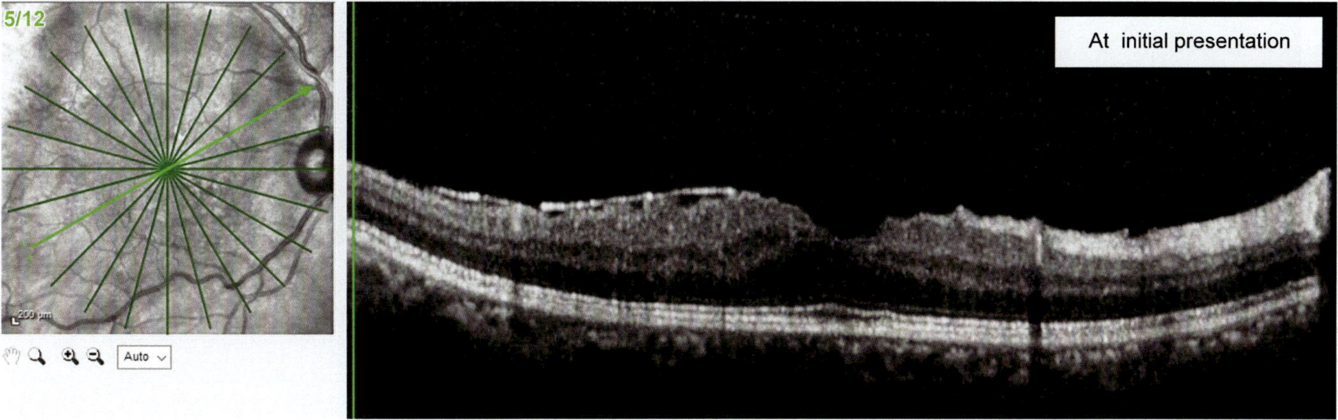

Fig. 1: RE-optical coherence tomography (OCT) shows epiretinal membrane (ERM) as a hyperreflective line on the inner retinal surface with normal foveal contour and well-defined retinal layers.

Treatment Plan

Observation and follow up with periodic OCTs

Thought Process

Decision	*Rationale*
Observe	• Observation and follow-up every 6 monthly with periodic OCTs • Many cases of ERM do not progress to require surgery **(Figs. 2A to D)**

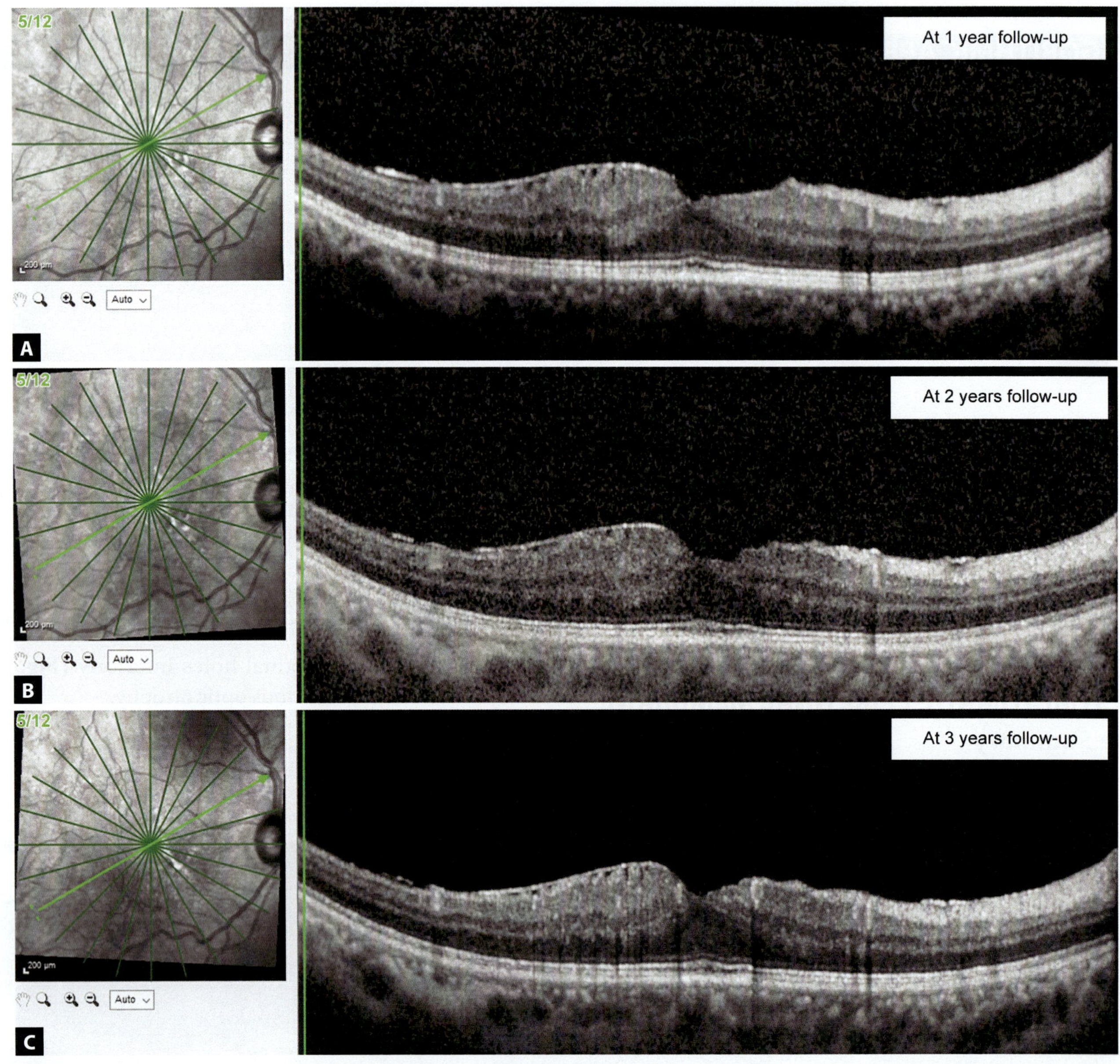

Figs. 2A to C

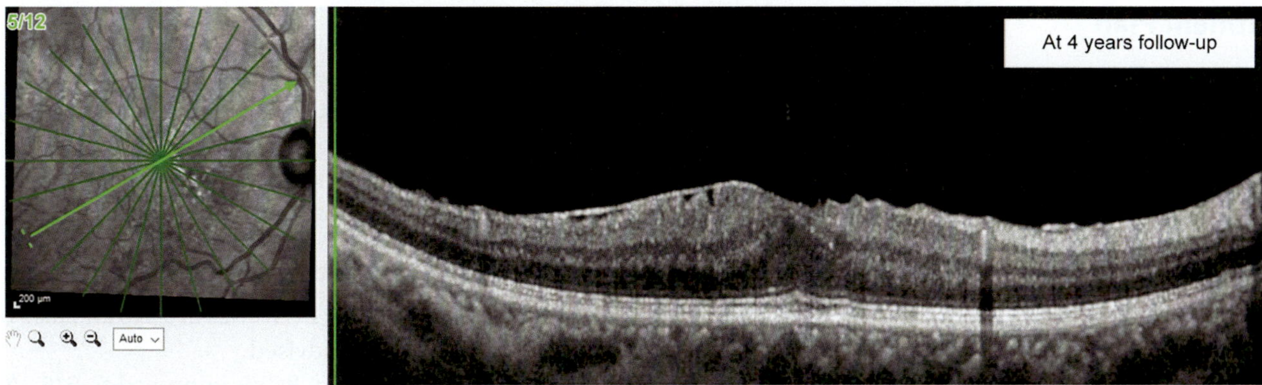

Fig. 2D

Figs. 2A to D: Serial optical coherence tomography (OCT) scans which shows presence of epiretinal membrane (ERM) and loss of foveal contour but outer retinal layers being intact and patient remained asymptomatic.

CASE SCENARIO 2: MANAGEMENT OF SYMPTOMATIC IDIOPATHIC EPIRETINAL MEMBRANE

Case Summary

A 72-year-old male, a known hypertensive, pseudophakic in both eyes presented with blurring of vision in LE associated with metamorphopsia for 1 month. Best-corrected visual acuity (BCVA) was 6/6, N6 in RE and 6/9P, N8 in LE. Fundus examination RE was WNL (within normal limits), LE showed ERM with macular pucker with PVD **(Fig. 3)**.

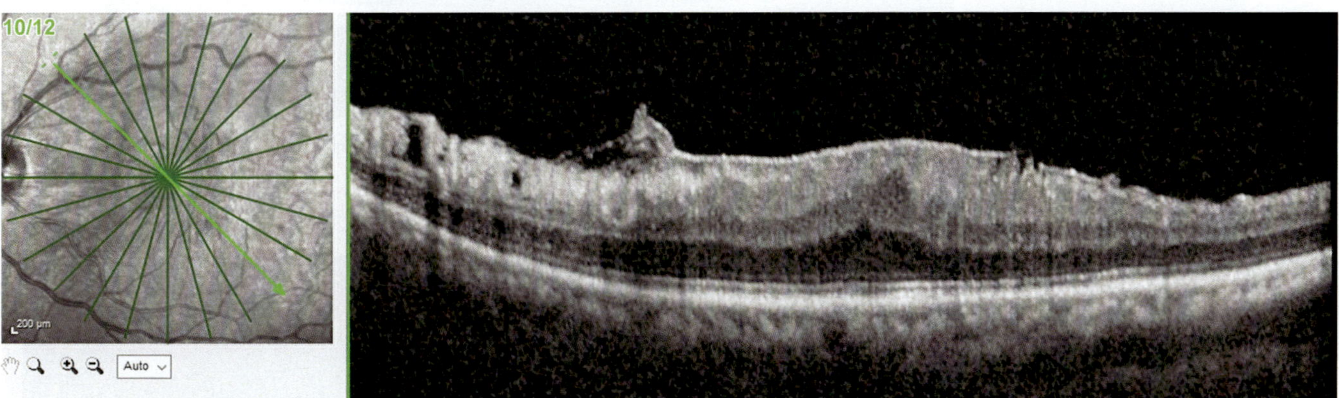

Fig. 3: LE-OCT showed macular ERM with alteration of foveal contour with ectopic inner foveal layers with distortion of inner retinal layers.

Treatment Plan

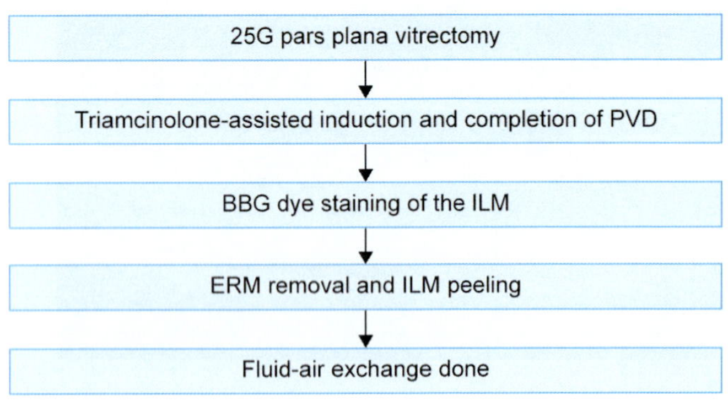

(BBG: brilliant blue G; ERM: epiretinal membrane; ILM: internal limiting membrane; PVD: posterior vitreous detachment)

Thought Process

Decision	*Rationale*
Vitrectomy advised	Patient symptomatic, though BCVA was 6/9
ILM peeling along with ERM removal	ILM peeling ensures complete removal of the ERM and the rate of recurrence of ERM postoperatively is significantly less

OUTCOME SUMMARY

Patient was asymptomatic, BCVA was 6/6, N6 and also one eyed. So observation was advised.

One month postsurgery BCVA improved to 6/6 , N6p **(Fig. 4)**.

VIDEO LEGEND

Video 12: Symptomatic ERM

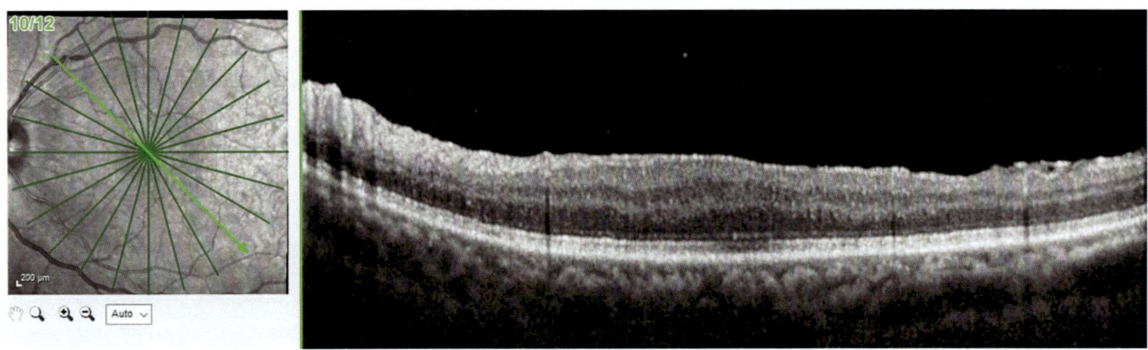

Fig. 4: LE OCT: Postoperatively 1 month showed better foveal contour.

CASE SCENARIO 3: MANAGEMENT OF SECONDARY EPIRETINAL MEMBRANE POSTVITRECTOMY

Case Summary

A 53-year-old lady came with complaint of diminution of vision LE for 15 days. BCVA was 6/6P in RE, hand movements in LE. She had undergone cataract surgery in both eyes 2 years back. Fundus RE was WNL, LE showed rhegmatogenous retinal detachment (RRD) with macula off with large HST temporally.

Figure 5 Ultra-widefield (UWF) photo of LE macula off rhegmatogenous retinal detachment (RRD) with large HST temporally. **Figure 6** LE-OCT shows macula off rhegmatogenous retinal detachment (RRD) with ORF.

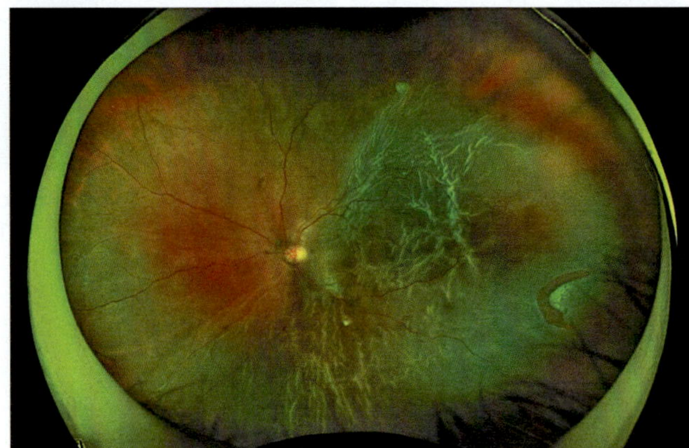

Fig. 5: Ultra-widefield (UWF) photo of LE showed macula off rhegmatogenous retinal detachment (RRD) with large HST temporally.

She underwent LE vitrectomy + FGE + EL + C3F8. Surgery was uneventful. 3 weeks postoperatively, BCVA in LE had improved to 6/15. Fundus LE showed attached retina with early macular ERM **(Fig. 7)**.

Two months postoperatively, BCVA in LE had decreased to 6/36. Fundus examination showed macular ERM with attached retina **(Fig. 8)**.

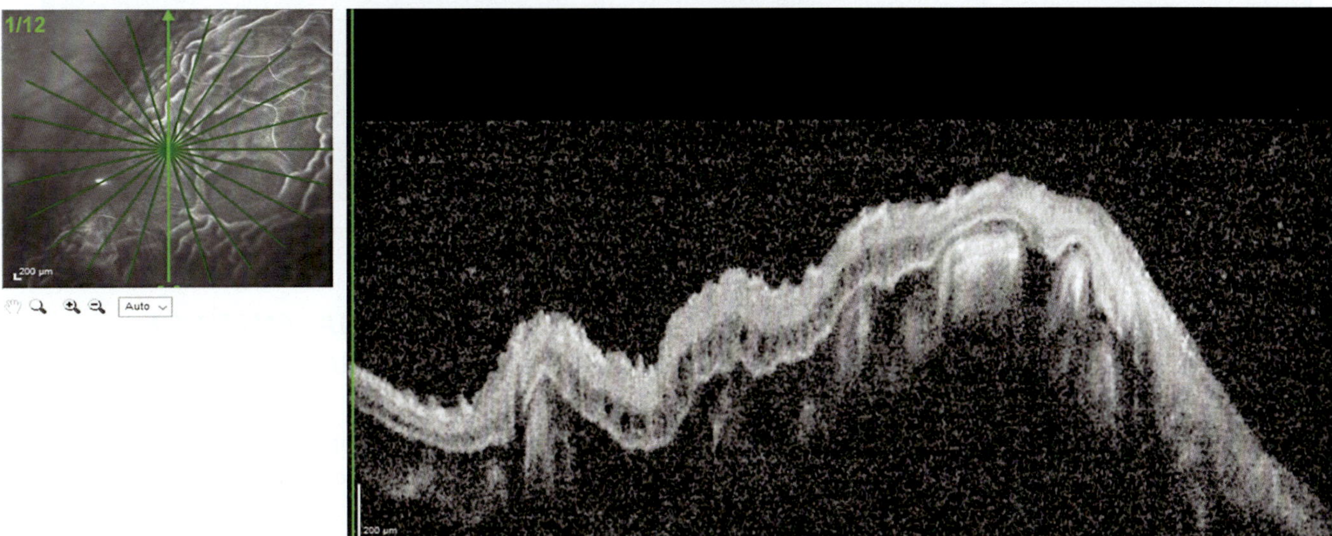

Fig. 6: LE-OCT showed macula off rhegmatogenous retinal detachment (RRD) with SRF (subretinal fluid).

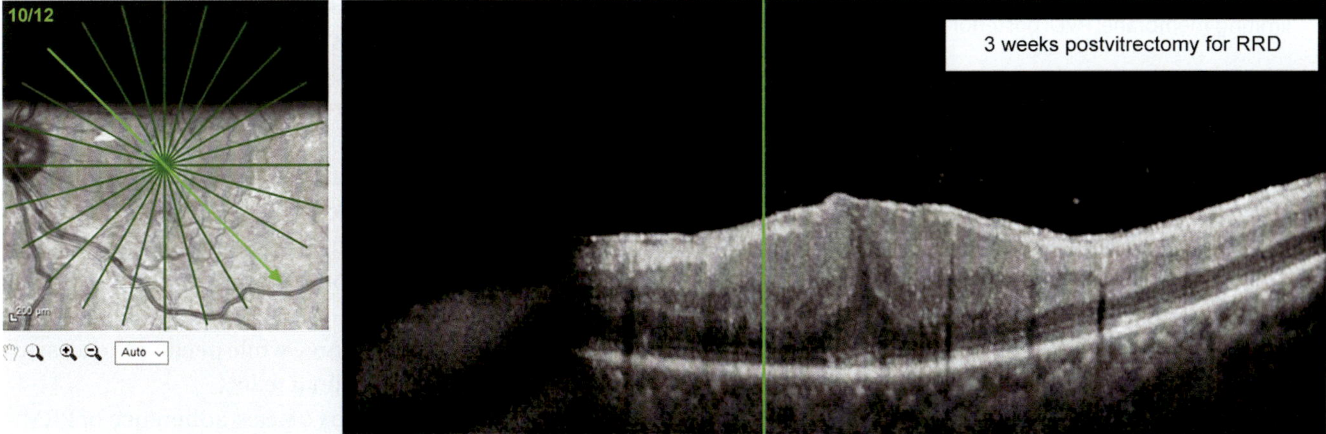

Fig. 7: LE-OCT—postoperatively 3 weeks—macula on with early epiretinal membrane (ERM) over macula.

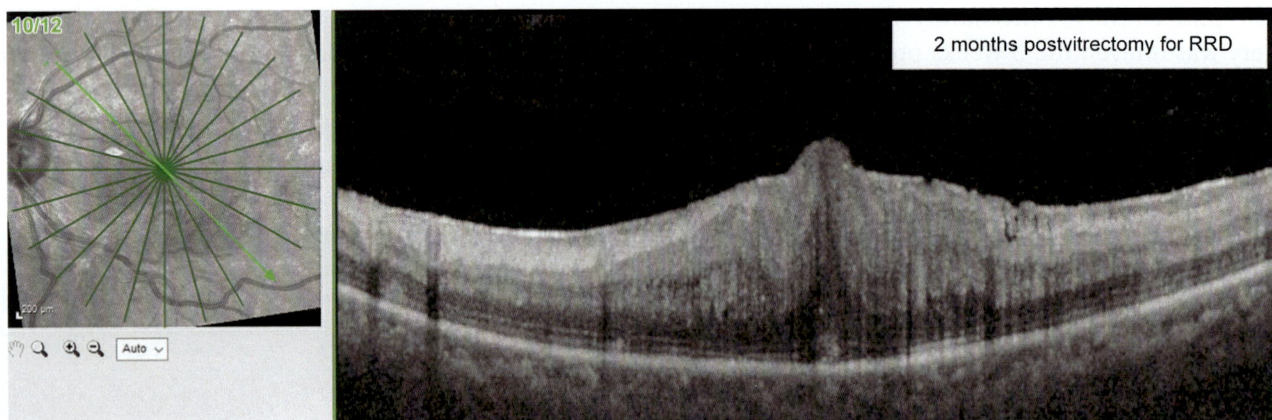

Fig. 8: LE-OCT showed macular ERM with elongated outer nuclear layer with distorted retinal layers.

Treatment Plan

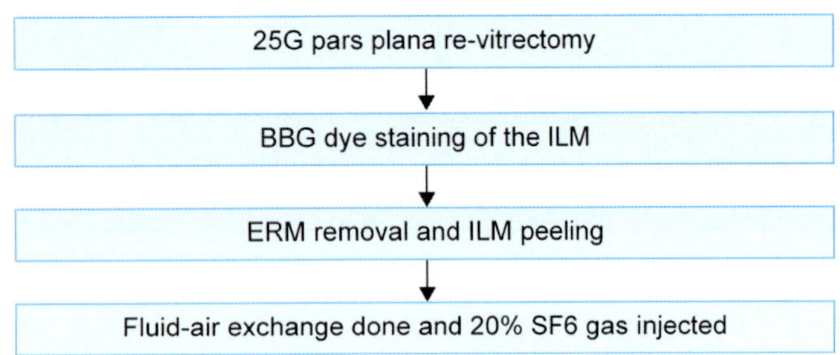

(BBG: brilliant blue G; ERM: epiretinal membrane; ILM: internal limiting membrane; PVD: posterior vitreous detachment)

Thought Process

Decision	*Rationale*
Surgery for ERM removal	Patient was symptomatic with reduced vision secondary to ERM formation postvitrectomy for RRD. The goal of surgery is not only to restore anatomy but to relieve functional traction before irreversible photoreceptor loss occurs. Early intervention after structural change gives better visual gain
ILM peeling along with ERM removal	ILM peel reduces recurrence of ERM

OUTCOME SUMMARY

She underwent LE ERM removal + ILM peeling + SF6 injection. 1 month later LE-BCVA was 6/9P **(Fig. 9)**.

KEY POINTS IN MANAGEMENT OF MACULAR EPIRETINAL MEMBRANE

- When not to operate:
  - Asymptomatic patient
  - Symptoms are not correlating with anatomical findings.
- *When to operate:* Visual symptoms like blurring of vision and metamorphopsia are interfering with daily activities
- *Points to note on OCT:* Foveal contour, presence/absence of foveal pit, distortion of retinal layers, elongation of outer nuclear layer, cotton ball sign, ectopic inner foveal layers, intraretinal fluid, areas of RNFL schisis, look for areas where there is safe plane for ERM peeling.
- Surgical Pearls in macular ERM surgery:
  - Always confirm PVD completion before membrane peeling—can use dilute triamcinolone for this.
  - Use high magnification lens while doing membrane peeling.
  - Use slow and steady force while peeling as excessive traction can cause retinal tears.
  - Start peeling from area of least adherence of ERM.
  - Avoid gripping directly over fovea.
  - While peeling the ERM, maintain view of ERM and the underlying retina—make sure not to grasp the retina.
  - ILM peeling along with ERM removal improves long-term stability but may cause microstructural changes.

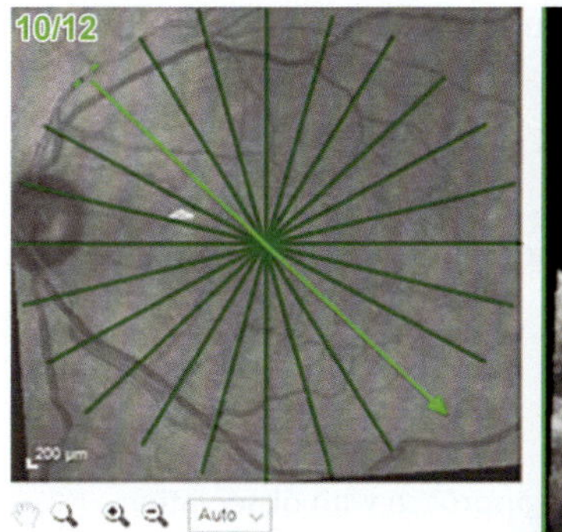

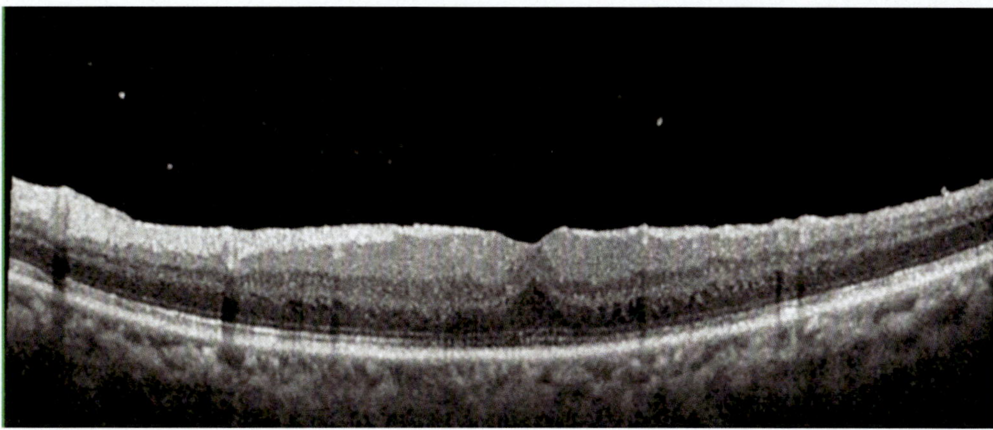

Fig. 9: LE-OCT showed much improvement of foveal contour.

- Visualization adjuvants like triamcinolone and brilliant blue can be used.

FURTHER READING

1. Fung AT, Galvin J, Tran T. Epiretinal membrane: A review. Clin Exp Ophthalmol. 2021;49(3):289-308.
2. Gass JD. Stereoscopic Atlas of Macular Diseases: Diagnosis and treatment, 2nd edition. St Louis: CV Mosby; 1977.
3. Smiddy WE, Maguire AM, Green WR, Michels RG, de la Cruz Z, Enger C, et al. Idiopathic epiretinal membranes. Ultrastructural characteristics and clinicopathologic correlation. Ophthalmology. 1989;96(6):811-20.

VIDEO LEGEND

Video 13: Secondary epiretinal membrane postvitrectomy

SURGICAL MANAGEMENT OF VITREOMACULAR TRACTION

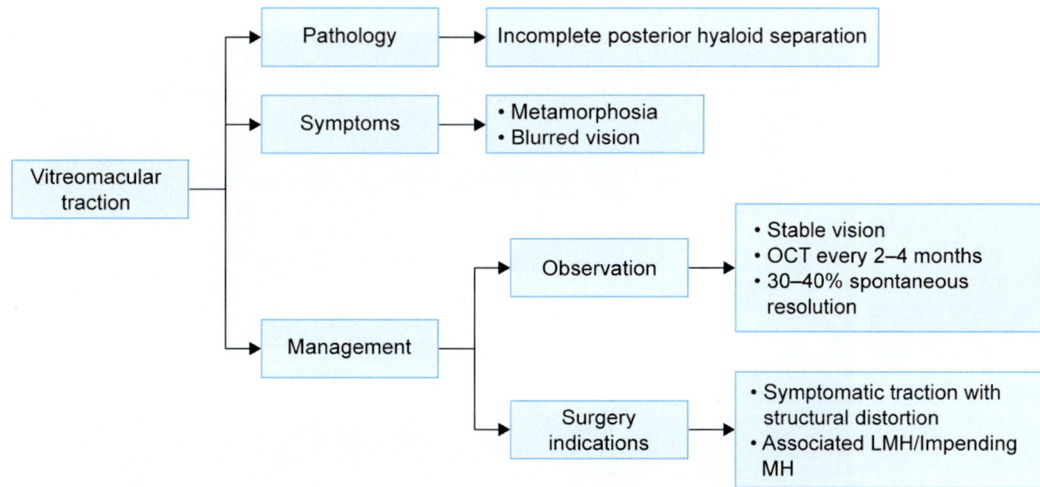

(ERM: epiretinal membrane; LMH: lamellar macular hole)

CASE SCENARIO 4: MANAGEMENT OF FOCAL VITREOMACULAR TRACTION WITH PRESERVED FOVEAL CONTOUR

Case Summary

A 60-year-old lady came for regular checkup. Her BCVA was 6/6, N6 in both eyes. LE-OCT showed vitreomacular traction (VMT) with near normal foveal contour **(Fig. 10)**.

Treatment Plan

She was advised observation and follow-up 6 monthly.

Thought Process

Decision	*Rationale*
Observation with periodic follow-up	Many cases of VMT remain stable without progression

CASE SCENARIO 5: MANAGEMENT OF FOCAL VMT WITH ALTERED FOVEAL CONTOUR

Case Summary

A 65-year-old female presented with complaint of floaters RE for 3 days. BCVA was 6/8, N6 in RE and 6/6, N6 in LE. Fundus RE showed macular ERM **(Fig. 11)** and LE was within normal limits.

Treatment Plan

Patient was advised observation and to review after 3 weeks.

Thought Process

Decision	*Rationale*
Observation with periodic OCTs	Conservative approach with observation and periodic follow-up is justified in patients with VMT with altered foveal contour with no or minimal symptoms as spontaneous resolution of VMT can occur

(OCT: optical coherence tomography; VMT: vitreomacular traction)

OUTCOME SUMMARY

At follow-up after 3 weeks, BCVA-RE had improved to 6/6, N6. Follow-up of OCT-RE after 3 weeks showed that the adhesion of the posterior hyaloid had released from the inner retinal surface with normalization of foveal contour with small cystoid spaces. Patient was advised to review after 3 months. Follow-up OCT after 3 months showed normal foveal contour. Patient was regularly followed up every 6 monthly thereafter. The BCVA was maintained at 6/6, N6 **(Figs. 12A and B)**.

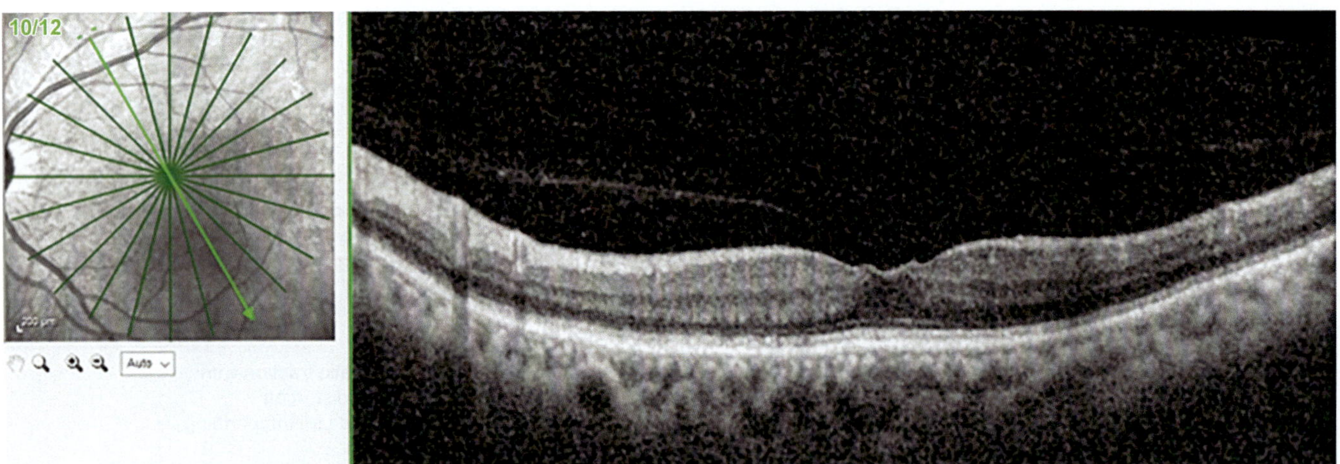

Fig. 10: LE-OCT showed vitreomacular traction (VMT) with near normal foveal contour.

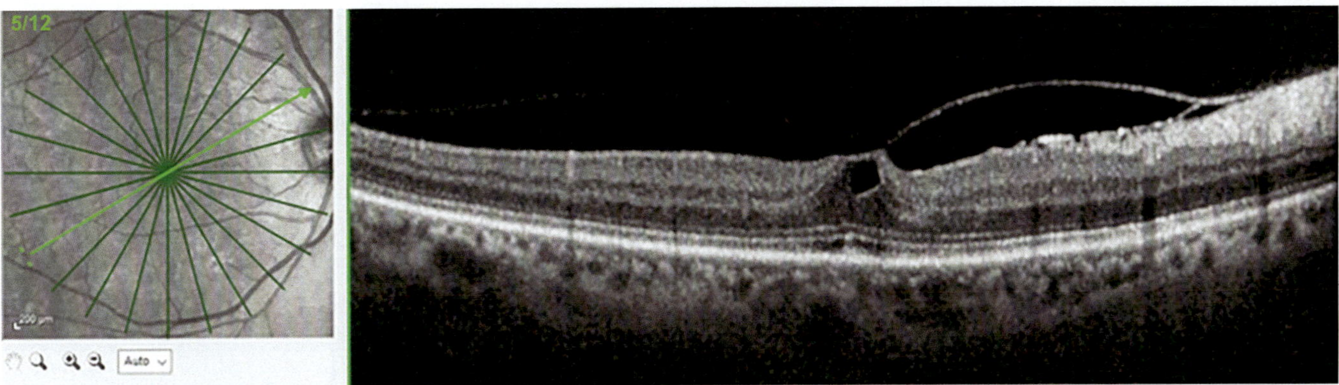

Fig. 11: RE-OCT showed alteration of foveal contour with vitreomacular traction (VMT) with small cystoid space and epiretinal membrane (ERM) with width of vitreomacular adhesion 476 µ.

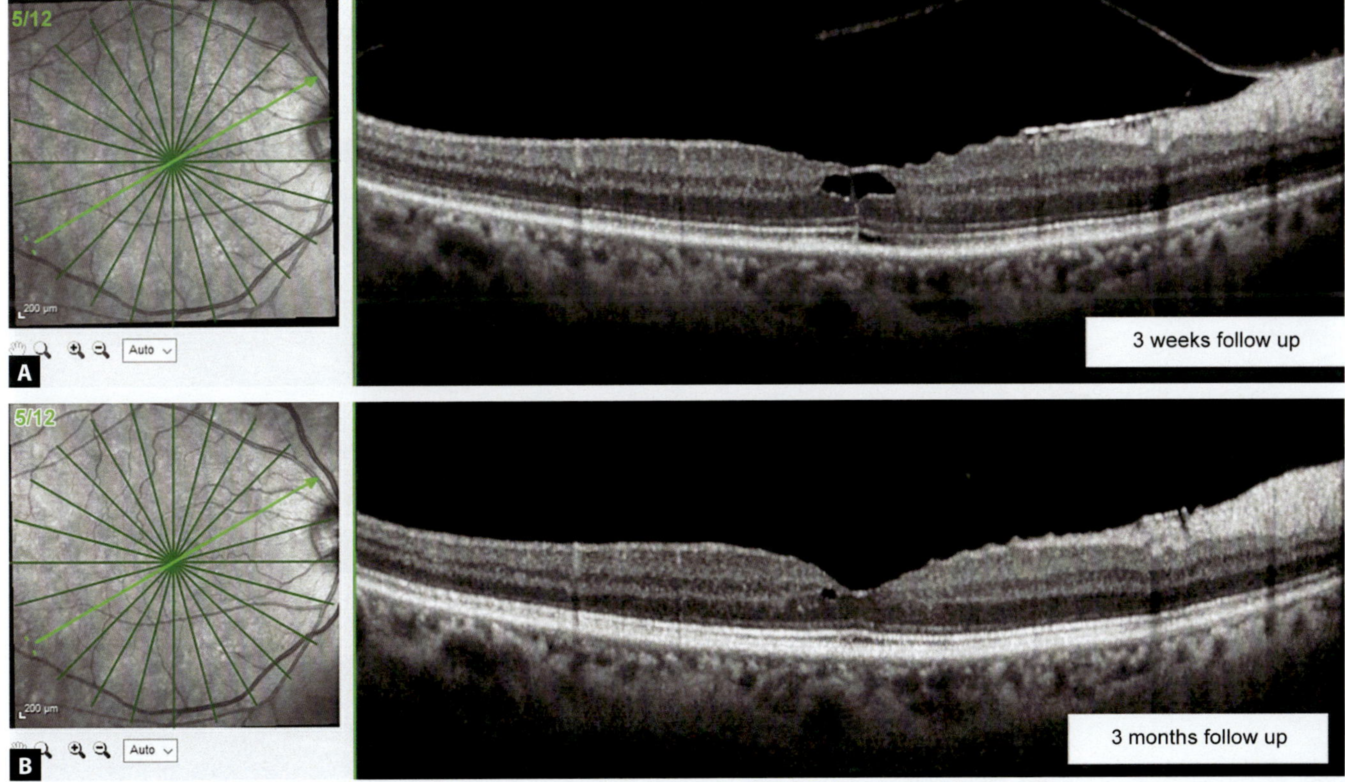

Figs. 12A and B: (A) Follow-up OCT-RE after 3 weeks showed that the adhesion of the posterior hyaloid had released from the inner retinal surface with normalization of foveal contour with small cystoid spaces; (B) Follow-up OCT after 3 months showed normal foveal contour.

CASE SCENARIO 6: MANAGEMENT OF SYMPTOMATIC FOCAL VITREOMACULAR TRACTION

Case Summary

An 85-year-old male, a known diabetic, came for routine check. BCVA was 6/8 in RE, CF 2 m in LE. Anterior segment of both eyes showed immature cataracts. Fundus RE OCT showed moderate NPDR with few drusen, LE showed moderate NPDR with scarred CNVM. RE OCT showed focal vitreomacular traction (VMT) with epiretinal membrane (ERM) **(Fig. 13)**.

As patient was asymptomatic and one eyed, he was advised observation and follow-up after 2 months. But, the patient came after 6 months with a complaint of RE-DOV. RE-BCVA was 6/12 p. RE-OCT showed increase in the traction at fovea with distorted foveal contour, CME, foveal detachment, and schitic vitreous **(Fig. 14)**.

Treatment Plan

Patient was advised RE cataract surgery + vitrectomy.

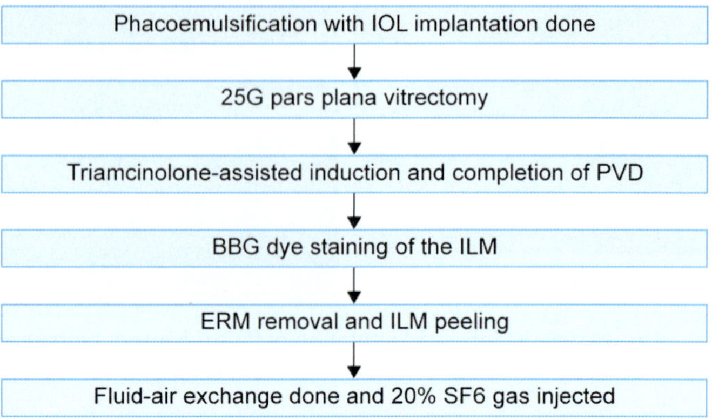

(BBG: brilliant blue G; ERM: epiretinal membrane; ILM: internal limiting membrane; IOL: intraocular lens; PVD: posterior vitreous detachment)

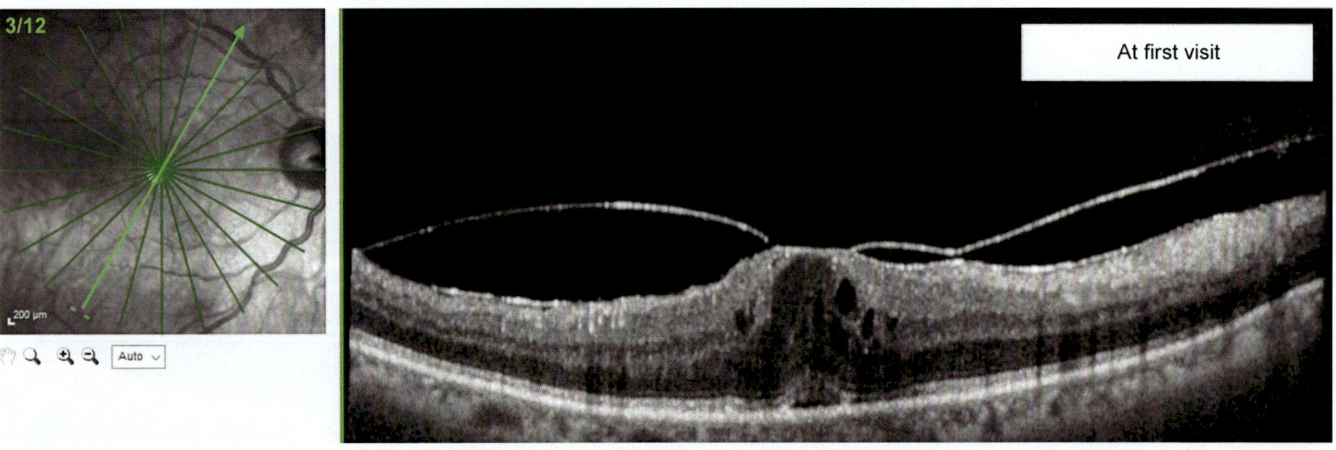

Fig. 13: RE-OCT showed focal vitreomacular traction (VMT) with epiretinal membrane (ERM).

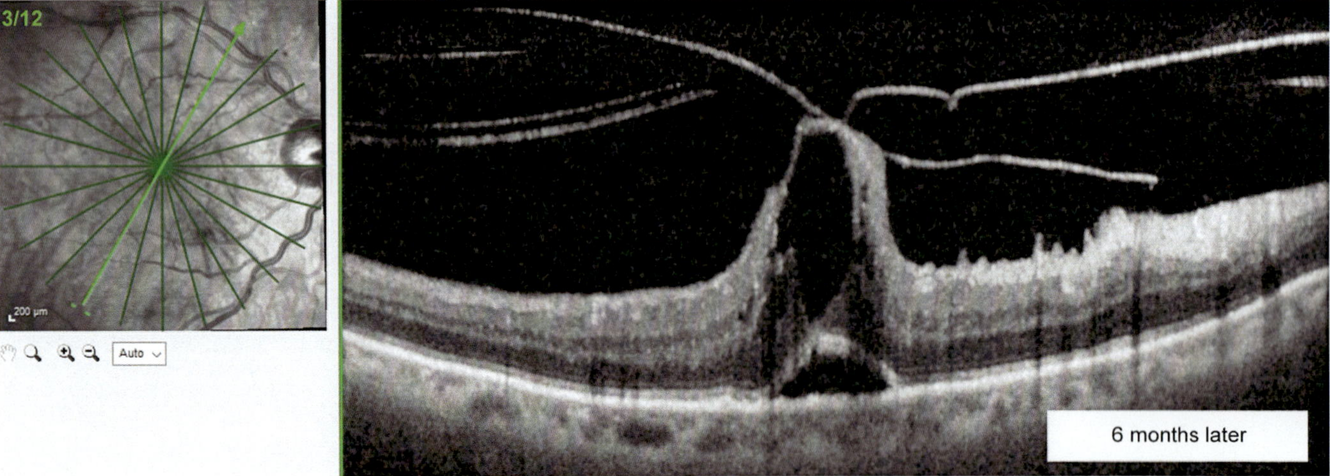

Fig. 14: RE-OCT showed increase in the traction at fovea with distorted foveal contour, CME, foveal detachment, and schitic vitreous.

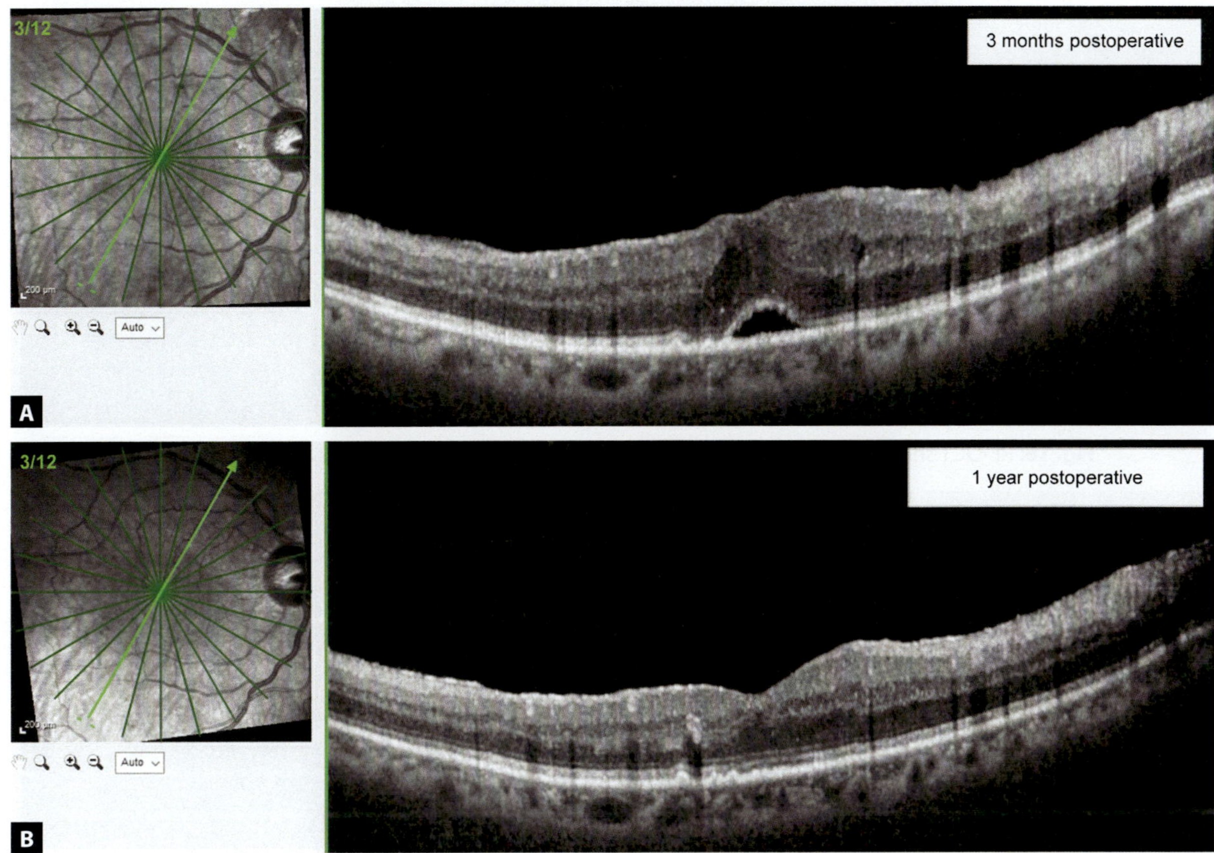

Figs. 15A and B: (A) RE-OCT showed improvement of foveal contour with small foveal detachment less than before; (B) At 1 year follow-up, RE-OCT showed normal foveal contour with resolution of foveal detachment.

Thought Process

Decision	*Rationale*
Surgery for VMT	Patient symptomatic with decrease in vision
Combined phaco with vitrectomy	To avoid second surgery in an 85-year-old patient with immature cataract and for clear visibility of posterior pole during ERM removal or ILM peeling
ILM peeling also to be done	To remove all traction at fovea

(ERM: epiretinal membrane; ILM: internal limiting membrane; VMT: vitreomacular traction)

OUTCOME SUMMARY

At follow-up after 3 months, BCVA had improved to 6/9, N6 **(Figs. 15A and B)**.

CASE SCENARIO 7: MANAGEMENT OF BROAD SYMPTOMATIC VITREOMACULAR TRACTION IN ONE EYE AND VITREOMACULAR TRACTION WITH SEVERE LOSS OF OUTER RETINAL LAYERS IN THE OTHER EYE

Case Summary

A 77-year-old lady presented with decrease in vision in RE for 4 years and LE for 4 months. She was pseudophakic in both eyes. BCVA was 6/60 RE and 6/12 LE. Fundus RE showed moderate NPDR with ERM with RPE alterations in fovea. LE showed moderate NPDR with ERM. BE-OCT was done **(Figs. 16 and 17)**.

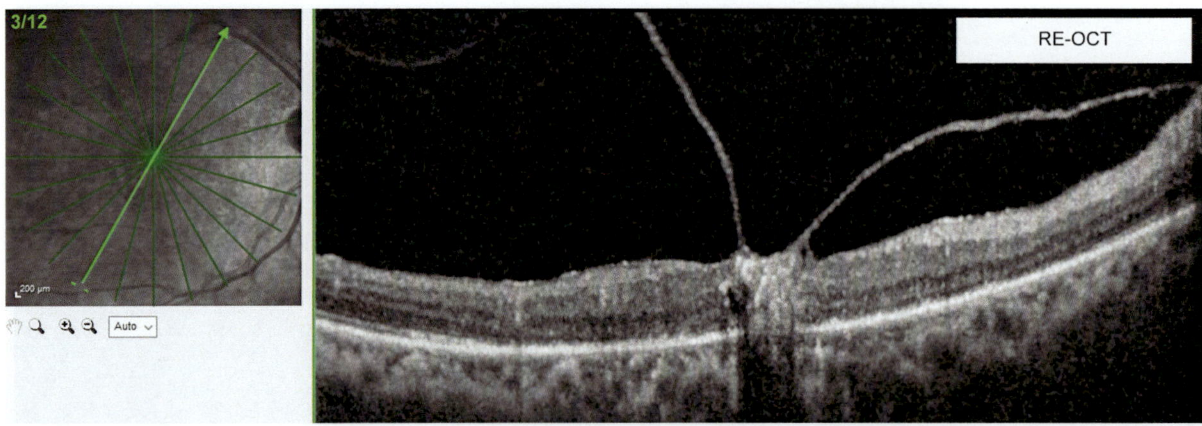

Fig. 16: RE-OCT showed vitreomacular traction (VMT) with loss of outer retinal layers in macula.

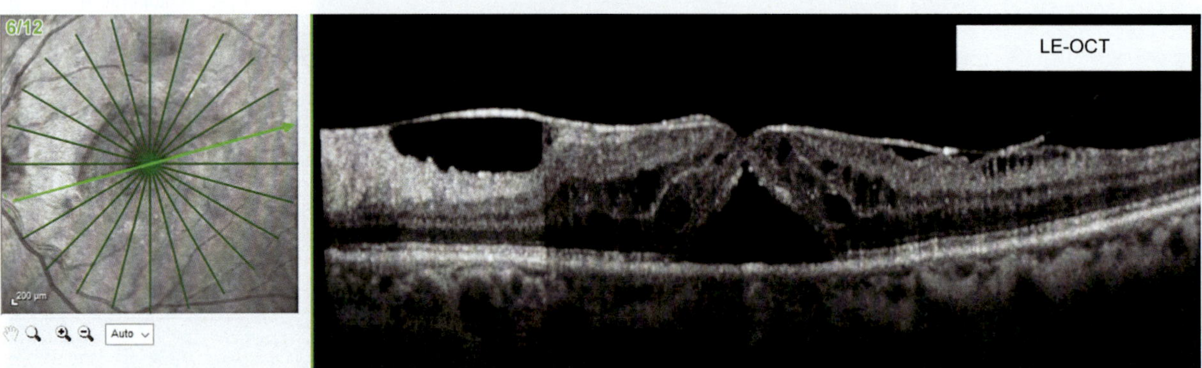

Fig. 17: LE-OCT showed broad vitreomacular traction (VMT) with width of VM adhesion 1,933 μ with foveal detachment.

Treatment Plan

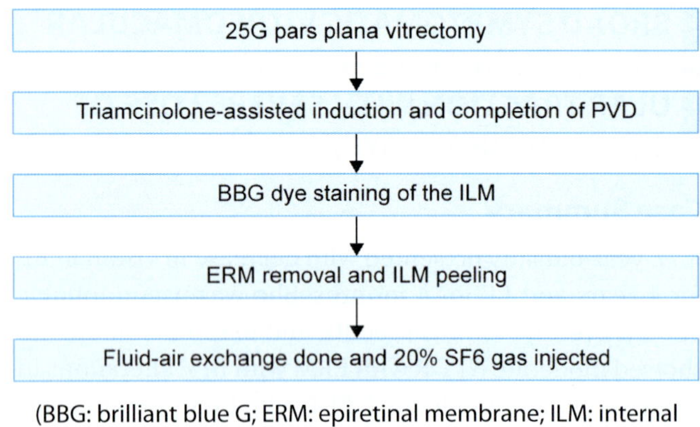

(BBG: brilliant blue G; ERM: epiretinal membrane; ILM: internal limiting membrane; PVD: posterior vitreous detachment)

Thought Process

Decision	*Rationale*
No vitrectomy for VMT in RE	Poor prognosis as loss of outer retinal layers in macula with long-standing poor vision
Vitrectomy for VMT in LE	Patient symptomatic with recent decrease in vision
ILM peeling with gas	To remove all traction on fovea and to prevent full thickness macular hole

(ILM: internal limiting membrane; VMT: vitreomacular traction)

OUTCOME SUMMARY

1 month postoperatively, there was improvement in BCVA to 6/9 as well as on OCT **(Fig. 18)**.

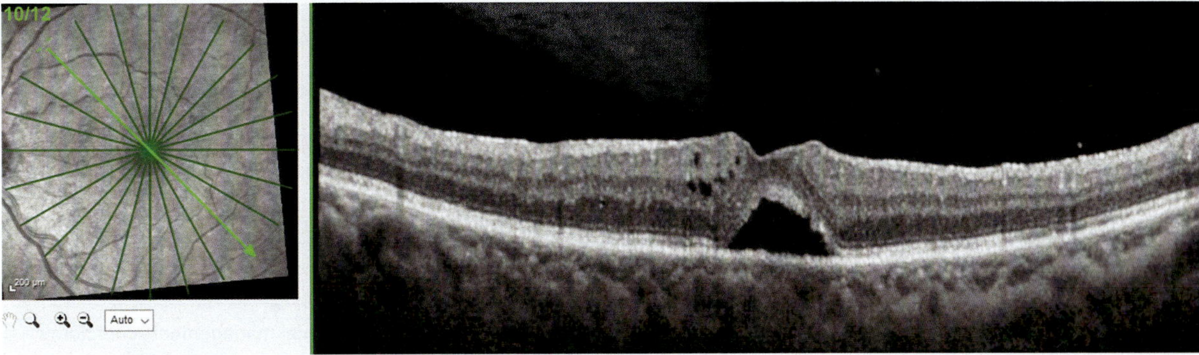

Fig. 18: LE-OCT showed better foveal contour with foveal detachment much less than before.

KEY POINTS

- Imaging-OCT-points to note include: Width of vitreomacular adhesion, intraretinal cystoid macular edema, ellipsoid zone (EZ) status, foveal detachment, impending macular hole, and associated ERM.
- Rationale for management for VMT:
  - Small focal adhesions with preserved foveal contour may resolve spontaneously.
  - Broad adhesions or associated ERM usually require surgical release of mechanical traction.
  - Early intervention prevents irreversible photoreceptor damage.

SURGICAL PEARLS IN VITREOMACULAR TRACTION SURGERY

- Always confirm presence and width of adhesion on OCT before planning surgery.
- Use triamcinolone to enhance visualization of posterior hyaloid.
- Begin separation away from the fovea to minimize trauma.
- Avoid excessive aspiration near the fovea; use gentle lift technique.
- Assess for ERM—it often coexists with VMT. If ERM is present, remove the ERM along with ILM.

FURTHER READING

1. Forte R, Pascotto F, de Crecchio G. Visualization of vitreomacular tractions with en face optical coherence tomography. Eye (Lond). 2007;21(11):1391-4.
2. John VJ, Flynn HW, Smiddy WE, Carver A, Leonard R, Tabandeh H, et al. Clinical course of vitreomacular adhesion managed by initial observation. Retina. 2013;34(3):442-6.
3. Yamada N, Kishi S. Tomographic features and surgical outcomes of vitreomacular traction syndrome. Am J Ophthalmol. 2005;139(1):112-7.

VIDEO LEGEND

Video 14: Symptomatic vitreomacular traction

MACULAR HOLE

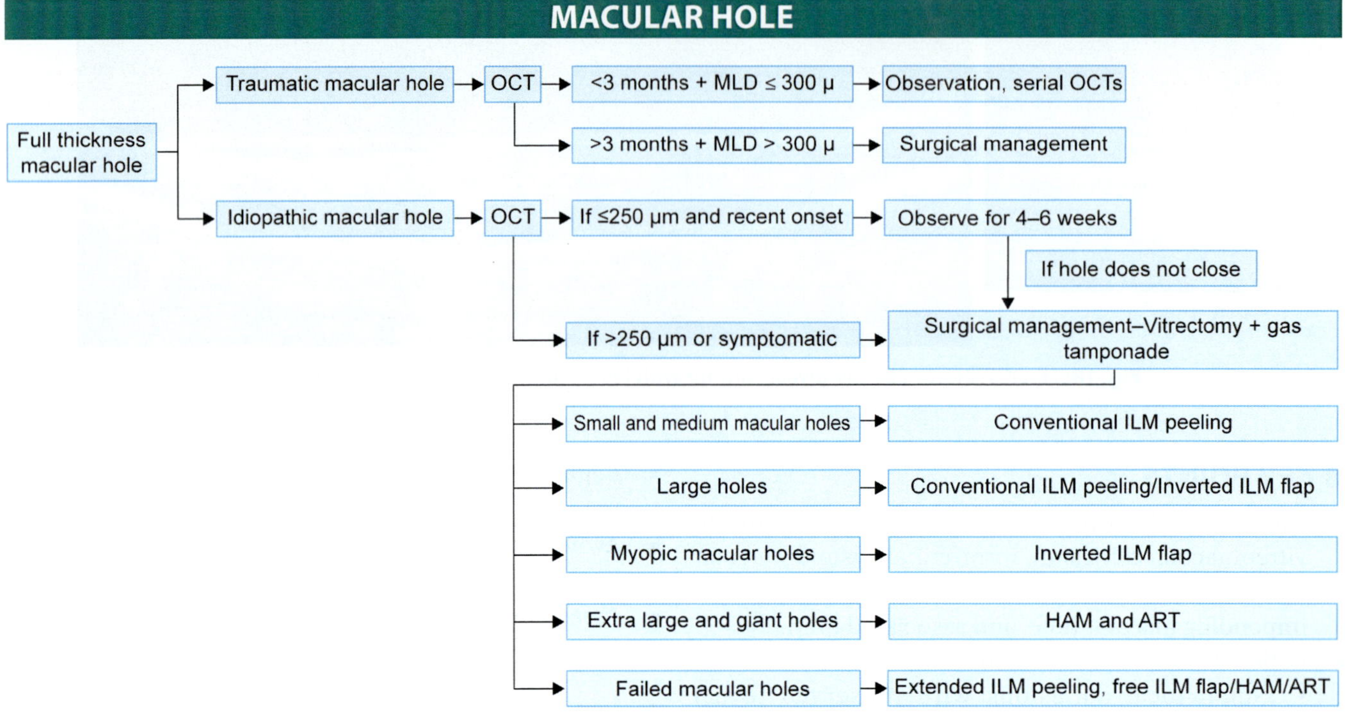

(ART: autologous retinal transplantation; HAM: human amniotic membrane; ILM: internal limiting membrane)

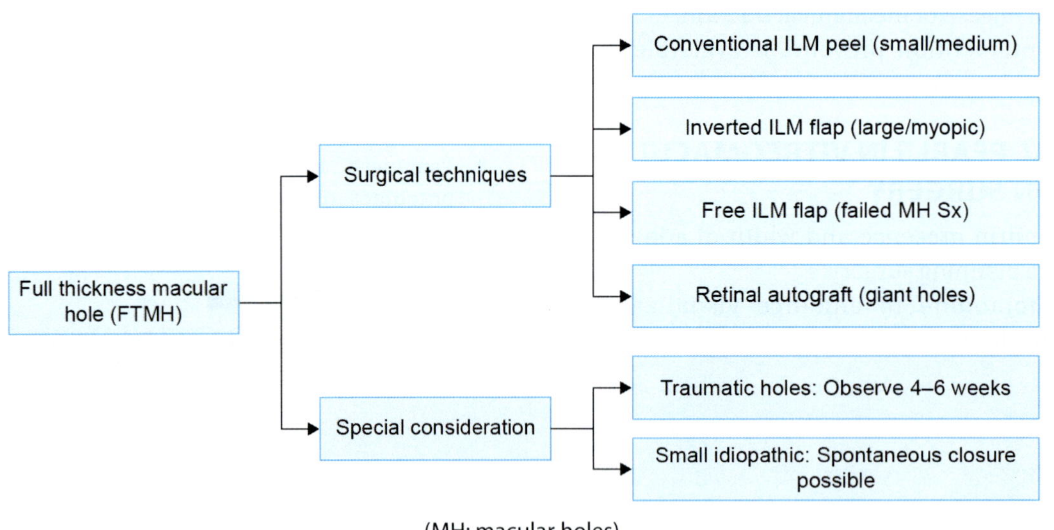

(MH: macular holes)

CASE SCENARIO 8: MANAGEMENT OF SMALL FRESH MACULAR HOLE

Case Summary

A 75-year-old male presented with decrease in vision in RE for 2 weeks. BCVA RE was 6/15, N18. Anterior segment showed immature cataract. Fundus examination showed small macular hole **(Fig. 19)**.

Treatment Plan

Observation and close follow-up.

Thought Process

Decision	*Rationale*
Observation of macular hole	Small macular holes can be observed for a short period with serial OCTs as spontaneous closure can occur

OUTCOME SUMMARY

Patient was advised observation and review after 3 weeks. At follow-up, BCVA had improved to 6/9, 6/9 RS **(Fig. 20)**.

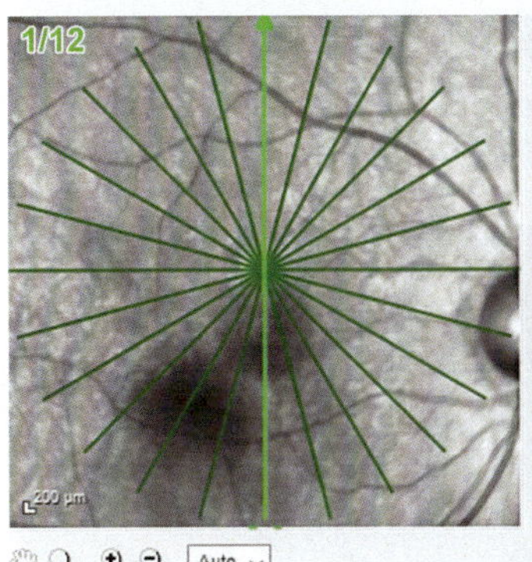

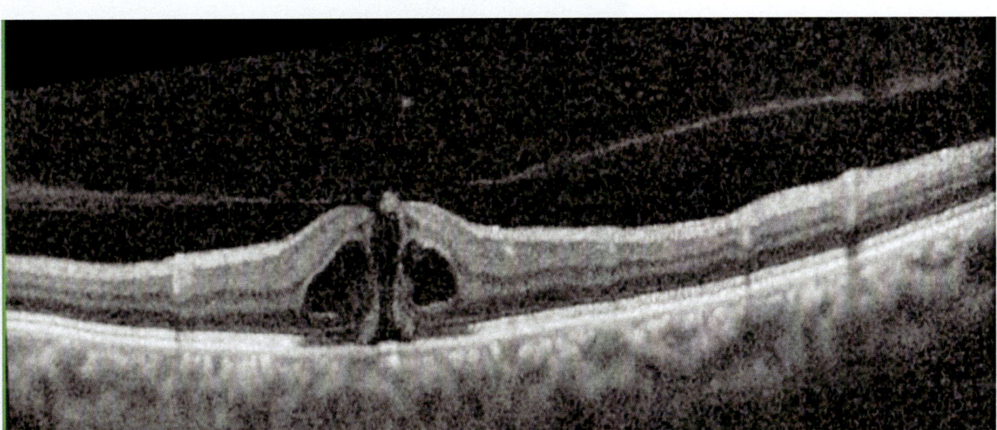

Fig. 19: RE-OCT showed small full thickness macular hole of size 171 μ.

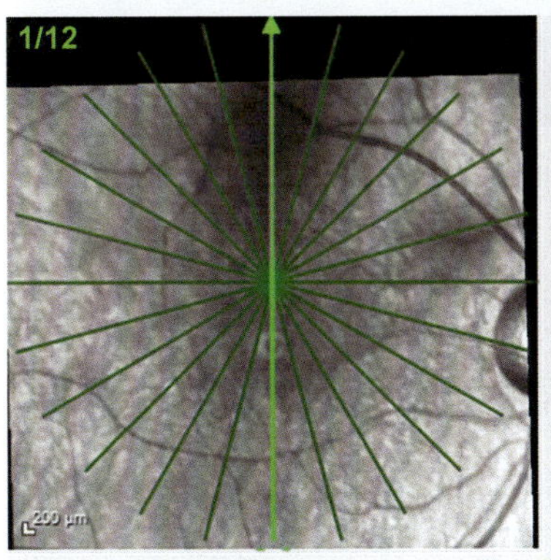

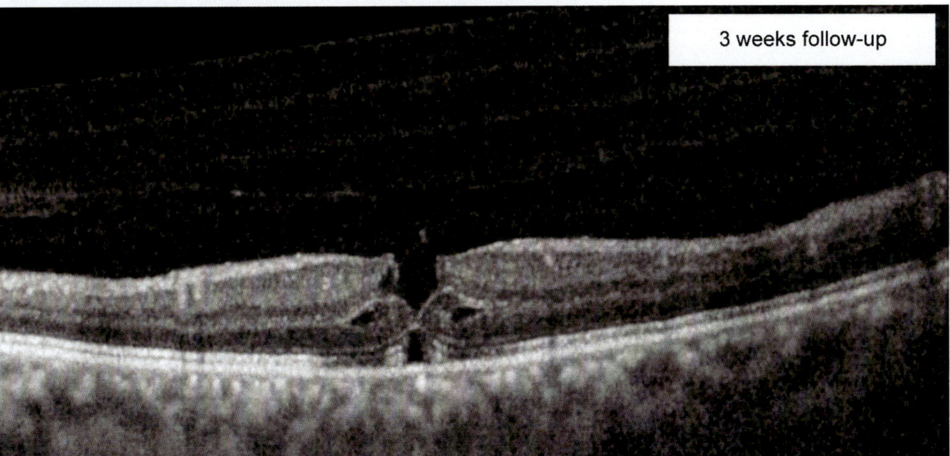

Fig. 20: RE-OCT showed a decrease in size of macular hole with approximation of outer retinal layers.

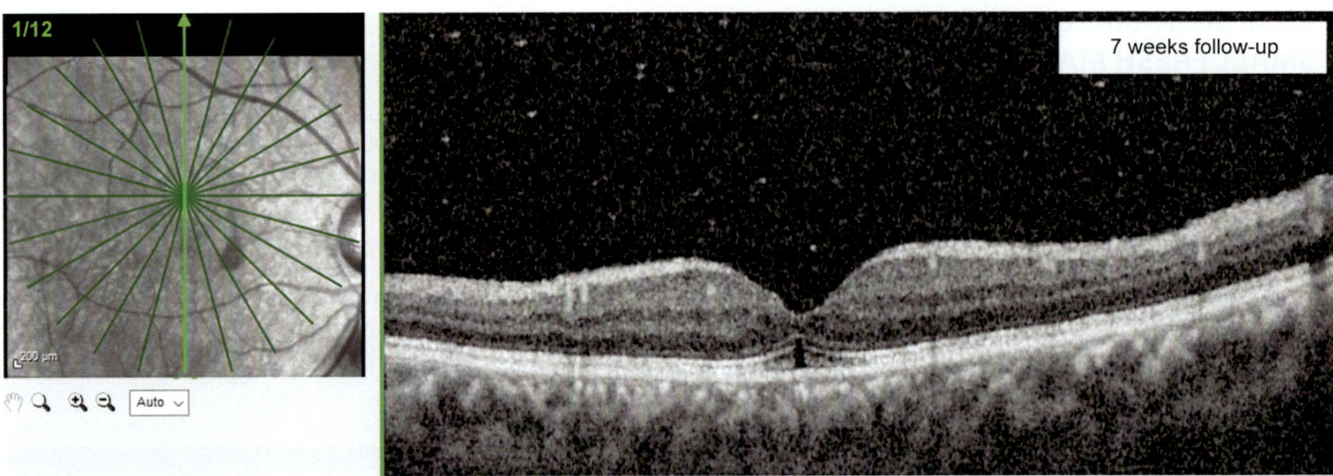

Fig. 21: RE-OCT showed type 1 spontaneous closure of macular hole with focal ellipsoid zone (EZ) defect.

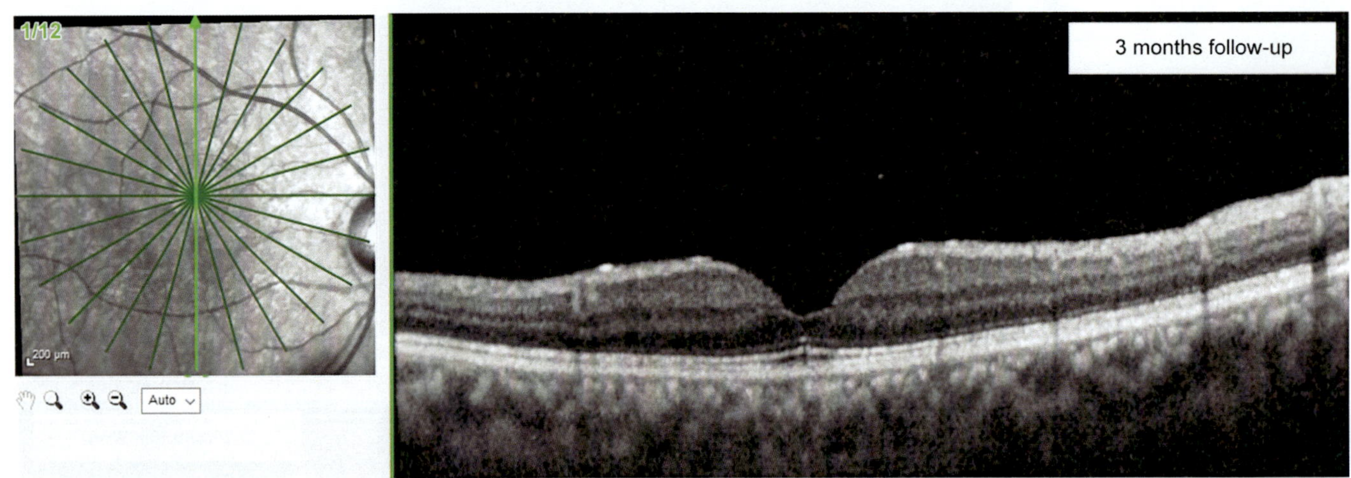

Fig. 22: Type 1 spontaneous closure with near normal foveal contour with decrease in ellipsoid zone (EZ) defect size.

He was advised to review after 1 month. At follow-up, BCVA was 6/9, 6/9 RS **(Fig. 21)**.

After 3 months, foveal contour was near normal with EZ defect much less than before **(Fig. 22)**.

CASE SCENARIO 9: MANAGEMENT OF MEDIUM-SIZED MACULAR HOLE, RECENT ONSET

Case Summary

A 65-year-old lady came with a complaint of DV LE for 1 month. BCVA was 6/9 P in RE and 6/36 P in LE. She had nuclear sclerosis grade 2 in BE. Fundus examination of LE showed macular hole **(Fig. 23)**.

Treatment Plan

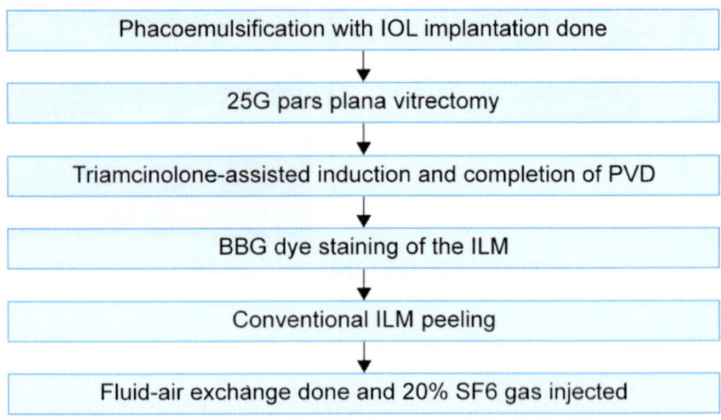

(BBG: brilliant blue G; ERM: epiretinal membrane; ILM: internal limiting membrane; IOL: intraocular lens; PVD: posterior vitreous detachment)

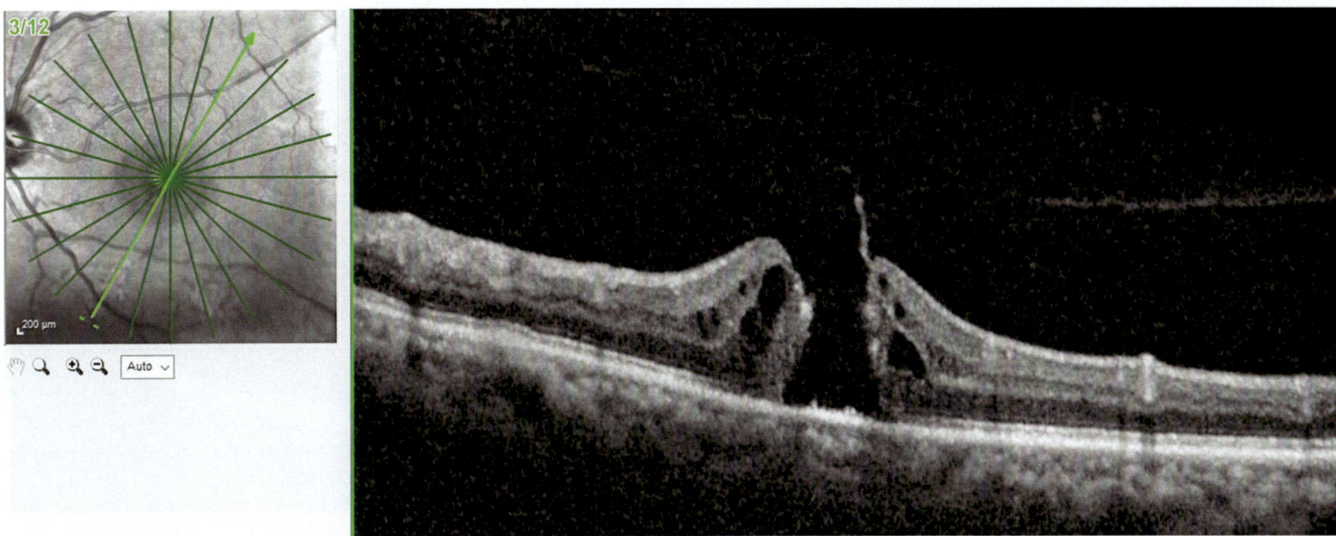

Fig. 23: LE-OCT showed full thickness of macular hole with MLD 390 µ. The posterior hyaloid was noted to be partially attached to the macula.

Thought Process

Decision	*Rationale*
Surgery for macular hole	Medium-sized macular hole and patient has come with decrease in vision
Combined phaco + vitrectomy	Significant cataract is present. Combined surgery will avoid one more surgery for the patient. Also, more vitreous can be removed and more gas fill is possible
Conventional ILM peeling	High success rate in medium-sized macular holes with conventional ILM peeling

(ILM: internal limiting membrane)

OUTCOME SUMMARY

Patient underwent combined phacoemulsification + IOL implantation with vitrectomy with ILM peeling with SF6 tamponade. At 1 month postoperatively, BCVA LE improved to 6/12p, N10P **(Fig. 24)**.

CASE SCENARIO 10: MANAGEMENT OF LARGE CHRONIC HOLE

A 74-year-old lady presented with complaint of decrease in vision in right eye for 1 year. She was pseudophakic in both eyes. BCVA-RE was 3/60, LE was 6/6. Fundus examination of RE showed old branch retinal vein occlusion with full thickness macular hole **(Fig. 25)**.

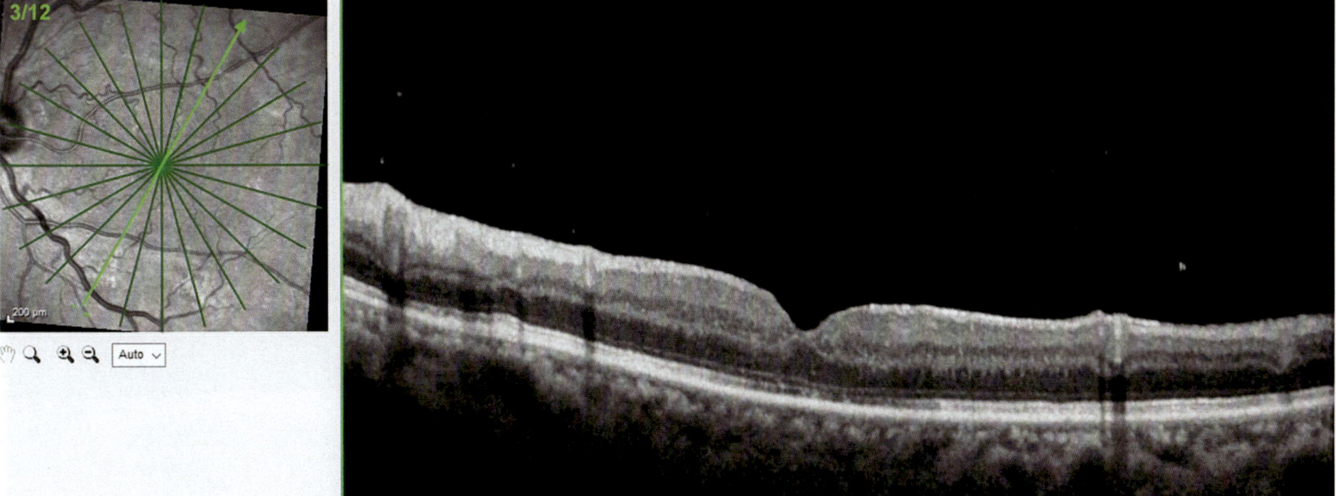

Fig. 24: LE-tOCT showed type 1 closure of macular hole.

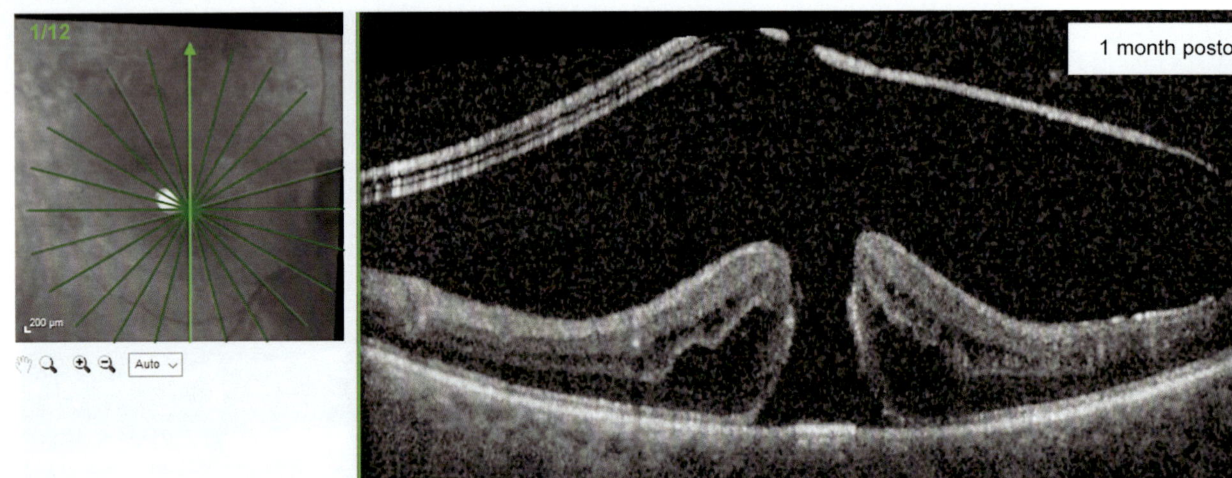

Fig. 25: RE-OCT showed full thickness macular hole with MLD 700 µ.

Treatment Plan

RE—vitrectomy with ILM flap with gas tamponade.

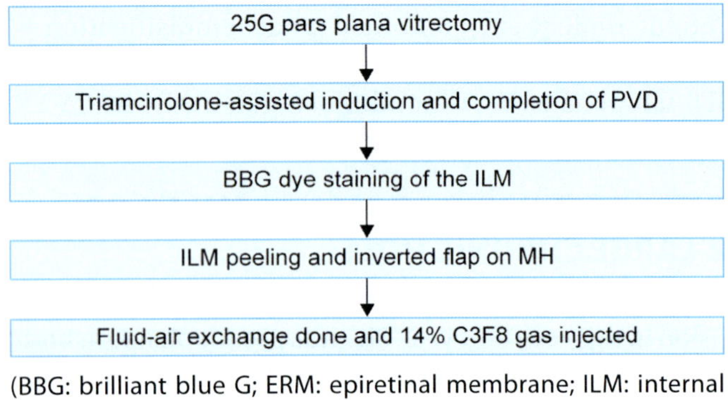

(BBG: brilliant blue G; ERM: epiretinal membrane; ILM: internal limiting membrane; IOL: intraocular lens; PVD: posterior vitreous detachment)

Thought Process

Decision	*Rationale*
Surgical intervention	Large macular hole requires surgery
Inverted ILM flap	Better chances of closure of large macular holes with inverted ILM flap
C3F8 tamponade	Longer tamponade desired

(ILM: internal limiting membrane)

OUTCOME SUMMARY

Patient underwent RE—vitrectomy with inverted ILM flap with C3F8 tamponade. At 1 month postoperatively, BCVA had improved to 6/75 with type 1 closure of macular hole noted on OCT **(Fig. 26)**.

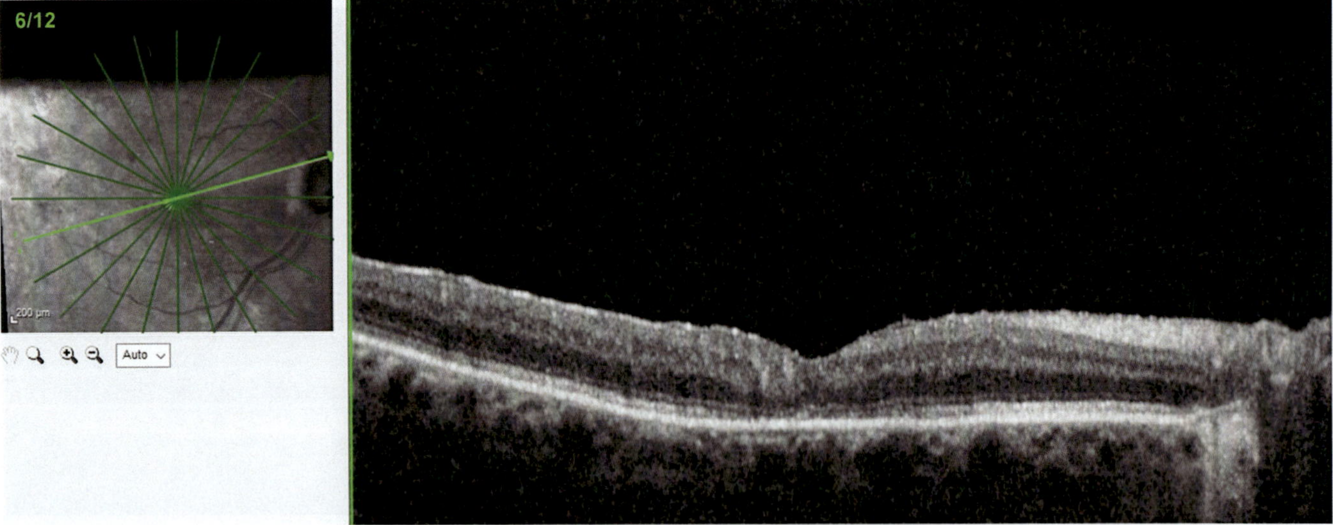

Fig. 26: RE-OCT showed type 1 closure of macular hole after 1 month.

CASE SCENARIO 11: MANAGEMENT OF FAILED MACULAR HOLE POSTVITRECTOMY

Case Summary

A 57-year-old female presented with RE persistent open macular hole following vitrectomy for macular hole. BCVA-RE was 6/30 **(Fig. 27)**.

Treatment Plan

RE—revitrectomy with free ILM flap.

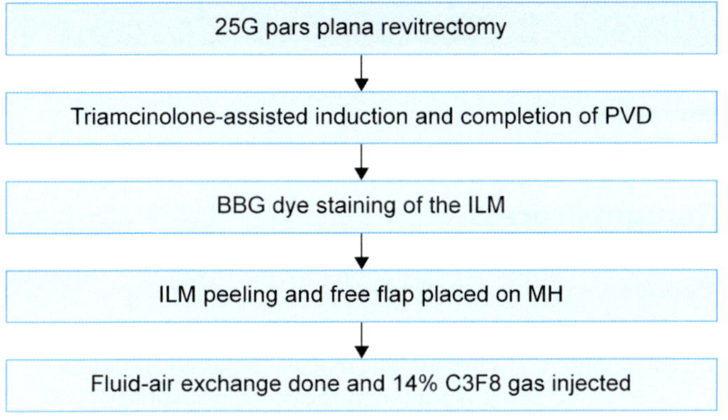

(BBG: brilliant blue G; ILM: internal limiting membrane; MH: macular holes; PVD: posterior vitreous detachment)

Thought Process

Decision	*Rationale*
Revitrectomy for failed macular hole	Chances of closure with re-surgery are good as cystoid changes in lips of hole
Check for extent of ILM peeling with BBG staining	If inadequate ILM peeling noted intraoperatively, to consider extended peeling
Free ILM flap decided	Extent of ILM peeling noted to be adequate, so further extension is not beneficial
Large ILM free flap	Make sure excess ILM flap over the macular hole to compensate for possible shifts during FAE
C3F8	Longer duration of tamponade required for failed macular hole

(BBG: brilliant blue G; ILM: internal limiting membrane; FAE: fluid-air exchange)

OUTCOME SUMMARY

After FGE, BBG was injected and then replaced with saline after 1 minute. Adequate ILM peeling around MH until the arcades were noted. So, a free ILM flap was taken from temporal to macula and then placed on the macular hole. Then, FGE was done followed by C3F8 injection. Prone position was advised postoperatively. At 3 weeks postoperatively, BCVA had improved to 6/24 **(Fig. 28)**.

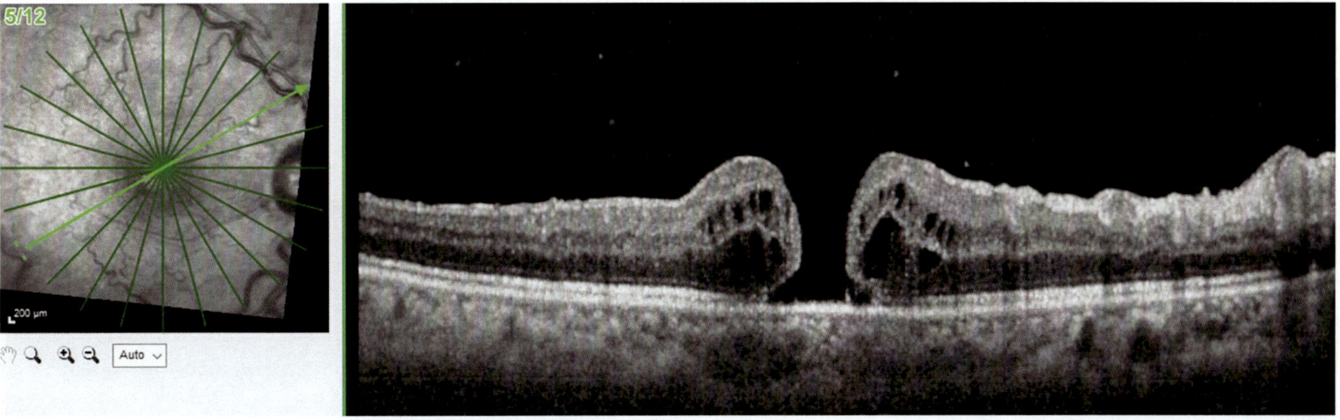

Fig. 27: RE-OCT showed open macular hole with cystoid spaces in lips of macular hole with MLD 800 µ.

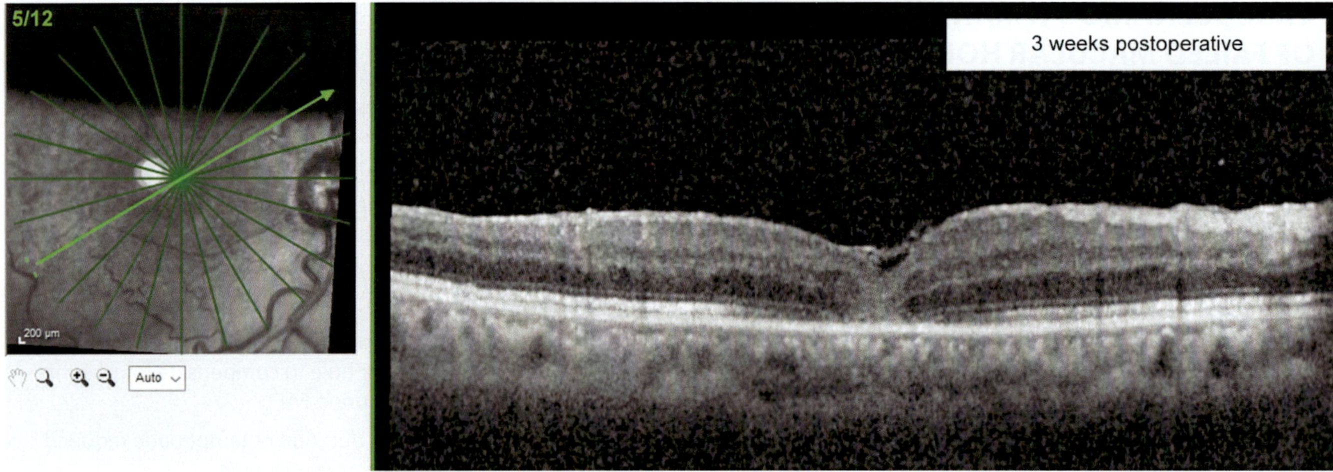

Fig. 28: At 3 weeks postoperatively, OCT showed type 1 closure of macular hole with internal limiting membrane (ILM) flap seen overlying the foveal center.

CASE SCENARIO 12: MANAGEMENT OF TRAUMATIC HOLE OF RECENT ONSET IN YOUNG PATIENT

Case Summary

A 31-year-old male presented with a complaint of DV RE for 1 day. He gave history of injury to RE with grinding wheel. BCVA was 6/120 in RE, 6/6 in LE. RE showed lid abrasion and AC cells 1+. Fundus of RE showed vitreous hemorrhage, subretinal hemorrhage inferiorly with retinal edema in posterior pole with macular hole **(Fig. 29)**.

Patient was advised to rest in head elevation, topical steroids and cycloplegics and observation for macular hole.

Thought Process

Decision	*Rationale*
Observation for macular hole	Short period of observation for post-traumatic macular holes is justified as spontaneous closure is possible

OUTCOME SUMMARY

He was reviewed 2 weeks later. BCVA had improved to 6/48. Fundus examination showed resolving vitreous hemorrhage with RPE alterations in fovea with closed macular hole **(Fig. 30)**.

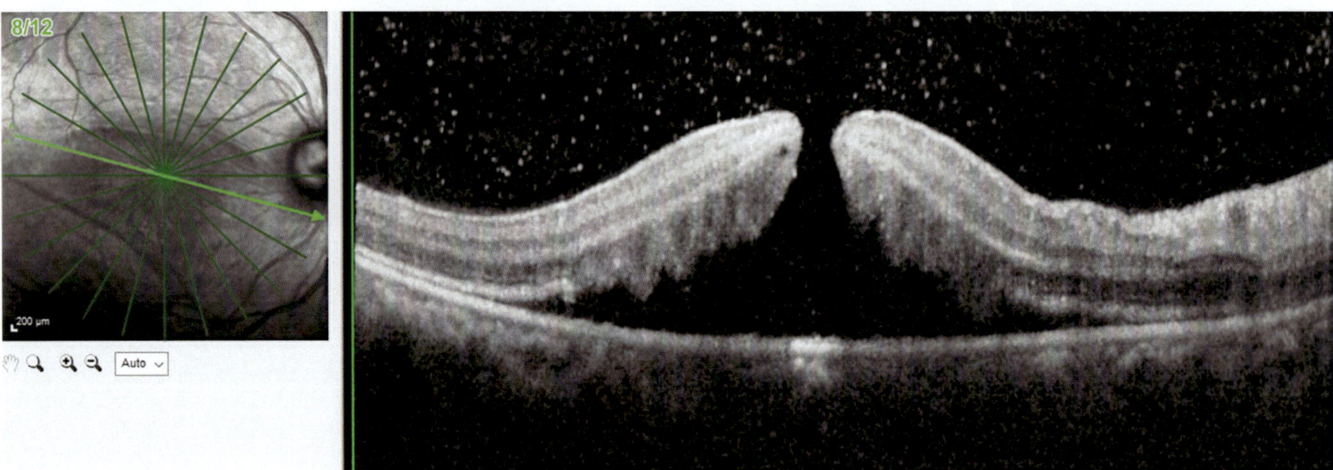

Fig. 29: RE-OCT shows full thickness of macular hole with localized retinal detachment in macula.

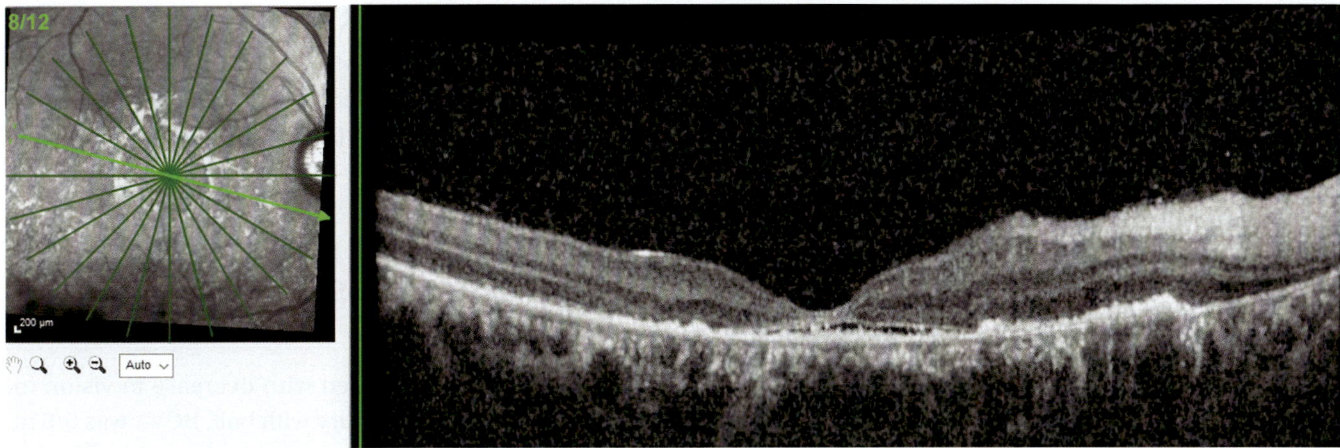

Fig. 30: RE-OCT shows closed macular hole with foveal thinning with minimal neurosensory detachment (NSD).

CASE SCENARIO 13: MANAGEMENT OF FAILED MACULAR HOLES POSTSURGERY

Case Summary

Patient had LE open MH postvitrectomy for MH done 1 month back. LE-BCVA was 6/24 **(Fig. 31)**. LE multimodal image showed eccentric ILP peel area as shown by yellow arrows on green and blue reflectance image **(Figs. 32A to D)**. Patient was advised resurgery.

Treatment Plan

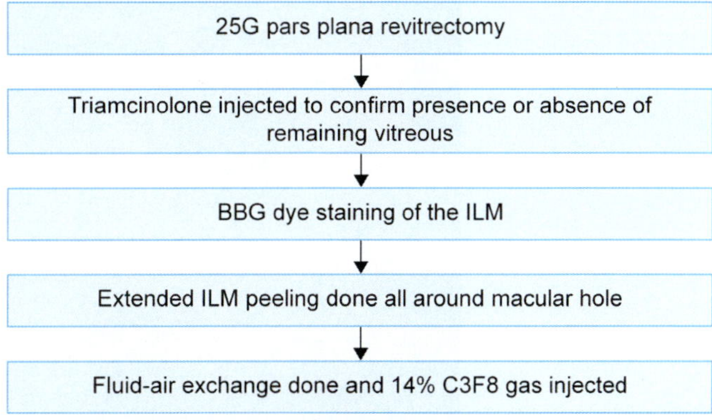

(BBG: brilliant blue G; ILM: internal limiting membrane; ERM: epiretinal membrane)

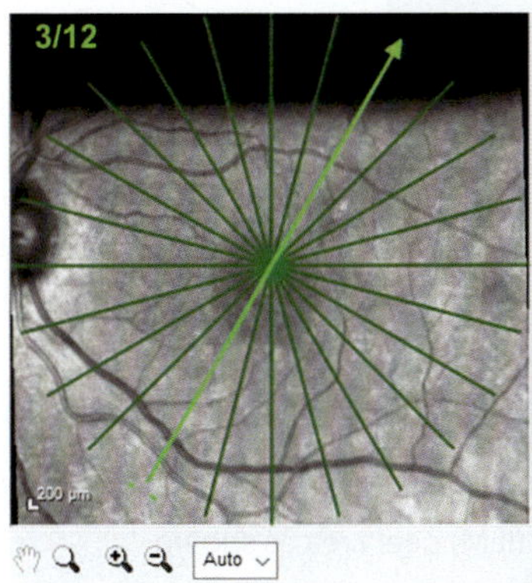

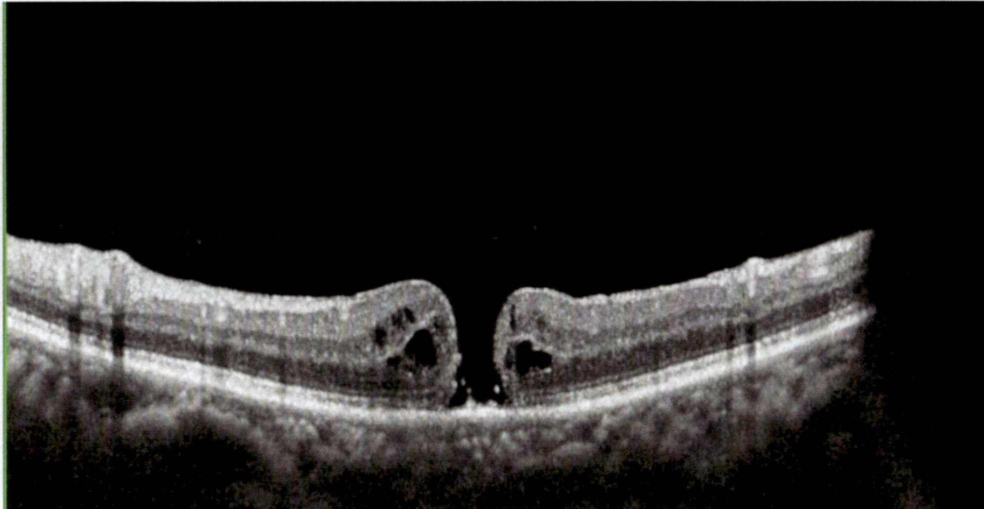

Fig. 31: LE-OCT shows small macular hole (MH).

Thought Process

Decision	*Rationale*
Use of IVTA	Triamcinolone helps to stain and visualize any remnant vitreous which may also be the cause of the nonclosure of the hole in the previous surgery. The crystals of TA also stick to the ERM which helps to delineate the margins of it
Extended ILM peeling	As the multicolor image showed the ILM peeled area was very small and eccentric around the macular hole, further extending the ILM peeling all around the hole will help to relieve the residual tangential traction

(ERM: epiretinal membrane; ILM: internal limiting membrane; IVTA: intravitreal triamcinolone acetonide)

OUTCOME SUMMARY

She underwent extended ILM peeling + C3F8 gas injection. 1 month postsurgery, the macular hole had closed and her BCVA had improved to 6/15 **(Figs. 32 to 34)**.

At 1 year postsurgery, LE-BCVA had improved to 6/9 p.

CASE SCENARIO 14: MANAGEMENT OF CHRONIC GIANT POST-TRAUMATIC HOLE

Case Summary

A 19-year-old male presented with decrease in vision in LE for >2 years following injury with ball. BCVA was 6/6 in RE and 6/60 in LE. Lens was clear in both eyes. LE fundus showed very large macular hole **(Fig. 35)**.

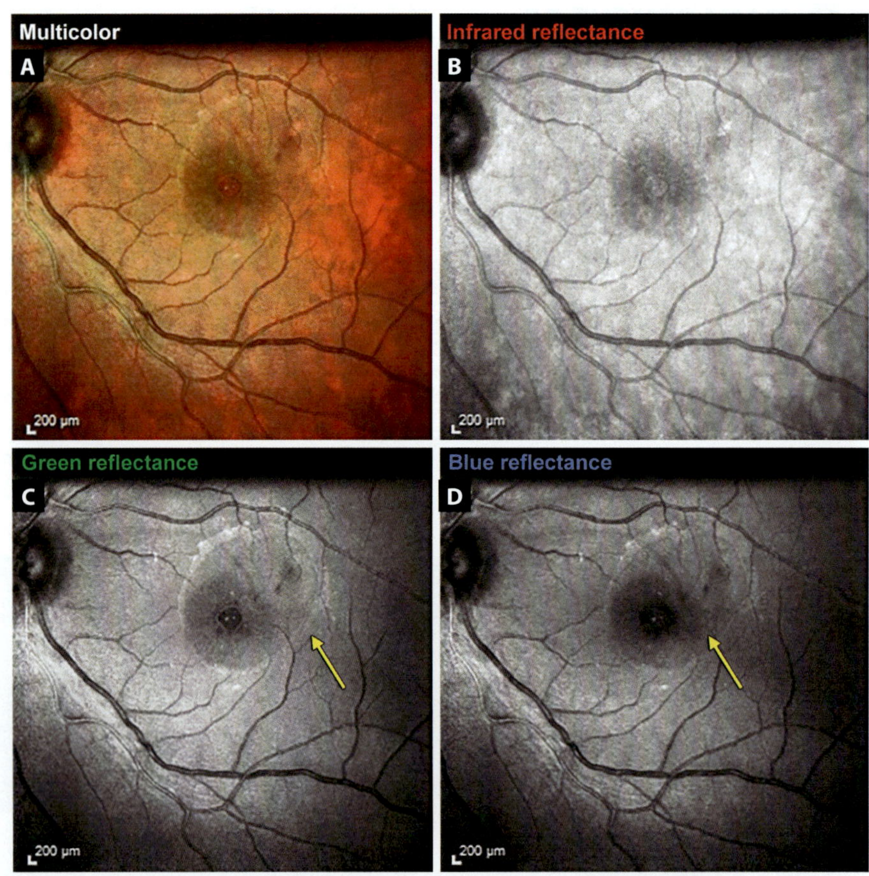

Figs. 32A to D: LE multicolor image (MCI) shows small, eccentric internal limiting membrane (ILM) peel area as shown by yellow arrows on the green and blue reflectance images.

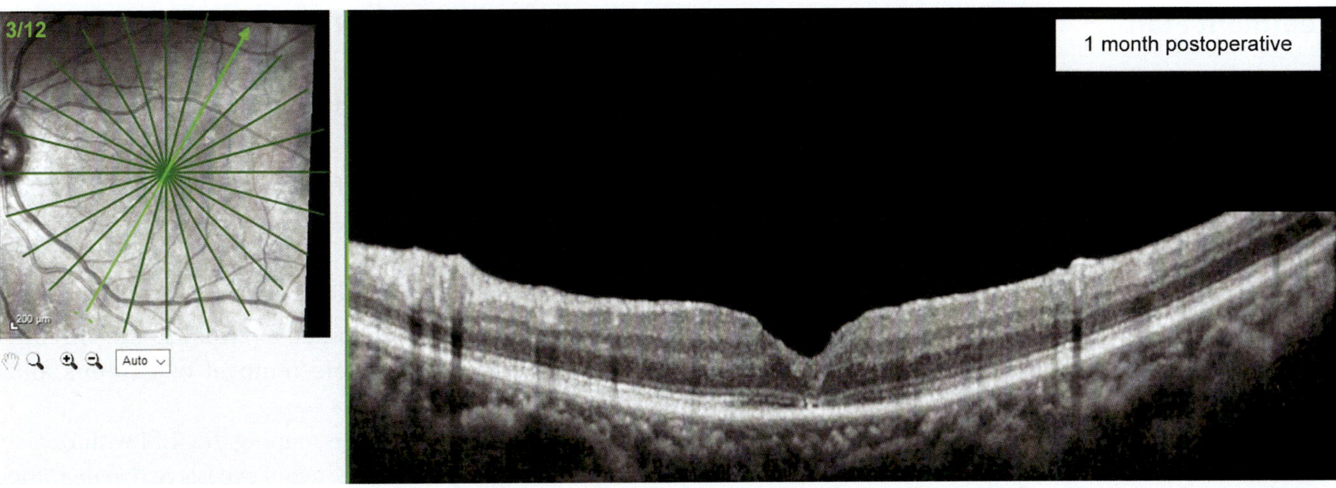

Fig. 33: LE-OCT shows type 1 closure of macular hole with ellipsoid zone (EZ) and external limiting membrane (ELM) disruptions.

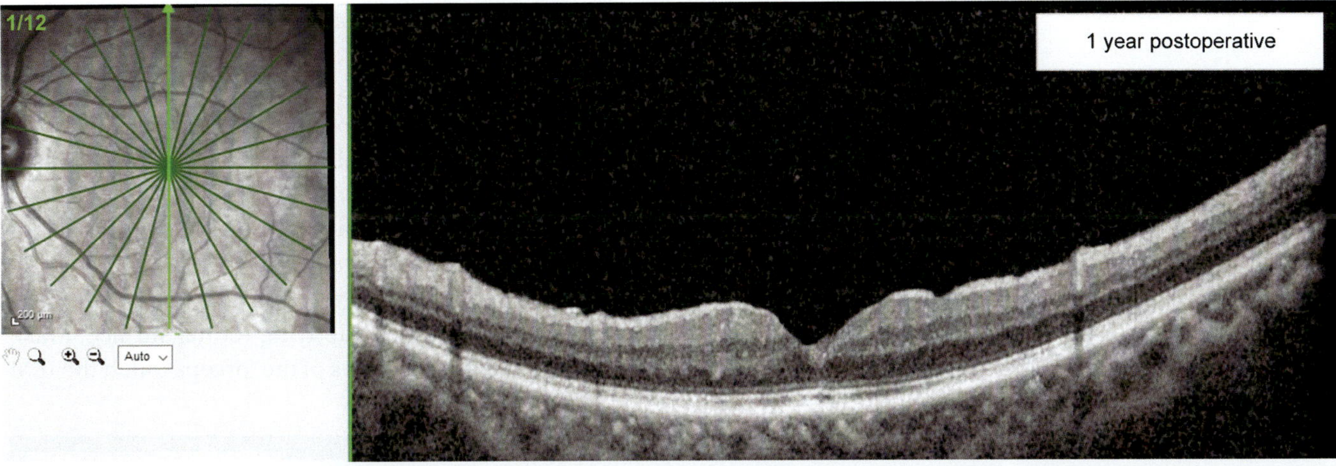

Fig. 34: LE-OCT shows closed macular hole with intact ellipsoid zone (EZ) and external limiting membrane (ELM) layers.

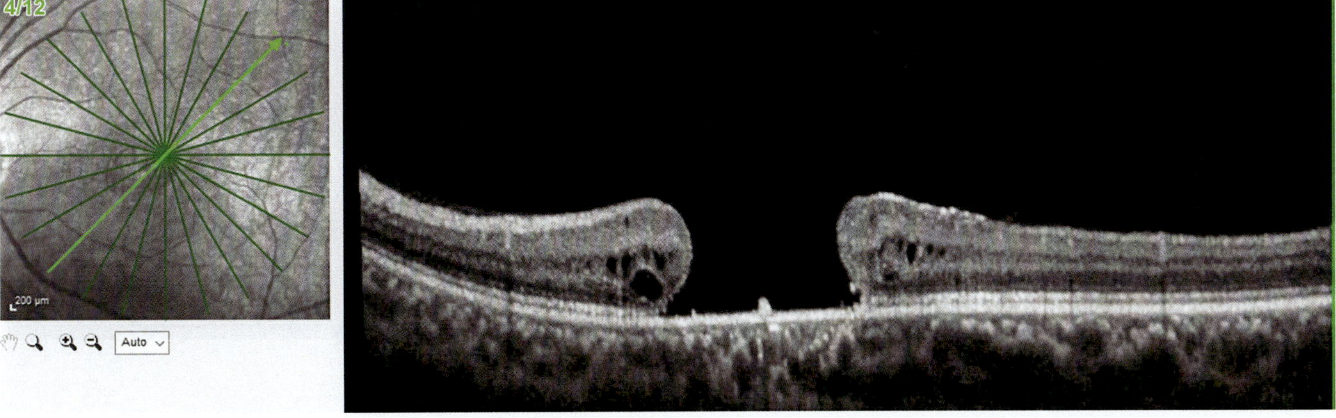

Fig. 35: LE-OCT shows very large full-thickness macular hole (FTMH) with MLD >2,000 µ.

Treatment Plan

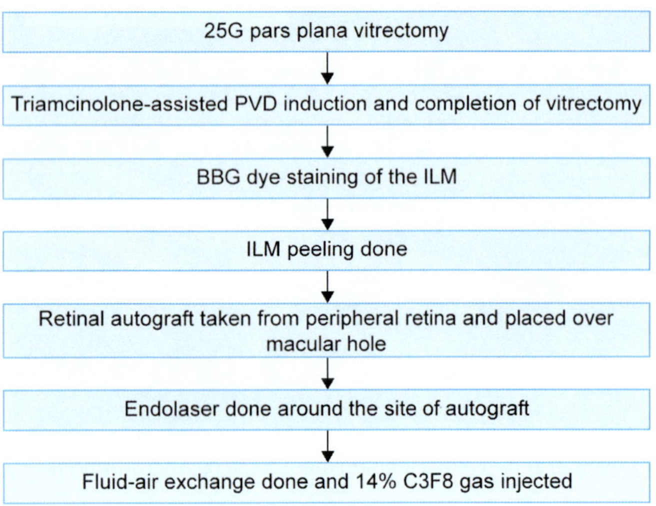

(BBG: brilliant blue G; ILM: internal limiting membrane; PVD: posterior vitreous detachment)

Thought Process

Decision	*Rationale*
Surgical intervention	Spontaneous closure is extremely unlikely in chronic post-traumatic holes
Retinal autograft to be placed over macular hole	Chances of closure of giant macular holes is better with retinal autograft and less with ILM peeling or inverted ILM flap

OUTCOME SUMMARY

Patient underwent LE vitrectomy + retinal autograft + Endolaser + C3F8 followed by prone positioning for 1 week.

Follow-up after 6 weeks LE fundus shows closed macular hole with improvement of visual acuity to 6/48 **(Fig. 36)**.

Surgical Pearls and Rationale

- Use triamcinolone acetonide to visualize the vitreous to enable more complete removal of vitreous and easier PVD induction.
- Points to remember while staining the ILM with BBG:
  - Stain lightly with BBG; avoid excessive dye near the fovea.
  - Staining can be done under air/saline.
- Staining under air has some advantages like:
  - Only small amount of dye is required and only for a short time.
  - Dye can be placed selectively over the required area.
  - There is no lens staining/loss of visualization.
- Peel initiation
  - Use ILM forceps/finesse loop/diamond dusted membrane scraper to initiate the peel. Pinch the ILM forceps and then let go. This enables the ILM to separate from underlying retinal surface. Make sure that both the jaws of the forceps touch the ILM

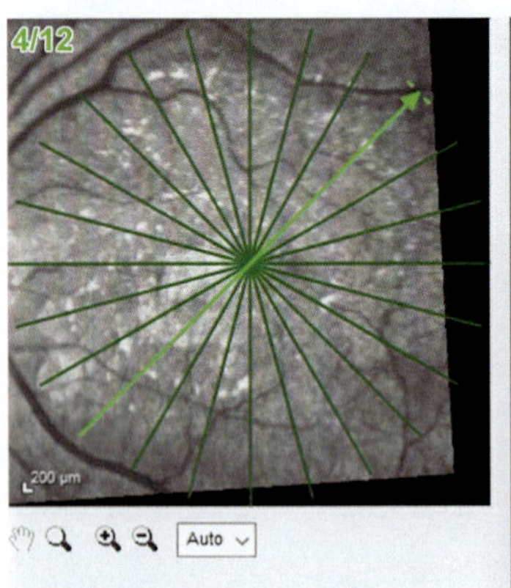

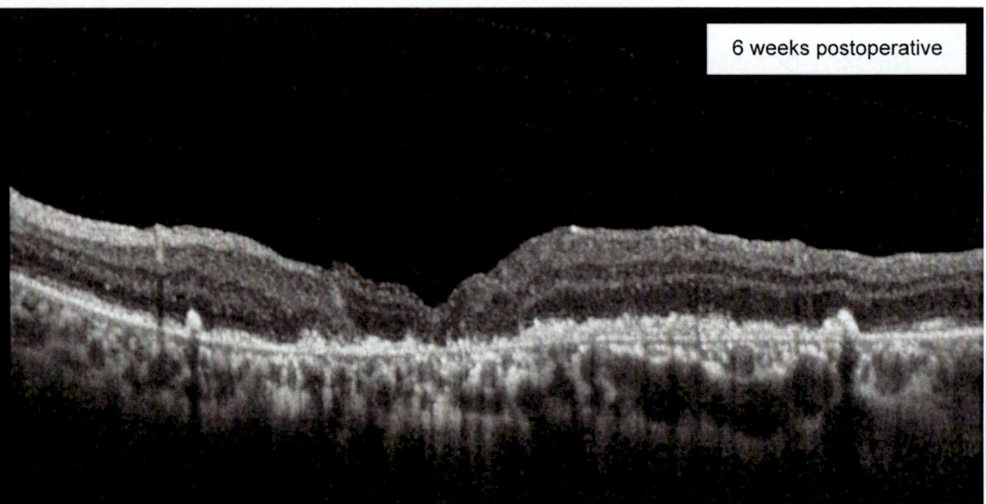

Fig. 36: LE-OCT shows closed macular hole.

at same time in order to make it easier to grab only the ILM without damaging the underlying retina.
  - Then, use the ILM forceps to regrasp the ILM and pull in a circumferential manner.
  - Begin ILM peeling away from the hole to prevent enlargement.
- Peel the ILM holding the edge nearest to the retina.
- Control the speed and direction of movement.
- To reduce risk of phototoxicity:
  - Keep the light directed away from fovea in an angled manner.
  - Also reduce the exposure time and the intensity of light.
- In large holes, create an inverted ILM flap hinged at temporal edge and gently drape over the hole. Doing temporally hinged flap is better than nasal as during FAE, the vector forces allow the flap to remain over the macular hole without need for additional manipulation.
  - Fluid-air exchange under low flow prevents flap dislodgment.
- Making the patient pseudophakic helps to maximize the amount of vitreous that can be removed which maximizes the size of gas bubble that can be injected.
- Strict postoperative positioning (face-down) for 5-7 days enhances closure.

FURTHER READING

1. Hu Z, Xie P, Ding Y, Zheng X, Yuan D, Liu Q. Face-down or no face-down posturing following macular hole surgery: a meta-analysis. Acta Ophthalmol. 2016;94(4):326-33.
2. Kuriyama S, Hayashi H, Jingami Y, Kuramoto N, Akita J, Matsumoto M. Efficacy of inverted internal limiting membrane flap technique for the treatment of macular hole in high myopia. Am J Ophthalmol. 2013;156(1):125-31.
3. Spiteri Cornish K, Lois N, Scott N, Burr J, Cook J, Boachie C, et al. Vitrectomy with internal limiting membrane (ILM) peeling versus with no peeling for idiopathic full-thickness macular hole (FTMH). Cochrane Database Syst Rev. 2014;121(3):649-55.

VIDEO LEGEND

Video 15: Retinal autograft for large macular hole

OPTIC DISC PIT MACULOPATHY

CASE SCENARIO 15: MANAGEMENT OF OPTIC DISC PIT MACULOPATHY

Case Summary

A 62-year-old gentleman presented with a history of recent-onset blurred vision in his right eye. He is a known diabetic, well controlled on oral hypoglycemic drugs. He had no similar complaints in the left eye.

Examination revealed that the right eye had a BCVA of 6/12 p on the Snellen chart, and the left eye had 6/6 vision. Both eyes showed early cataractous changes, and the intraocular pressure was within the normal range.

Fundus examination of the right eye showed an optic disc pit at the temporal edge with maculopathy involving the fovea (**Fig. 37A**, red-free image). Optical coherence tomography (OCT) confirmed a schisis-like change in the fovea with foveal detachment **(Figs. 37B and C)**. The left eye fundus was normal.

A diagnosis of right eye optic disc pit maculopathy with age-related cataract was made, and vitrectomy surgery was planned as the primary treatment.

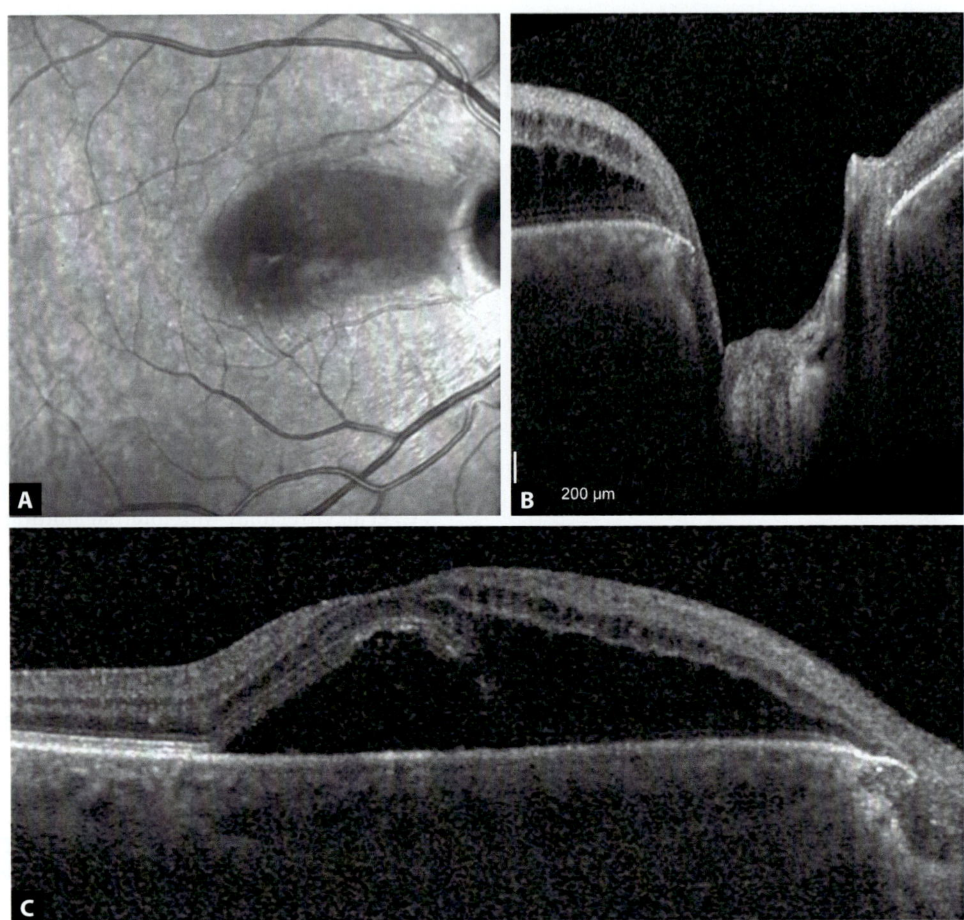

Figs. 37A to C: Red-free image of the right eye showing a disc pit with adjacent maculopathy (A). OCT scan passing through the disc (B) and macula (C) showing pit morphology.

Treatment Plan

25G pars plana vitrectomy

↓

Triamcinolone-assisted PVD induction and completion of vitrectomy

↓

BBG dye staining of the ILM at disc and macular area

↓

Stained abnormal tissue over the pit area was carefully removed using ILM peeling forceps

↓

Small strip of ILM was harvested adjacent to the disc pit and stuffed into the pit

↓

Fibrin glue (optional) was applied over the pit area to secure the stuffed ILM

↓

Air or SF6 tamponade was used at the end of the procedure

(BBG: brilliant blue G; ILM: internal limiting membrane; PVD: posterior vitreous detachment)

Thought Process

Decision	*Rationale*
Surgical intervention	Recent onset vision loss and less likely it resolves spontaneously
No laser to PMB area	As the detachment of neurosensory retina is significant, effective laser adhesions of outer and inner retina and RPE may not be possible
Limited ILM peeling	As the maculopathy is limited to smaller area, large ILM peel is avoided and not necessary
ILM stuffing into pit	To ensure adequate pit closure
Use of glue	Glue over pit area is optional to avoid long-term tamponade and added side effects of tamponade

(ILM: internal limiting membrane; RPE: retinal pigment epithelium)

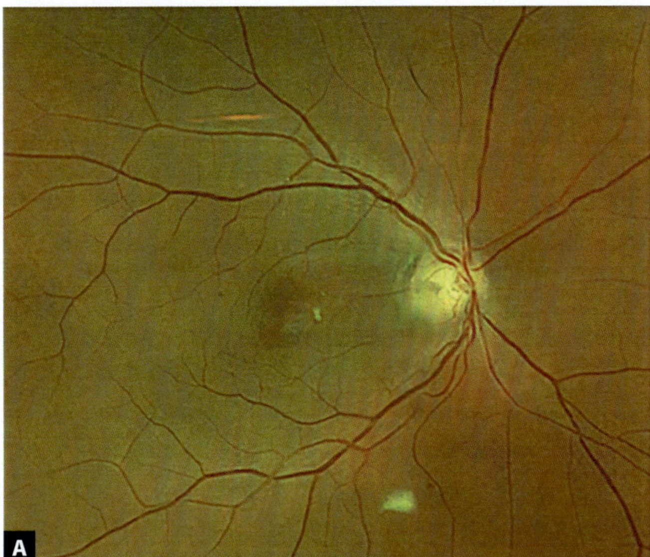

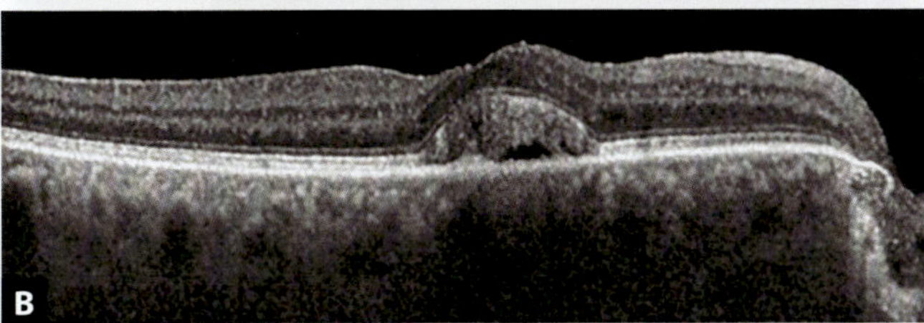

Figs. 38A and B: 2 weeks postsurgery showing fundus picture postvitrectomy surgery with resolving maculopathy (A). OCT shows resolving schitic detachment (B).

OUTCOME SUMMARY

At the 6-weeks postoperative follow-up, the retinal schisis had completely resolved and the neurosensory detachment had significantly reduced **(Figs. 38A and B)**. Vision improved from 6/12 p to 6/6 p.

KEY POINTS

- Vitrectomy is the standard surgical approach for optic disc pit maculopathy with significant vision loss.
- ILM peeling can be restricted to the papillary area, and the macula can be spared.
- Fibrin glue can be effectively utilized in these cases to reduce the need for prolonged gas or oil tamponade.

FURTHER READING

1. Almeida DRP, Chin EK, Arjmand P, Velez G, Evans LP, Mahajan VB. Fibrin Glue and Internal Limiting Membrane Abrasion for Optic Disc Pit Maculopathy. Ophthalmic Surg Lasers Imaging Retina. 2018;49(12):e271-7.
2. Soni A, Singh SR, Chhablani J. Fibrin glue for treatment of optic disc maculopathy. Saudi J Ophthalmol. 2021;34(3):227-9.

VIDEO LEGEND

Video 16: Optic disc pit maculopathy

CASE SCENARIO 16: MANAGEMENT OF MACULOPATHY ASSOCIATED WITH COLOBOMA AND OPTIC DISC PIT

Case Summary

A 32-year-old lady presented with diminished vision in her right eye for 1 year. The vision had worsened over the last 2 weeks. There was no history of similar complaints in the fellow eye.

Her best-corrected visual acuity was 6/48 in the right eye and 6/6 in the left eye. The anterior segment was essentially normal in both eyes.

Fundus examination of the right eye showed a disc coloboma involving the temporal aspect, with adjacent retinal detachment of the macula extending 8–10-disc diameters **(Fig. 39)**. A small disc pit was noted at the temporal edge of the disc along with the colobomatous defect.

OCT through the disc and macula revealed macular detachment with a schitic macula and a presumed ICM break at the coloboma margin, along with a concurrent pit within it **(Figs. 40A to C)**.

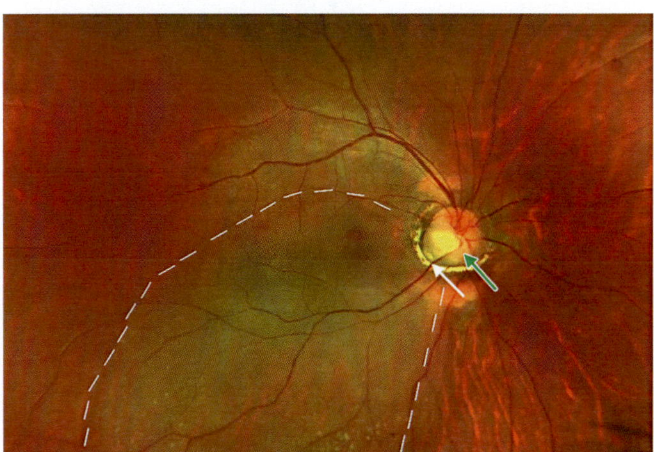

Fig. 39: Ultra-widefield (UWF) image of the right eye showing disc coloboma (green arrow) and disc pit at the temporal edge (white arrow). The dashed line indicates the extent of subretinal fluid.

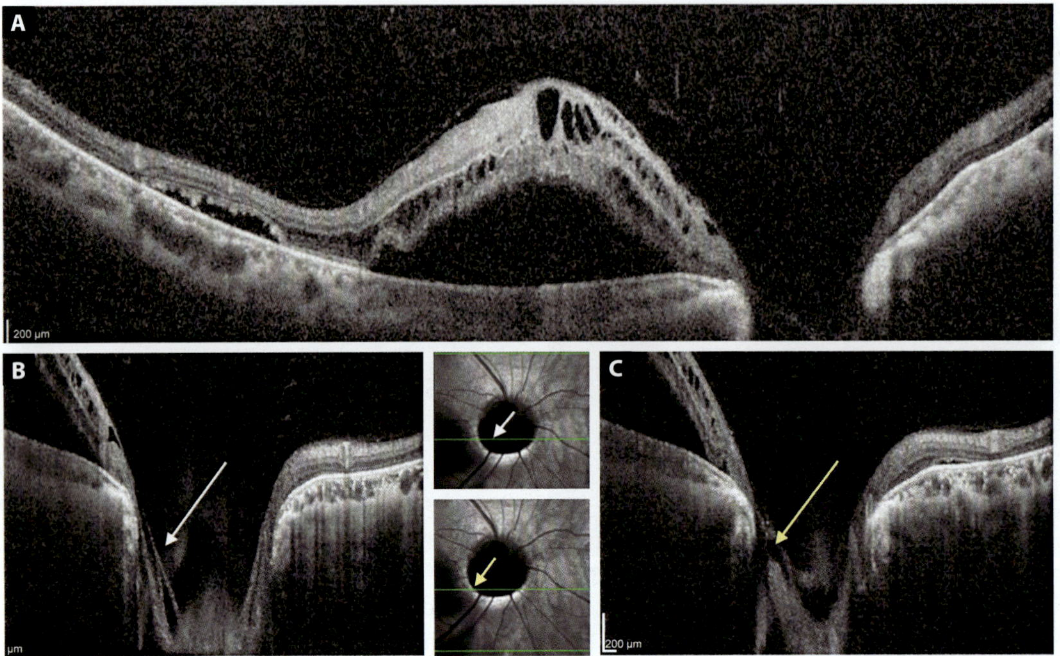

Figs. 40A to C: Composite OCT images through the disc and macula: (A) Schitic macula with neurosensory detachment; (B) White arrow showing colobomatous tissue at the temporal disc area; (C) Presumed disc pit (yellow arrow).

Treatment Plan

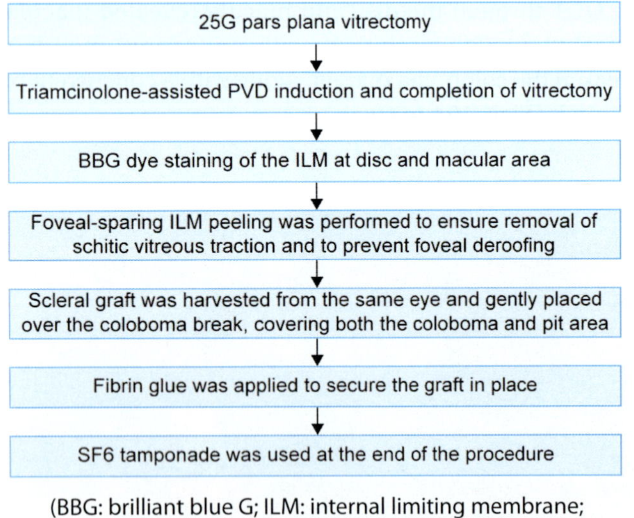

(BBG: brilliant blue G; ILM: internal limiting membrane; PVD: posterior vitreous detachment)

Thought Process

Decision	*Rationale*
Surgical intervention	Recent worsening of vision suggestive of progression of retinal detachment
Likely combined pathology	Likely the schitic macula could be secondary to pit and recent worsening of vision due to retinal detachment secondary to possible break in coloboma
Limited ILM peeling	Not mandatory, can be planned to ensure removal of residual hyaloid if any
Scleral graft	To ensure adequate closure of pit and coloboma break
Use of glue	Glue prevents graft dislodgment and is optional to avoid long-term tamponade and added side effects of tamponade

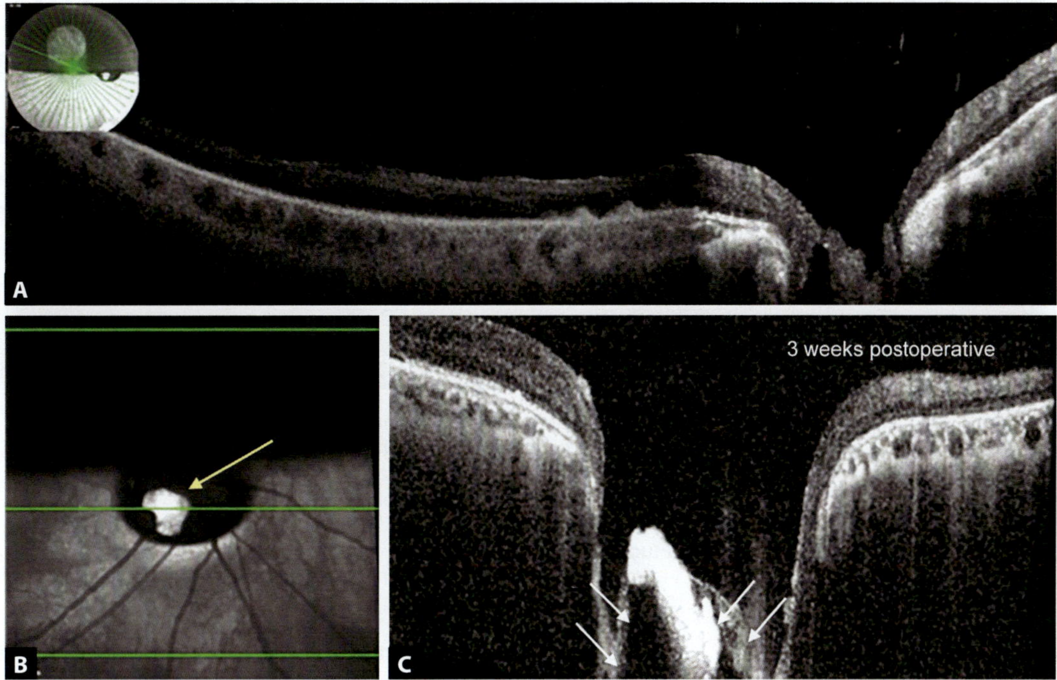

Figs. 41A to C: Composite postoperative OCT pictures showing (A) Resolution of SRF and (B and C); Scleral graft becoming integral part of disc covering the defect (yellow and white arrows).

OUTCOMES SUMMARY

Postoperatively, vision improved to 6/12. OCT through the macula confirmed resolution of subretinal fluid **(Fig. 41A)**. The graft became an integral part of the disc, covering the defects **(Figs. 41B and C)**.

KEY POINTS

- A break at the coloboma edge of the disc can present with maculopathy or macular detachment.
- Concomitant occurrence of disc coloboma and pit must be addressed during treatment.
- Scleral grafts and glue application are effective adjuncts in such cases and help to avoid laser and prolonged tamponade.

FURTHER READING

1. Babu N, Kohli P, Ramasamy K. Comparison of various surgical techniques for optic disc pit maculopathy: vitrectomy with internal limiting membrane (ILM) peeling alone versus inverted ILM flap 'plug' versus autologous scleral 'plug'. Br J Ophthalmol. 2020;104(11): 1567-73.
2. Kannan NB, Sarkar AD, Vallinayagam M, Jena S, Shah S, Ramasamy K. Anatomical and functional outcome of surgical correction of optic disc pit maculopathy using autologous scleral patch graft: a long-term retrospective analysis. BMC Ophthalmol. 2024;24(1):519.

VIDEO LEGEND

Video 17: Maculopathy

CHAPTER 11

Decision Making in Surgical Management of Coloboma Detachments

Matthew GJ Trese, Antonio Capone Jr

LASER RETINOPEXY FOR PROPHYLAXIS OF CHORIORETINAL COLOBOMA-RELATED RETINAL DETACHMENTS

Identification of a chorioretinal coloboma

↓

Routine monitoring at 6–12–month intervals: Including clinical exam and multimodal imaging

Any combination of the below may be employed at each visit:

- **Widefield fundus photography:**
  - Peripheral retinal characterization and evaluation of apex fibrosis
- **Optical coherence tomography:**
  - Evaluation of the intercalary membrane and the coloboma margin
- **Fluorescein angiography:**
  - If choroidal neovascular membrane is suspected and to evaluate posterior ciliary arteries vs retinal arteries
- **Ultrasonography:**
  - B scan: monitoring for elevation of and/or breaks in the intercalary membrane
  - UBM: characterization of the coloboma apex if needed

↓

If intercalary membrane detachment develops, a clear Intercalary membrane break is seen, atypical features of the locus minoris resistentiae develop consider laser prophylaxis

↓

Possible clinical scenarios:

1. If coloboma margin is juxtafoveal → close observation (or potentially laser prophylaxis with foveal skip)
2. If coloboma margin encompasses the optic nerve but not the fovea → consider laser prophylaxis
3. If coloboma margin encompasses the fovea and optic nerve → highly consider laser prophylaxis
4. If coloboma margin is peripheral not involving the fovea/optic nerve fovea→ laser prophylaxis is recommended

CASE SCENARIO 1

A 26-year-old, monocular female without past medical history presents as a referral from her general ophthalmologist for monitoring of a chorioretinal coloboma. The patient has a history of severe microphthalmia, no light perception vision, and a prosthetic shell for cosmesis in her left eye. Her right eye has an Ida Mann Type 5 chorioretinal coloboma that is not involving the fovea or the optic nerve. However, the locum minoris resistentiae has large cystic changes and an area of pigmentary changes suggestive of previous subretinal fluid.

A type 5 Ida Mann coloboma in an asymptomatic, monocular patient. The coloboma displays atypical margin anatomy, including a cyst at 4 o'clock with pigmentary changes suggestive of possible old subretinal fluid After a discussion, the patient elected to proceed with laser prophylaxis **(Fig. 1)**.

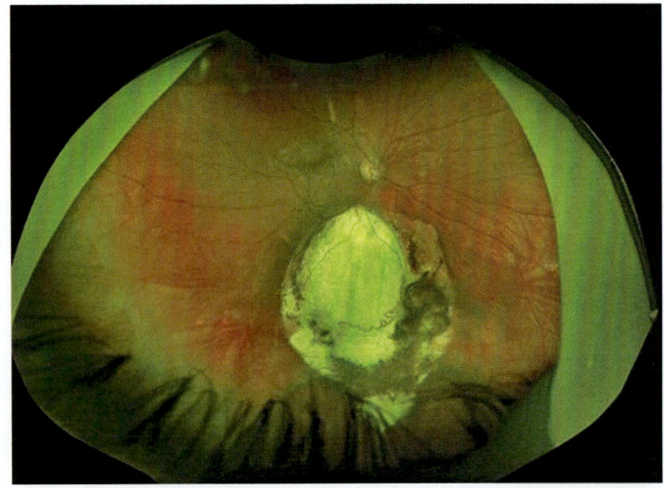

Fig. 1: Coloboma with atypical margin anatomy including a cyst and pigmentary changes extending beyond the coloboma margin.

Treatment Plan

Prophylactic laser retinopexy around the coloboma

↓

Reassess in 2–4 weeks to ensure adequate laser

Thought Process

Decision	*Rationale*
Proceed with prophylactic laser retinopexy	Atypical features of the margin of the coloboma, monocular patient, and suboptimal success rates for retinal detachment repair in eyes with chorioretinal colobomas
Consider red laser	Deeper burn to avoid vitreoretinal interface
Laser into good retina	Avoid contraction of the locum minoris resistentiae
Avoid glial apex of the coloboma	This tissue when present has abnormal vitreoretinal and lenticular adhesions

OUTCOME SUMMARY

Laser was applied to isolate the coloboma and the patient has been stable for >2 years. Care was taken to apply the laser into "good" retina to avoid contraction of the locum minoris resistentiae. Further, a wide berth to the coloboma margin was given inferiorly, as there was glial tissue that appeared to have vitreoretinal traction as well as an abnormal connection to the lens capsule **(Fig. 2)**. The patient tolerated the procedure well and with >2 years of follow-up a retinal detachment has not developed.

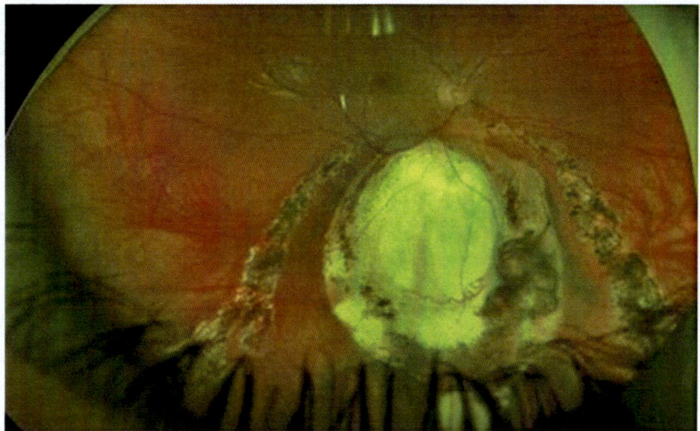

Fig. 2: Coloboma with atypical margin anatomy status post indirect laser prophylaxis. The laser was placed further away from the margin of the coloboma to mitigate issues regarding laser related complications.

KEY POINTS

- Individuals with chorioretinal colobomas are more likely to have syndromes (such as CHARGE and others) and central nervous system abnormalities, thus a systemic workup may be required.
- Eyes with chorioretinal colobomas are more likely to develop retinal detachments.
- These detachments are notoriously hard to fix, regardless of the approach taken.
- The judicious use of prophylactic laser, guided by multimodal imaging, may confer a protective effect in patients with atypical coloboma margin features, elevation of the intercalary membrane, and those with monocular status.

FURTHER READING

1. Tripathy K, Chawla R, Sharma YR, Venkatesh P, Sagar P, Vohra R, et al. Prophylactic laser photocoagulation of fundal coloboma: Does it really help? Acta Ophthalmol. 2016;94(8):e809-10.
2. Uhumwangho OM, Jalali S. Chorioretinal coloboma in a paediatric population. Eye (Lond) 2014;28(6):728-33.

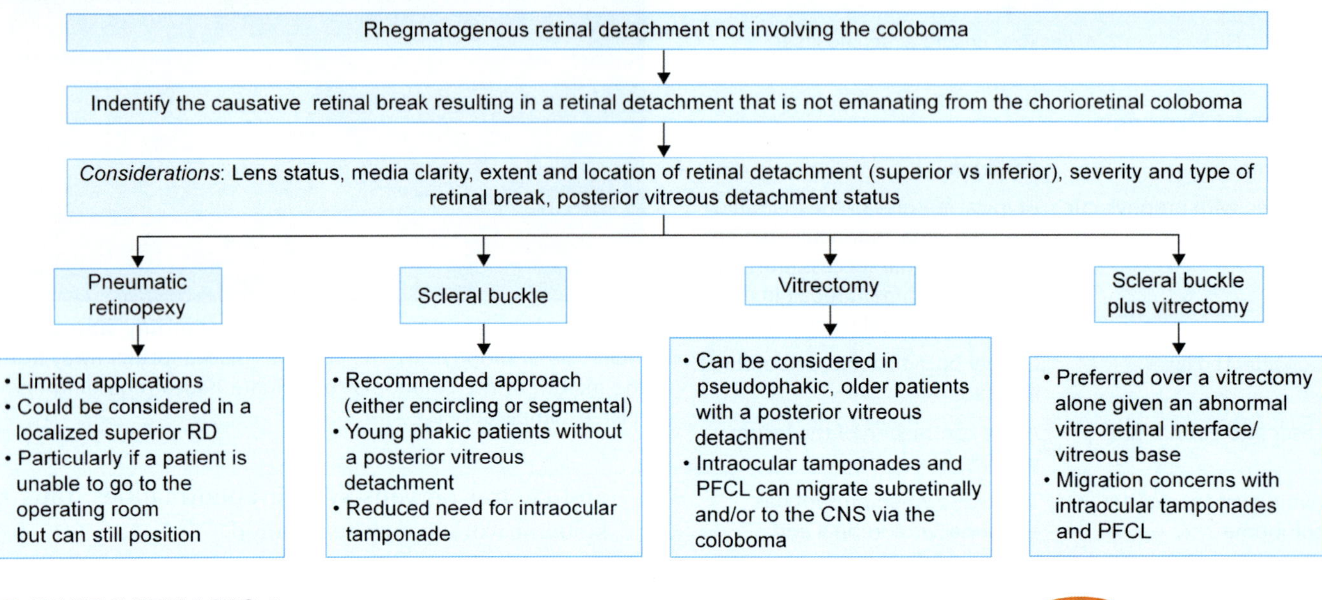

CASE SCENARIO 1

A 38-year-old female presents for an annual eye examination to their comprehensive ophthalmologist. The patient is asymptomatic, but on routine examination was found to have an inferior localized retinal detachment with two small retinal breaks in the peripheral retina away from the coloboma. Subretinal fluid extended from the breaks to the inferior coloboma, but the margin of the coloboma was intact and subretinal fluid was not emanating from the coloboma itself.

No preoperative images were obtained prior to the patient's surgery. However, this is a drawing from the chart which shows the location of the localized retinal detachment, which is adjacent to, but not emanating from the discontinuous Type 5 coloboma. Further, there is a note regarding the B scan interpretation which shows subretinal fluid was seen on ultrasonography **(Fig. 3)**. Given the configuration of the retinal detachment, it was decided to perform a primary scleral buckle.

Treatment Plan

Repair the retinal detachment with a scleral buckle, but inform the patient that a vitrectomy may be needed

↓

Follow the patient postoperatively to ensure that the retina reattaches and does not require additional surgery

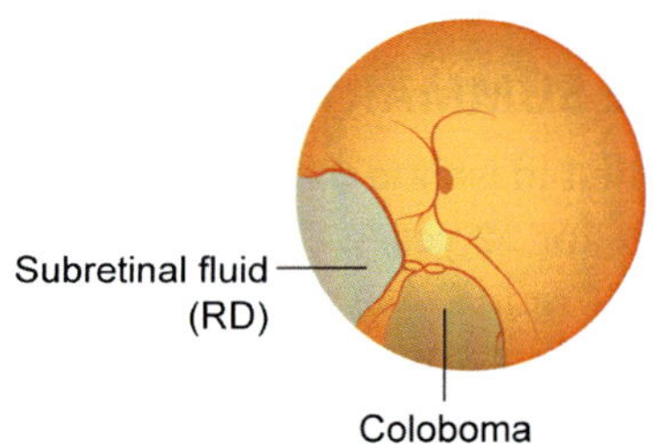

Fig. 3: Fundus drawing of a colobomatous retinal detachment (RD) with fluid abutting the coloboma but not emanating from it. In addition, the preoperative note states that there were retinal tears adjacent to the coloboma.

Thought Process

Decision	*Rationale*
Scleral buckle	Young, phakic, inferior retinal detachment (RD), no posterior vitreous detachment (PVD), obvious causative break seen, known abnormal vitreoretinal interface in patients with colobomas, thus there is a preference for an external approach
No external drainage	Localized RD with minimal fluid

OUTCOME SUMMARY

The patient is now 48 years old (i.e., 10 years after the primary buckle) and the retina remains attached fundus showed adequate scleral indentation from the buckle **(Fig. 4)**. There has been an interval worsening of the

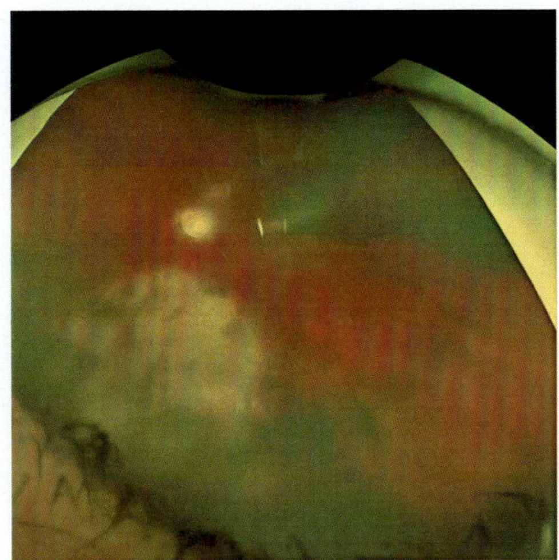

Fig. 4: Color fundus photograph displaying an attached retina, a discontinuous coloboma, and the indentation of an encircling scleral buckle.

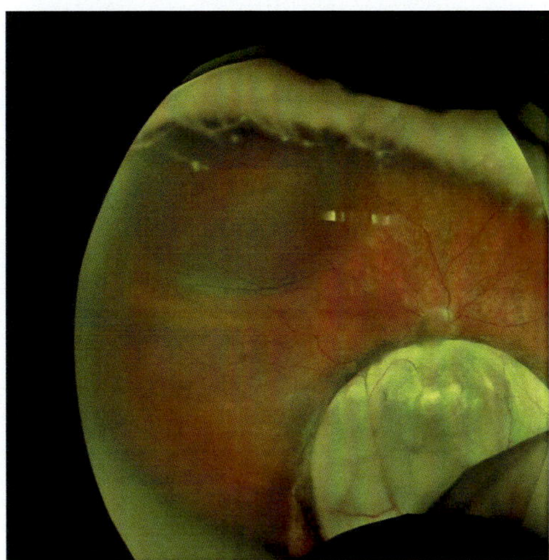

Fig. 5: Fundus image shows horseshoe tear with superior retinal break and a macula on retinal detachment from 9 to 12 o'clock. Careful examination also shows a retinal tear at 11 o'clock.

patient's cataract resulting in suboptimal visualization on examination and imaging, but she remains 20/30 and is happy with her vision currently and the retina remains attached.

CASE SCENARIO 2

A pseudophakic, 48-year-old, monocular male presents with a 2-day history of new floaters and a new inferior curtain. Examination found a horseshoe tear with superior retinal break and a macula on retinal detachment from 9 to 12 o'clock. Careful examination also shows a retinal tear at 11 o'clock **(Fig. 5)**. After a discussion it was decided to perform a primary vitrectomy.

Treatment Plan

Primary vitrectomy with short-term gas tamponade

Thought Process

Decision	*Rationale*
Primary vitrectomy with 20% sulfur hexafluoride gas tamponade	Pseudophakic, posterior vitreous detachment (PVD), and superior retinal detachment with clear retinal tear

OUTCOME SUMMARY

Two weeks after primary vitrectomy, the retina redetached. There was no obvious break on examination. The original break was well treated. On examination, subretinal fluid now extended from the temporal periphery to the previously lasered coloboma margin **(Fig. 6)**. It was decided to take the patient back to the operating room to perform a scleral buckle with vitrectomy and silicone oil tamponade.

Treatment Plan

Scleral buckle, vitrectomy, and silicone oil tamponade

Thought Process

Decision	*Rationale*
Scleral buckle, vitrectomy, and silicone oil	Recurrent retinal detachment in a monocular patient with a chorioretinal coloboma requires additional vitreous base support
Plan for peripheral laser to the abnormal vitreous base	Facilitate vitreous base support and barricade any small pseudophakic breaks
Silicone oil tamponade	Silicone oil will allow this monocular patient to remain functional and provide stability while retinal reattachment occurs

OUTCOME SUMMARY

This 48-year-old male presented with a rhegmatogenous retinal detachment. Given his pseudophakic status, posterior vitreous detachment, superior location, and identifiable causative retinal tear, the patient underwent primary vitrectomy. There was recurrence of the retinal detachment, which required placement of a scleral buckle,

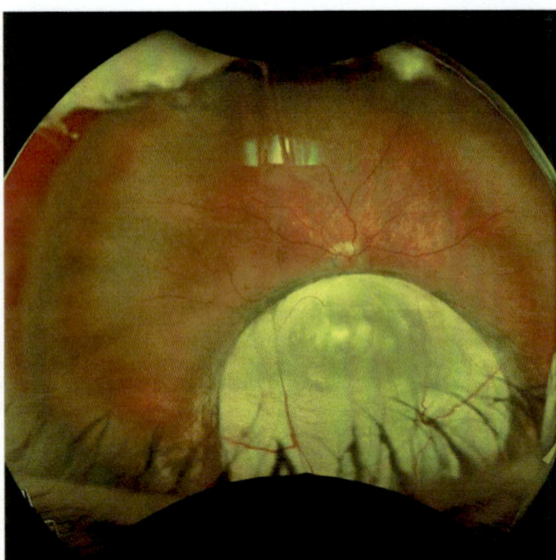

Fig. 6: Fundus image showing subretinal fluid now extended from the temporal periphery to the previously lasered coloboma margin.

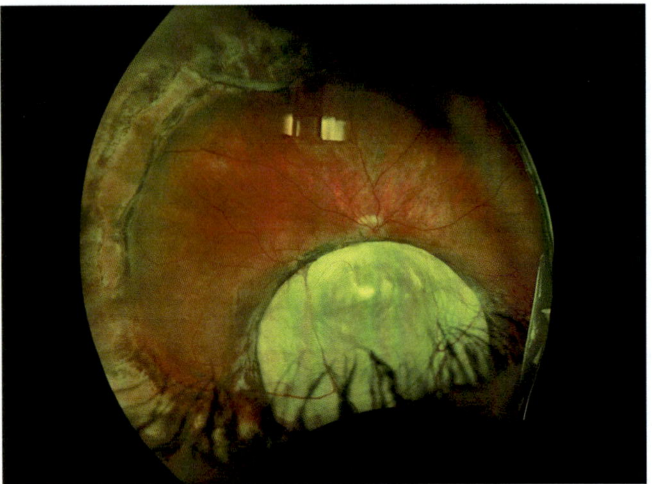

Fig. 7: A color fundus images showing an attached retina with a peripheral coloboma that had remained stable under silicone oil for 6 months.

repeat vitrectomy, and silicone oil tamponade. The oil remained in the eye for 6 months and was subsequently removed. The patient has remained attached for 6 months and has maintained excellent visual acuity **(Figs. 7 and 8)**.

KEY POINTS

- A rhegmatogenous retinal detachment in an eye with a chorioretinal coloboma behaves differently than a routine rhegmatogenous retinal detachment. This is likely because the congenital malformation (i.e., failure of the optic fissure to close), results in an abnormal vitreoretinal interface as well as other intraocular anomalies.
- Although traditional considerations such as age, lens status, posterior vitreous detachment status, and location of retinal detachment (RD) should be considered. When possible, an external approach (scleral buckle) is preferred and can result in long-term retinal reattachment.
- It is reasonable to attempt a staged surgical approach, meaning a primary scleral buckle followed by vitrectomy if retinal reattachment fails.
- Vitrectomy can also be performed successfully in eyes with rhegmatogenous retinal detachment that are not emanating from the chorioretinal coloboma; however, vitreoretinal interface abnormalities, zonular abnormalities, and intercalary membrane disruption can be encountered.
- The role of pneumatic retinopexy for the repair of rhegmatogenous retinal detachments in eyes with chorioretinal colobomas is less well defined.

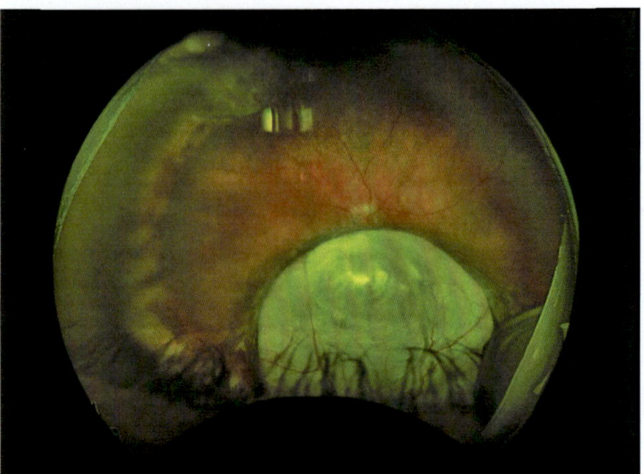

Fig. 8: The same eye, 6 months after removing silicone oil. The retina remains attached and the patient has excellent visual acuity.

FURTHER READING

1. Abouammoh MA, Alsulaiman SM, Gupta VS, Younis A, Chhablani J, Hussein A, et al. Surgical Outcomes and Complications of Rhegmatogenous Retinal Detachment in Eyes with Chorioretinal Coloboma: The results of the KKESH international collaborative retina study group. Retina. 2017;37(10):1942-7.
2. Gopal L, Badrinath SS, Sharma T, Parikh SN, Shanmugam MS, Bhende PS, et al. Surgical management of retinal detachments related to coloboma of the choroid. Ophthalmology. 1998;105(5):804-9.
3. Hussain RM, Abbey AM, Shah AR, Drenser KA, Trese MT, Capone A Jr. Chorioretinal coloboma complications: Retinal detachment and choroidal neovascular membrane. J Ophthalmic Vis Res. 2017;12(1):3-10.
4. Uhumwangho OM, Jalali S. Chorioretinal coloboma in a paediatric population. Eye. 2014;28(6):728-33.

CHORIORETINAL COLOBOMA-RELATED RETINAL DETACHMENTS

Every attempt must be performed to identification of the retinal break in a CC–RDs

↓

Common locations for retinal break include:
- Central intercalary membrane
- Locus minoris resistentiae
- Unidentifiable (presumed to be within the coloboma

↓

If the break is within the coloboma then vitrectomy, with or without scleral buckle, is required to repair the retinal detachment

↓

Vitrectomy consideration:
- Meticulous hyaloid elevation without damage to the intercalary membrane must be performed
- Retinotomy may be used to limit the use of heavy liquids as posterior migration of PFCL (and silicone oil) have been reported
- Silicone oil tamponade may be considered as long-term tamponaded is often required
- An abnormal vitreous base is commonly encountered, scleral buckle and/or encircling laser may provide additional support

CASE SCENARIO 1

An 18-year-old female without past medical history presents with worsening central and peripheral vision in her right eye and states that objects "look slanted." She states her symptoms started 1 month ago, but she ignored this because the right eye has always been her worse seeing eye. Her baseline best corrected visual acuity is 20/800 OD and 20/20 OS. On presentation she was hand motion OD and remained 20/20 OS. She is aware that she has a chorioretinal coloboma in the right eye and feels that she is losing usable peripheral vision. Examination showed a normal anterior segment. However, the posterior segment displayed a total retinal detachment.

Examination showed a chorioretinal coloboma-related retinal detachment. No obvious retinal break was seen on examination **(Fig. 9)**. After discussion with the patient, it was decided to attempt surgical repair.

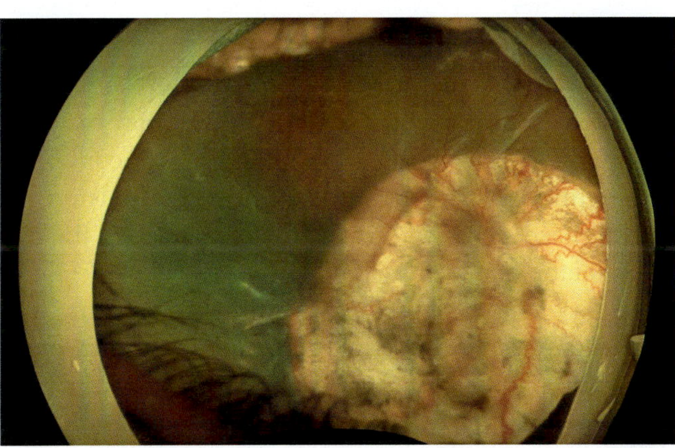

Fig. 9: This color fundus photograph shows a total retinal detachment in an 18-year-old child; at the time of this photograph no break could clearly be identified and it was assumed that the retinal detachment was emanating from the coloboma.

Treatment Plan

Vitrectomy with silicone oil tamponade

Thought Process

Decision	*Rationale*
Vitrectomy with a plan for silicone oil to repair a total retinal detachment without obvious retinal break	Vitrectomy performed because the lack of a clear retinal break combined with the detachment configuration suggests that the detachment is emanating from the coloboma

Contd...

Contd...

Decision	*Rationale*
Retinotomy for retinal reattachment	Perfluorocarbon liquid (PFCL) must be used with caution in eyes with chorioretinal colobomas, particularly those that involve the optic nerve, as migration into the central nervous system (CNS) have been reported
Peripheral 360° endolaser	360° laser performed given the abnormal vitreoretinal interface as well as the posteriorly inserted vitreous base
Silicone oil tamponade	Silicone oil provides long-term endotamponade. However, there are also reports of CNS migration and must be used judiciously

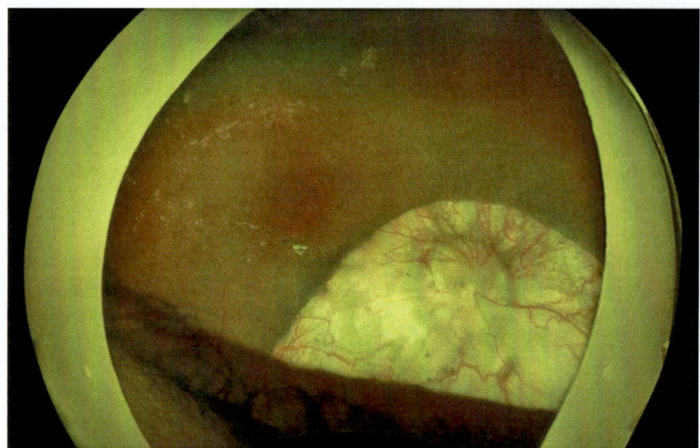

Fig. 10: A postoperative color fundus image showing complete retinal reattachment under silicone oil. The patients visual acuity improved from hand motion to count fingers.

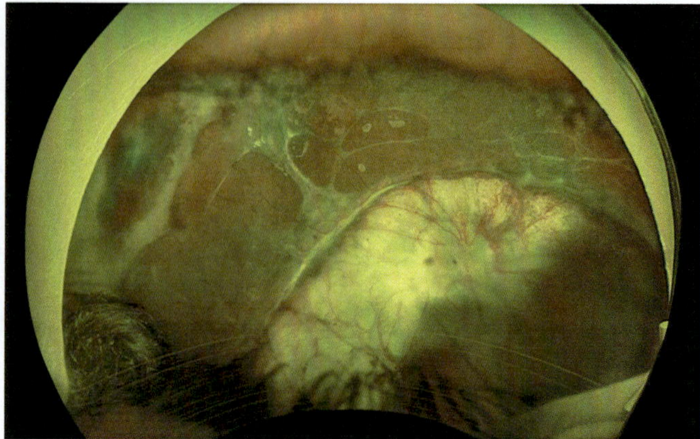

Fig. 11: Color fundus image showing a recurrent total retinal detachment with pre and subretinal proliferative vitreoretinopathy (PVR).

OUTCOME SUMMARY

After careful vitrectomy with meticulous posterior hyaloid elevation and retinotomy, the retina was able to be flattened. However, a peripheral break could not be identified. Next, endolaser was used to bolster the vitreous base 360°, and silicone oil was placed in the eye for endotamponade. Intraoperative visual acuity declined secondary to lens opacification, thus a lensectomy was performed. Despite this, visual acuity improved from hand motion to count fingers **(Fig. 10)**.

Unfortunately, 3 weeks after successful retinal detachment repair the patient developed a recurrent retinal detachment with extensive pre and subretinal proliferative vitreoretinopathy (PVR). Her visual acuity again declined to light perception. The patient again felt that her peripheral vision was compromised, and she elected to attempt a second surgical repair. After 3 years the retina has remained partially attached **(Fig. 11)** under silicone oil with a physiologic intraocular pressure (IOP), however her visual acuity never recovered.

KEY POINTS

- Chorioretinal coloboma-related retinal detachments are notoriously difficult to repair and often require multiple surgeries to achieve anatomic success. Even when anatomic success is achieved, visual outcomes are often poor. Despite this, patients often value their peripheral vision as evidenced by our patients' desire for multiple surgeries regardless of a long-standing history of poor visual acuity.
- Retinal break localization, when possible, is essential and may facilitate surgical approaches which improve patient outcomes and reduce the need for multiple surgical interventions. In eyes without an identifiable retinal break, and where subretinal fluid is in contact with coloboma margin, it is assumed that a break exists at the locum minoris resistentiae most often in conjunction with an intercalary membrane break.
- The judicious use of heavy liquids and silicone oil must be considered as posterior migration in the central nervous system have been reported. Retinotomy with subretinal fluid drainage under air represents a promising technique which may be beneficial in cases where posterior migration is a concern.
- Laser around the coloboma margin, even if the coloboma margin involves the macula, may be required to achieve retinal attachment.
- The development of classification systems and surgical techniques which better address CC-RDs are required to improve patient outcomes.

FURTHER READING

1. Abouammoh MA, Alsulaiman SM, Gupta VS, Younis A, Chhablani J, Hussein A, et al. Surgical Outcomes and Complications of Rhegmatogenous Retinal Detachment in Eyes with Chorioretinal Coloboma: The results of the KKESH international collaborative retina study group. Retina. 2017;37(10):1942-7.

2. Daufenbach DR, Ruttum MS, Pulido JS, et al. Chorioretinal colobomas in a pediatric population. Ophthalmology. 1998;105(8):1455-8.
3. Gopal L, Badrinath SS, Sharma T, Parikh SN, Shanmugam MS, Bhende PS, et al. Surgical management of retinal detachments related to coloboma of the choroid. Ophthalmology. 1998;105(5):804-9.
4. Hussain RM, Abbey AM, Shah AR, Drenser KA, Trese MT, Capone A Jr. Chorioretinal coloboma complications: Retinal detachment and choroidal neovascular membrane. J Ophthalmic Vis Res. 2017;12(1):3-10.
5. Jesberg DO, Schepens CL. Retinal detachment associated with coloboma of the choroid. Arch Ophthalmol. 1961; 65163-73.
6. Maumenee IH, Mitchell TN. Colobomatous malformations of the eye. Trans Am Ophthalmol Soc. 1990;88123-5.
7. Schubert HD. Structural organization of choroidal colobomas of young and adult patients and mechanism of retinal detachment. Trans Am Ophthalmol Soc. 2005;103457–72.
8. Uhumwangho OM, Jalali S. Chorioretinal coloboma in a paediatric population. Eye. 2014;28(6):728-33.

CHAPTER 12

Decision Making in Surgical Management of Drop Nucleus and Secondary Intraocular Lens

CK Nagesha, Chaitra Jayadev

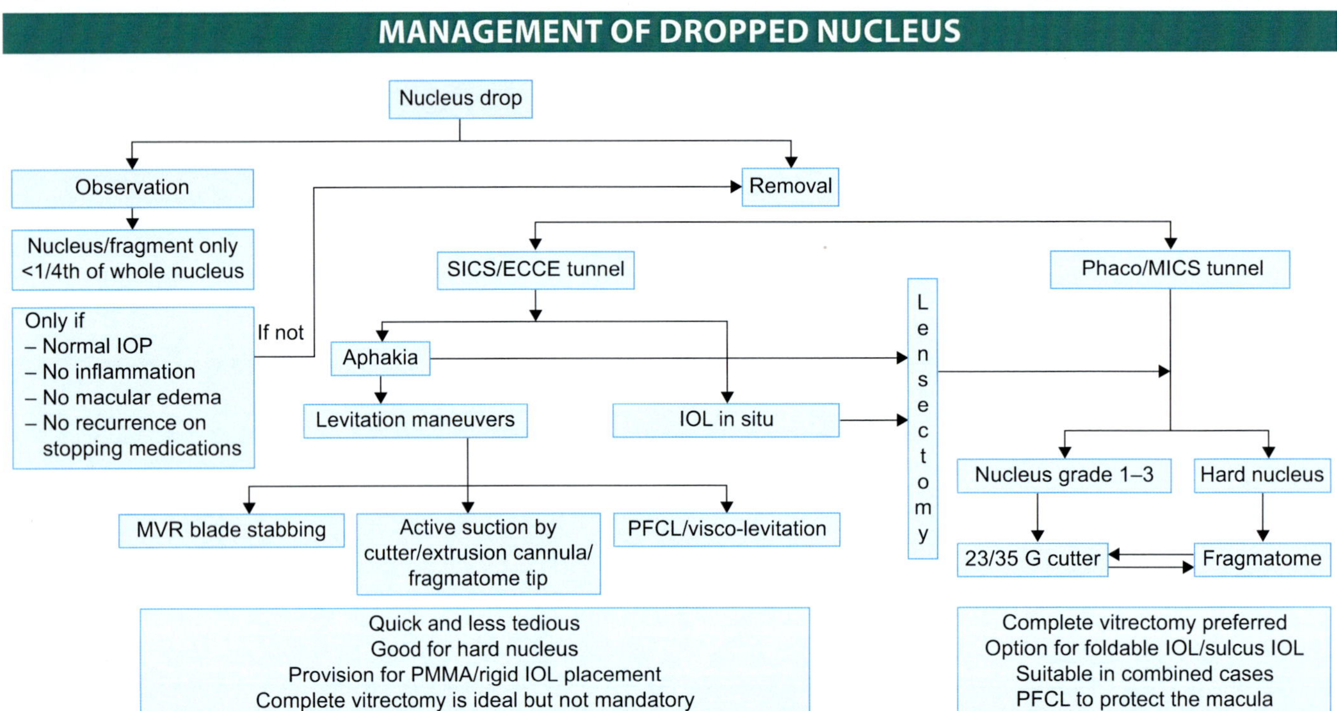

(IOL: intraocular lens; MICS: Microincision cataract surgery, MVR: microvitreoretinal; PFCL: perfluorocarbon liquid)

CASE SCENARIO 1: VITRECTOMY AND IOL MANIPULATION IN MANAGEMENT OF NUCLEUS DROP SECONDARY TO PHACOEMULSIFICATION

Case Summary

A 60-year-old patient, on anti-glaucoma medications (AGM), underwent microincision phacoemulsification surgery for a hard cataract. Posterior capsular dehiscence during nucleus sculpting led to a nucleus drop. All anterior cortical remnants were removed, retaining the anterior capsular rim intact and leaving the posterior capsular tear untouched. A plate-haptic intraocular lens (IOL) was placed in the sulcus over the anterior capsular rim **(Fig. 1A)**.

The patient was seen 2 days post-cataract surgery with IOL implantation. The best corrected distance visual acuity was 6/60, and the intraocular pressure was 26 mm Hg on two AGMs. Anterior chamber cells were Grade 2+. Fundus examination showed uncleared lens fragments of more than two-thirds of the size with a cortical shell **(Fig. 1B)**. The media was clear, and the retina appeared healthy with a normal peripheral fundus examination.

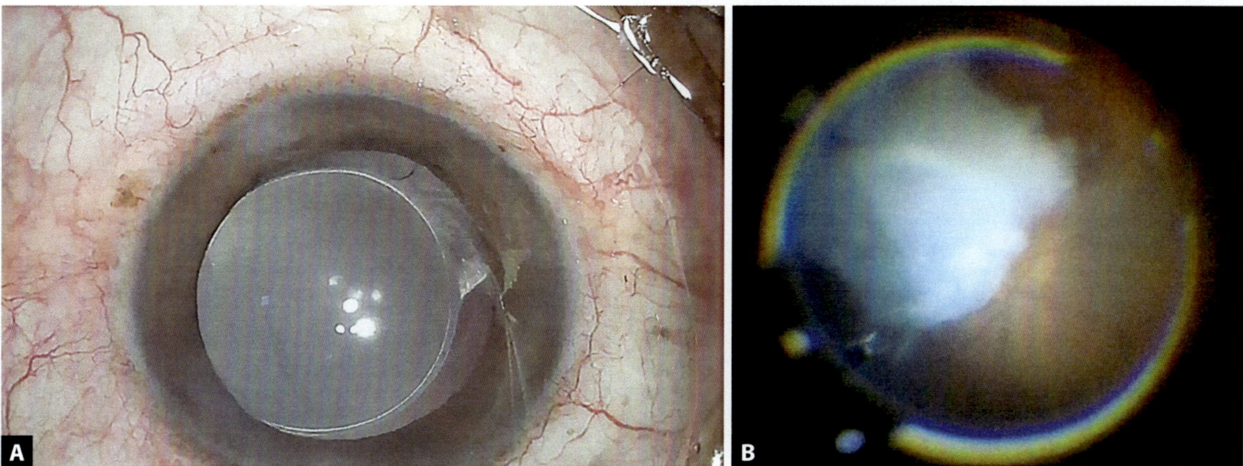

Figs. 1A and B: (A) Anterior segment image of the plate-haptic intraocular lens, slightly decentered; (B) Intraoperative fundus photograph showing lens fragments in the vitreous cavity.

Treatment Plan

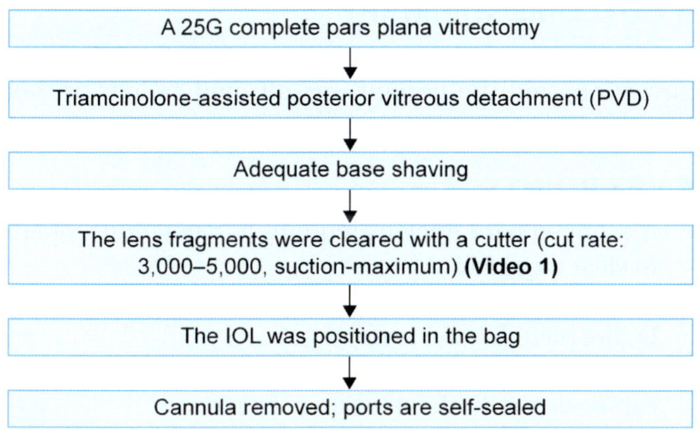

Thought Process

Decision	*Rationale*
Lensectomy	Media clear, nucleus is of Grade 2–3 with IOL in situ
Complete vitrectomy	With premium IOLs, the risk of cystoid macular edema reduces ideal visual outcomes
Avoid the fragmatome, prefer the vitreous cutter	Advantage of sutureless sclerotomies, patient already on two AGMs—need to secure a healthy conjunctiva for the possibility of glaucoma surgery
Move the sulcus plate haptics IOL into the bag	The large surface area of plate haptics in the sulcus causes iris chafing. Place into the bag if possible; if not, replace with a foldable 3-piece IOL

(AGM: anti-glaucoma medication; IOL: intraocular lens)

OUTCOME SUMMARY

During the postoperative period, the IOP normalized without AGMs, and the vision improved to 6/6 with correction. The patient was stable after 8 weeks of topical medications.

KEY POINTS

- Dropped nuclear material causes significant inflammation and a rise in intraocular pressure.
- A vitrectomy cutter or a framatome is used based on the hardness of the nucleus.
- Large haptics IOLs need to be placed within the bag, if feasible, to prevent iris contact.

VIDEO LEGEND

Video 18: Vitrectomy and IOL manipulation in management of nucleus drop secondary to phacoemulsification

CASE SCENARIO 2: MANAGEMENT OF DECENTERED IOL AND NUCLEUS FRAGMENT DROP

Case Summary

A patient was referred to us for management of a dropped nucleus following routine phacoemulsification surgery. A limited anterior vitrectomy had been performed, and a 3-piece IOL had been placed in the sulcus during the primary surgery.

On Day 2 examination, the patient's best-corrected distance visual acuity was 3/60. There was minimal corneal haze, a deep anterior chamber, and a decentered 3-piece IOL in the sulcus **(Fig. 2A)**. The IOP was normal with one

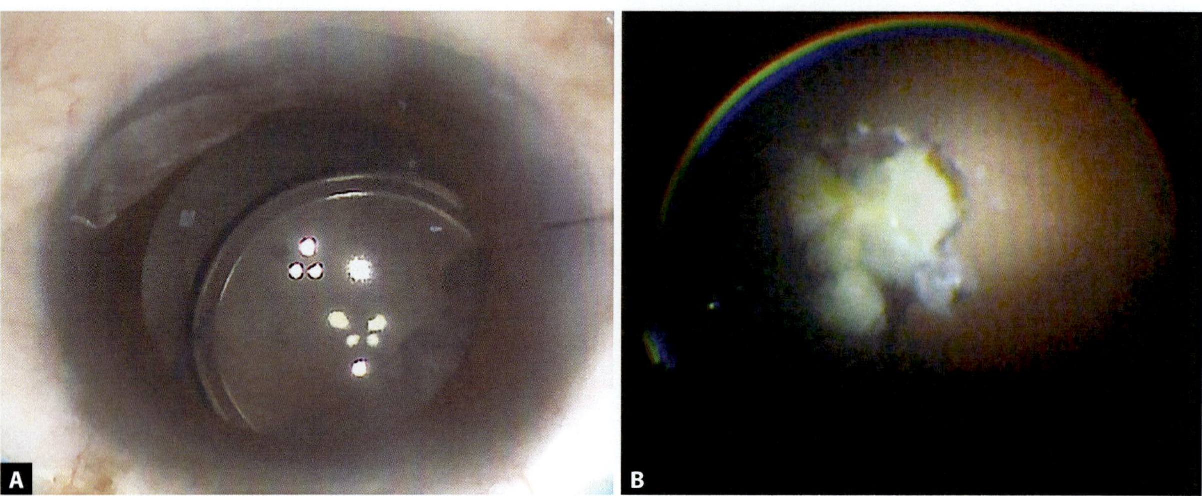

Figs. 2A and B: (A) Anterior segment image of the decentered intraocular lens in the sulcus; (B) Intraoperative fundus photograph showing nuclear fragments and cortical matter in the vitreous cavity.

AGM. The fundus examination revealed a partially cracked nucleus, Grade 3-4, along with some cortical matter **(Fig. 2B)**.

Treatment Plan

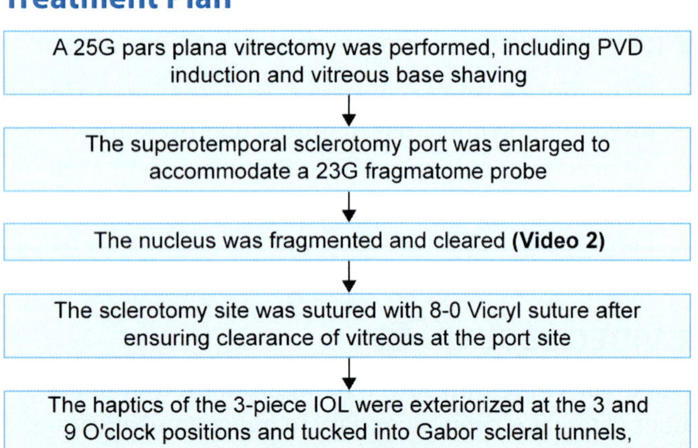

Thought Process

Decision	*Rationale*
Nucleus removal	Size more than 2/3rd, associated with cortical matter
Framatome is preferred	Brown nucleus
Vitrectomy	Complete vitrectomy is good to prevent vitreous pull during phacofragmentation
IOL centration	A decentered IOL will lead to astigmatism and chronic inflammation secondary to iris touch and off axis. Need to attain good centration

(IOL: intraocular lens)

OUTCOME SUMMARY

Postoperatively, the vision improved to 6/6 with correction, and the patient was off medications at the 6-week follow-up.

KEY POINTS

- A dropped hard nucleus requires a fragmatome, often to clear it quickly.
- A full PVD and complete vitreous removal is required before planning the fragmatome.
- The decentered 3-piece IOL need to be centered, and can be done by scleral tucking of haptics.

VIDEO LEGEND

Video 19: Management of decentered IOL and nucleus fragment drop

CASE SCENARIO 3: MANAGEMENT OF NUCLEUS DROP IN A HARD CATARACT

Case Summary

The patient was referred with a history of being operated on for a hard cataract, with the entire nucleus being dislocated into the vitreous cavity. Initially, a small incision cataract surgery was planned with the intention of manually removing the nucleus and implanting a 3-piece IOL in the bag. However, due to the dislocation of the nucleus, an adequate anterior vitrectomy was done, and the patient was left aphakic at the time of referral.

Examination revealed a best-corrected distance visual acuity of 1/60 and an IOP of 32 mm Hg. Corneal haze was minimal, and the anterior chamber was deep **(Fig. 3A)**.

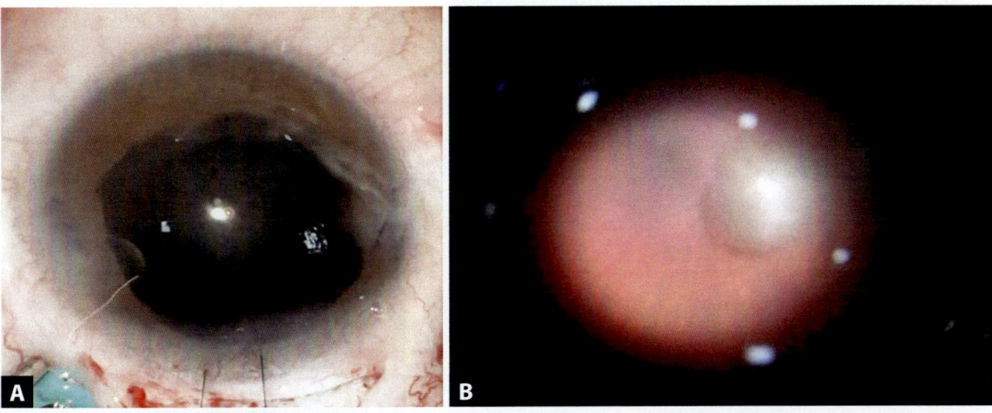

Figs. 3A and B: (A) Anterior segment image with a sutured sclerocorneal tunnel and aphakia; (B) Intraoperative fundus photograph showing the entire nucleus in the vitreous cavity.

The vitreous showed the nucleus in toto, and the retina appeared normal **(Fig. 3B)**.

Treatment Plan

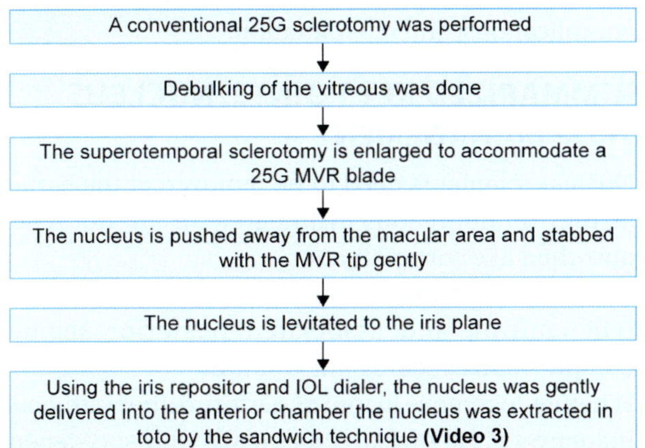

Thought Process

Decision	*Rationale*
Preoperative IOP management	Good IOP control preoperatively improves corneal clarity and prevents intraoperative choroidal detachment and bleeding
Whole lens removal	Good option, as the sclerocorneal tunnel was large enough to facilitate nucleus removal by the levitation method
Vitrectomy	A bed of vitreous over the retina is preferred during maneuvers when using PFCL bubble, or can leave cushion of vitreous when stabbing method is used to prevent retinal injury
Large-diameter PMMA IOL placement	A large tunnel provides an opportunity to place a rigid or foldable 3-piece IOL

(IOP: intraocular pressure; IOL: intraocular lens; PFCL: perfluorocarbon liquid; PMMA: polymethyl methacrylate)

OUTCOME SUMMARY

Postoperatively, vision improved to 6/9 with residual astigmatism, which remained stable during a 6-month follow-up period.

Key Points

- Levitation techniques are a safe, quick, and effective way to remove the nucleus in toto.
- The nucleus brought into the anterior chamber can be cleared with phaco or removed through a small incision cataract surgery (SICS) tunnel.
- Suitable for harder nuclei and when the fragmatome is unavailable.
- Pressure injury to the retina during stabbing or remnants of perfluorocarbon liquid (PFCL) are the main concerns.

VIDEO LEGEND

Video 20: Management of nucleus drop in a hard cataract

CASE SCENARIO 4: CONSERVATIVE MANAGEMENT IN NUCLEUS DROP

Case Summary

This patient was referred for the management of the entire lens in the vitreous cavity. History revealed that the right eye had been operated on 30 years ago in a surgical camp setup. No documents about the previous surgery were available. The patient was asymptomatic with unrelated symptoms in the other eye secondary to a pterygium.

Examination revealed a best-corrected distance visual acuity of 6/24 and an IOP of 18 mm Hg. The IOL appeared stable with a mid-dilated and fixed pupil and no signs of a pupillary block **(Fig. 4A)**. There was no anterior chamber inflammation, and it was free of any vitreous remnants.

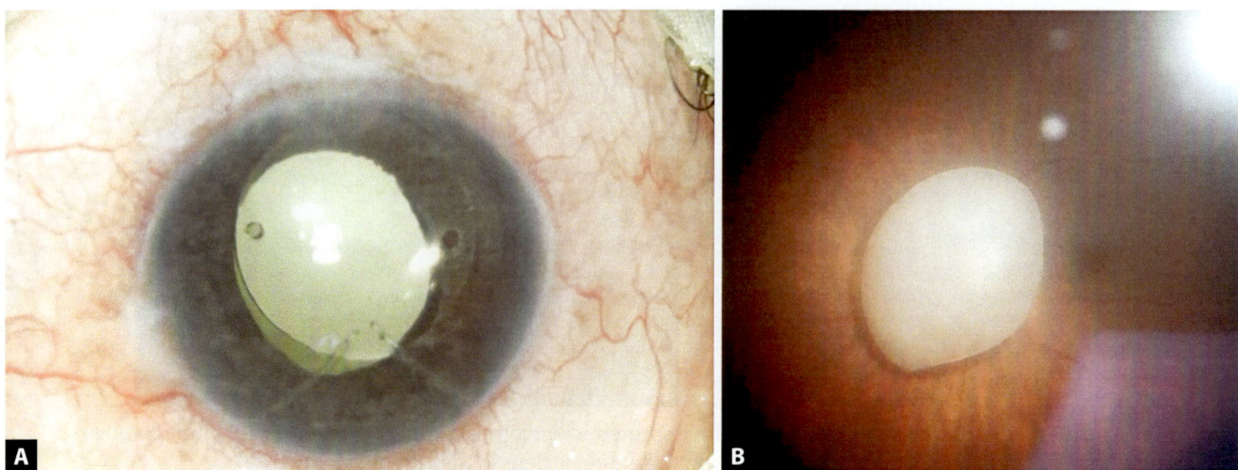

Figs. 4A and B: (A) Anterior segment image of a stable IOL with a mid-dilated and fixed pupil; (B) Fundus photograph showing the entire crystalline lens in the vitreous cavity. (IOL: intraocular lens)

Fundus examination revealed a clear vitreous, and the entire lens with an intact capsule was observed lying in the inferior fundus **(Fig. 4B)**. The retina and peripheral fundus appeared normal.

Treatment Plan

No intervention was done

↓

Follow-up was advised every 3 months or as and when required

Thought Process

Decision	*Rationale*
No active intervention	Asymptomatic for the last 3 decades, no signs of active or past inflammation
Close follow-up	Chances of protein leak due to bag dehiscence or increased IOP and inflammation secondary to progressive lens protein decay
Surgical intervention, if complications occur	Vitrectomy and lensectomy

(IOP: intraocular pressure)

OUTCOME SUMMARY

The eye remained stable over the 2-year follow-up period.

KEY POINTS

- Dislocation of the whole lens can be observed, provided no secondary complications develop.
- Often seen in eyes with syndromic myopia with weak zonules and rarely spontaneously dislocated hypermature cataract.
- The need for surgical intervention solely depends on the guiding principles of inflammation, retinal complications, and rehabilitation.

SUMMARIZED KEY POINTS: NUCLEUS DROP MANAGEMENT

- Nuclear fragments need to be removed at the earliest, as they do not readily disintegrate or are not readily absorbed like cortical matter.
- The ideal timing is dictated by media clarity, IOP control, and associated posterior segment complications needing intervention.
- Whether to remove in toto or perform other intraocular maneuvers is at the surgeon's discretion and depends on the presence of an IOL.
- Surgical techniques are available to levitate the dropped nucleus using PFCL, a microvitreoretinal (MVR) blade, a suction cannula, and vitrectomy cutter suction.
- Often, dropped nucleus management can be combined with an IOL placement.

FURTHER READING

1. Merani R, Hunyor AP, Playfair TJ, Chang A, Gregory-Roberts J, Hunyor AB, et al. Pars plana vitrectomy for the management of retained lens material after cataract surgery. Am J Ophthalmol. 2007;144(3):364-70.
2. Schutz JS, Mavrakanas NA. Posterior-assisted levitation in cataract surgery. Curr Opin Ophthalmol. 2010;21:50-4.
3. Sahay P, Goel S, Maharana PK, Sharma N, Titiyal JS. Sequelae of neglected hypermature senile cataract. Indian J Ophthalmol. 2019;67(10):1707-8.

MANAGEMENT OF DISLOCATED INTRAOCULAR LENSES AND SECONDARY INTRAOCULAR LENSES

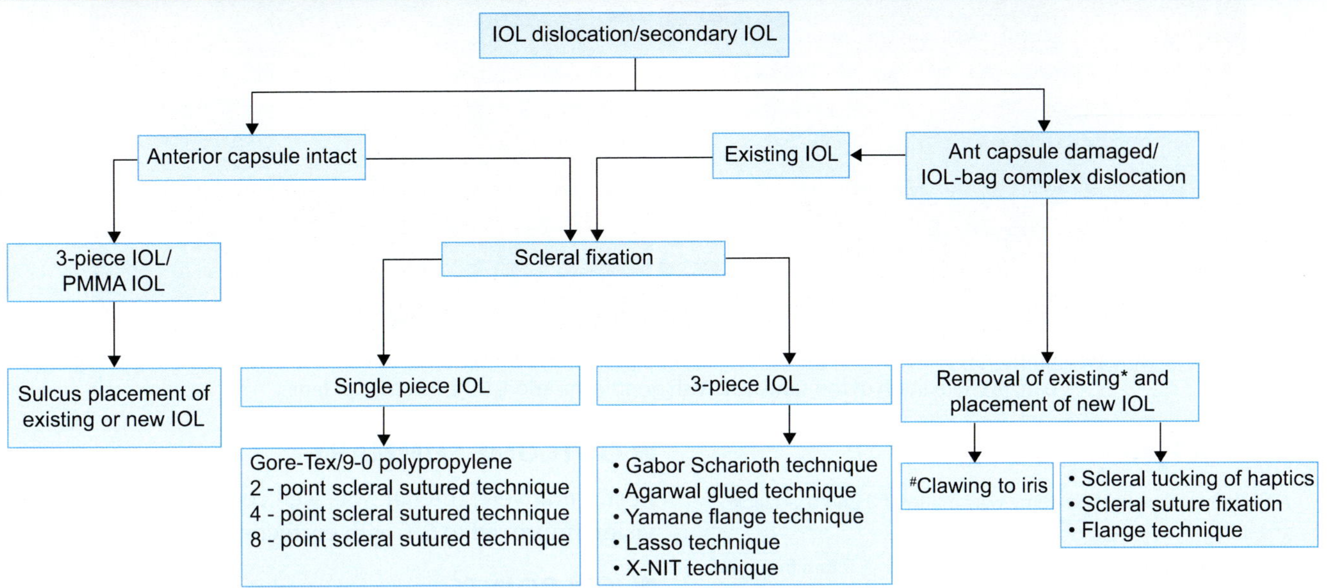

*Indications to remove existing IOL; Damaged/opacified IOL; Not amenable to refixation; Postcataract surgery refractive surprise
#Indicatied when large white-to-white diameter; Scleral thinning/diseases
(IOL: intraocular lens; PMMA: polymethyl methacrylate)

CASE SCENARIO 5: IOL REFIXATION USING GABOR SCHARIOTH TECHNIQUE

Case Summary

A 54-year-old patient had undergone a microincision phacoemulsification for a Grade 2 soft nuclear cataract. A posterior capsular dehiscence was noted during epinucleus removal with vitreous loss. A foldable 3-piece IOL had been placed in the sulcus, which had descended through the inferior posterior capsular rent into the anterior vitreous. When referred to us, a large plate of epinucleus was seen covering the entire nasal capsular bag area, with the dislocated IOL suspended in the anterior vitreous phase.

The right eye had a best-corrected distance visual acuity of 4/60, and intraocular pressure was 24 mm Hg on a single AGM. The cornea was clear, and the AC was well formed. The IOL was partially in the sulcus, with a major part of it in the anterior vitreous **(Fig. 5A)**. The epinucleus remnant in the bag was noted in the nasal quadrant, and the zonular loss with temporal displacement of the capsular bag was observed. The anterior vitreous appeared clear with no nuclear or cortical matter. The fundus was grossly normal with a limited field of view.

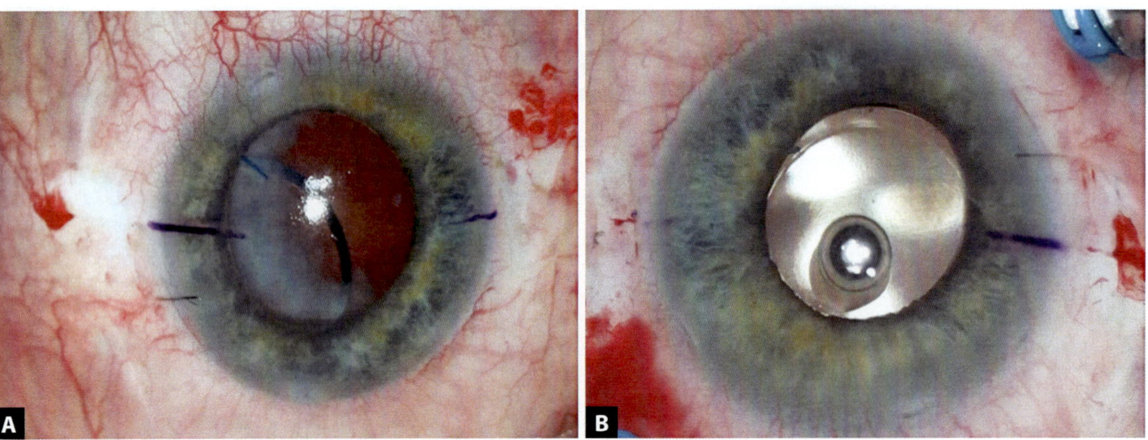

Figs. 5A and B: (A) Inferotemporally dislocated 3-piece IOL. A large epinucleus remnant was noted in the nasal part of the capsular bag; (B) Refixation of the same IOL with good centration. (IOL: intraocular lens)

Treatment Plan

A limited conjunctival peritomy was made at 3 and 9 O'clock

↓

Gabor Scharioth scleral pockets were made 1–1.5 mm from and parallel to the limbus

↓

A limited anterior vitrectomy was done through 25G sclerotomies, and the retained epinucleus was removed

↓

The haptics of the IOL were docking into a 26G needle

↓

The haptics are exteriorized at 3 and 9 O'clock and inserted into scleral tunnels **(Video 20)**

Thought Process

Decision	*Rationale*
To take up for revision surgery immediately	The cornea was clear enough for adequate visualization. Intraocular pressure was in the near-normal range, and the IOL was still in the anterior vitreous
Plan to remove the entire capsular bag remnant along with the retained epinucleus	The anterior capsular margin was poorly delineated, and more than 180° of nasal zonular dehiscence was noted along with a displaced capsular bag
Existing IOL refixation	As the sulcus placement of the IOL was not stable, the haptics can be exteriorized at 3 and 9 o'clock and tucked into the sclera (Gabor technique)
Limited anterior vitrectomy	As the vitreous and underlying retina appeared grossly normal, no or a limited vitrectomy suffices

(IOL: intraocular lens)

OUTCOME SUMMARY

Postoperatively, the IOL was well centered **(Fig. 5B)**, and vision improved to 6/6 with correction.

KEY POINTS

- IOLs placed in the sulcus can subluxate over the anterior capsule.
- Converting a 3-piece sulcus IOL to a scleral-tucking SFIOL (scleral fixation of intraocular lens) is a viable option.
- If a significant capsular rim is present, reverse optic capture prevents decentration or subluxation.

VIDEO LEGEND

Video 21: IOL refixation using Gabor Scharioth technique

CASE SCENARIO 6: EXPLANATION OF DISLOCATED IRIS CLAW LENS IN A PSEUDOPHAKIC EYE

Case Summary

A 56-year-old female was referred from elsewhere with a PMMA rigid IOL placed in the anterior chamber after an attempt to fix an iris claw lens had failed. The patient was referred for IOL removal and scleral fixation of a newer IOL, as the primary surgeon had removed the damaged capsular bag.

The right eye had a best-corrected distance visual acuity of 6/60 with a rigid single-piece IOL in the anterior chamber **(Fig. 6A)**. The intraocular pressure was 18 mm Hg with one AGM. The pupil was dilated and not reacting to light. The fundus view was hazy with minimal vitreous hemorrhage and no apparent iatrogenic retinal injuries.

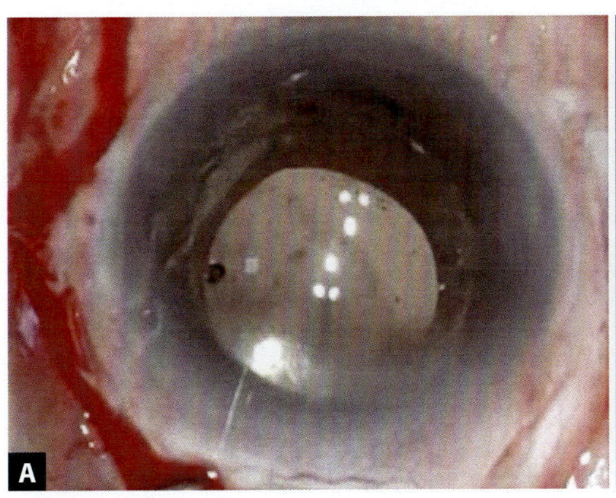
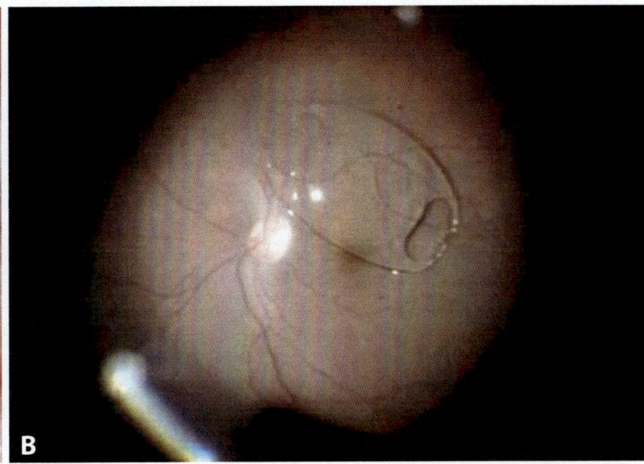

Figs. 6A and B: (A) Anterior segment image showing a rigid PMMA IOL placed in the anterior chamber; (B) Fundus image of the same eye with the dislocated iris claw IOL on the retina. (IOL: intraocular lens; PMMA: polymethyl methacrylate)

An intact iris claw IOL was noted to be posteriorly dislocated **(Fig. 6B)**.

Treatment Plan

The existing corneoscleral incision was opened

↓

The rigid PMMA IOL in the anterior chamber was guided out using a MacPherson forceps and iris repositor

↓

25G sclerotomies were made, and a complete vitrectomy was done

↓

Low infusion pressure was preferred to prevent turbulence and vigorous flow currents inside the vitreous cavity to prevent movement of the posteriorly dislocated IOL

↓

After grasping with an IOL holding forceps, it was levitated up to the iris plane and exteriorized using the handshake technique through the corneoscleral tunnel

↓

After placing an SFIOL using an ab-externo 4-exit 2-point fixation, the tunnel was sutured with 10-0 prolene **(Video 5)**

Thought Process

Decision	*Rationale*
IOL removal through the existing corneoscleral incision	Rigid IOL with a large diameter
Complete vitrectomy before IOL removal	To prevent complications like retinal detachment
First option: Placing SFIOL in the same sitting	The existing corneoscleral incision can be used for a sutured SFIOL. Better to avoid an iris claw IOL due to damaged iris tissue from previous placement
Second option: Deferred IOL placement	To analyze postoperative residual astigmatism at a later date and plan SFIOL with accurate power

(IOL: intraocular lens; SFIOL: scleral fixation of intraocular lens)

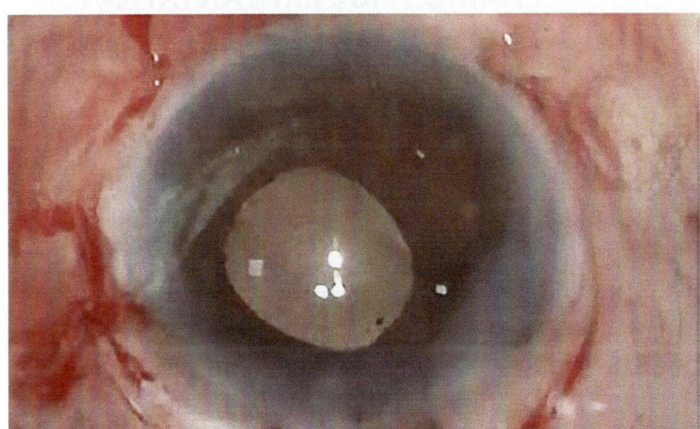

Fig. 6C: Post-scleral fixation of a PMMA IOL by the 4-exit 2-point ab-externo fixation technique. (IOL: intraocular lens; PMMA: polymethyl methacrylate)

OUTCOME SUMMARY

Postoperative 1-month follow-up revealed a well-centered IOL **(Fig. 6C)**. The vision improved to 6/9 with astigmatism correction of 1.75 DC.

KEY POINTS

- Iris claw IOLs are a good choice for aphakics with healthy iris tissue.
- Placement of a PMMA in-the-bag IOL in the anterior chamber can risk inflammation and IOP elevation.
- The best options in such cases are scleral fixation of a PMMA IOL with eyelets or a 3-piece rigid IOL with scleral tucking.

VIDEO LEGEND

Video 22: Explanation of dislocated iris claw lens in a pseudophakic eye

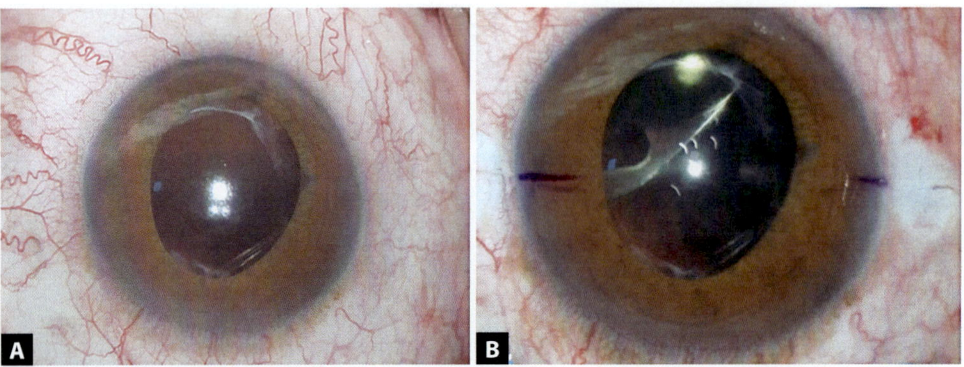

Figs. 7A and B: (A) Anterior segment image shows an intact anterior capsular rim and aphakia; (B) part of the single-piece foldable IOL. (IOL: intraocular lens)

CASE SCENARIO 7: IOL EXPLANTATION THROUGH CORNEAL TUNNEL

Case Summary

A 51-year-old male underwent phacoemulsification in his right eye 2 years ago and has had a best-corrected distance visual acuity of 6/9 since then. He presented with a sudden decrease in vision for 3 days. He denied any preceding events, including a history of trauma. He mentioned that a foldable IOL had been placed during the surgery and was on postoperative medications for >3 months. Currently, he was not on any medications and had not visited for a regular checkup post-surgery.

The best-corrected distance visual acuity in his right eye was 6/6 with +11DS. The cornea was clear, and the anterior chamber was deep. An intact anterior capsular rim was noted, and the posterior capsule was largely deficient **(Fig. 7A)**. The IOL appeared to be suspended in the anterior vitreous and was partly seen off the visual axis upon tilting the globe **(Fig. 7B)**. The fundus examination was unremarkable.

Treatment Plan

Scleral grooves and Gabor Scharioth scleral tunnels were made at 3 and 9 O'clock

↓

A clear corneal 2.8-mm entry was made

↓

The existing IOL was grasped with a MacPherson forceps, maneuvered into the anterior chamber, and exteriorized using an iris repositor

↓

The damaged capsular remnant was removed in toto

↓

The rest of the surgery was carried out with the Gabor Scharioth scleral tucking of a 3-piece IOL **(Video 6)**

Thought Process

Decision	*Rationale*
Single-piece IOL removal	Single piece IOLs are not suitable when significant posterior capsule defect is present Sulcus placement of these lenses are avoided as the large haptic surface might come in contact with iris
Anterior approach to remove the IOL	As the IOL was suspended in the anterior vitreous, it was removed through a corneal tunnel with easy maneuvers
2.8 corneal entry to remove the IOL	Since it was intended to place a foldable 3-piece IOL, a small corneal entry suffices to remove the existing IOL and insert the newer one
Limited or complete vitrectomy	Surgeon preference in this case. Complete vitrectomy is optional
Sulcus placement of IOL	If the capsular rim is intact, a 3-piece IOL in the sulcus is the simplest option
If the capsule is significantly damaged	The existing 3-piece IOL haptic is exteriorized, and the haptics are inserted into scleral pockets

(IOL: intraocular lens)

OUTCOME SUMMARY

Immediate postoperative period examination revealed a well-centered 3-piece IOL with adequate intrascleral haptic length **(Fig. 7C)**. The best corrected vision improved to 6/6p at 6-week follow-up.

KEY POINTS

- Single-piece IOLs cannot be placed on the sulcus if the capsular bag is compromised.
- Ideally, they should be removed and replaced with an appropriate lens (PMMA/3-piece IOL) in the sulcus.

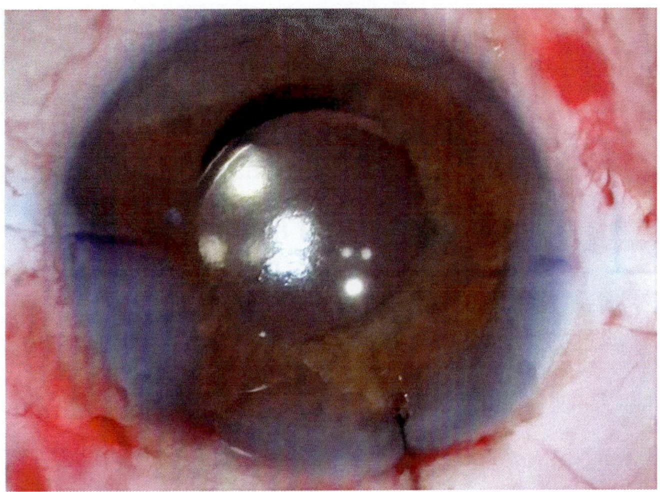

Fig. 7C: Postoperative picture of the newly placed 3-piece IOL using the Gabor Scharioth scleral tucking method. (IOL: intraocular lens)

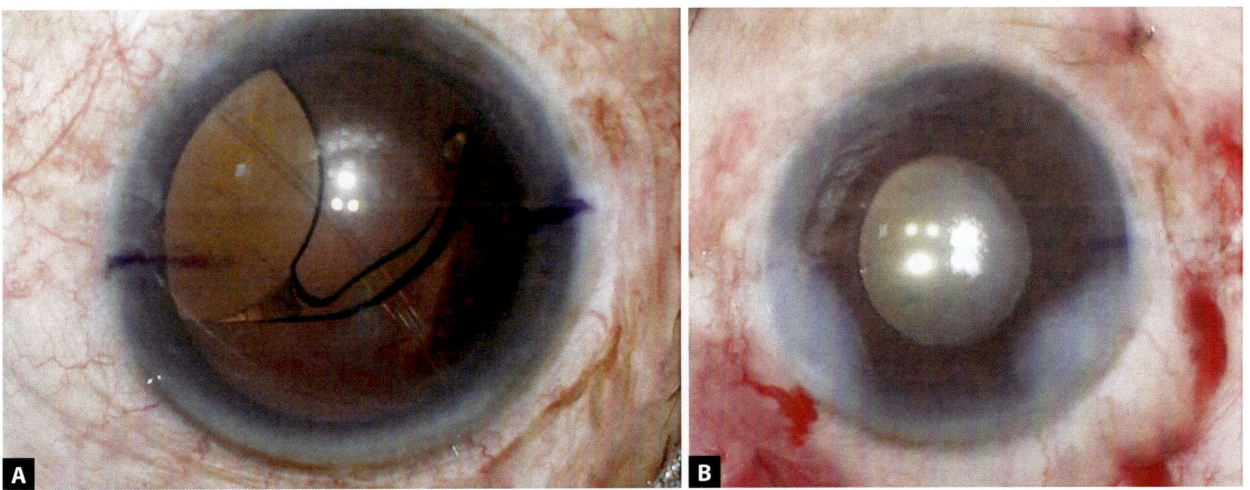

Figs. 8A and B: (A) Subluxated single-piece IOL with a compromised capsule; (B) postoperative anterior segment image showing a pierced IOL with good centration. (IOL: intraocular lens)

- Alternatively, a 3-piece IOL can be fixed with the Gabor Scharioth technique.

VIDEO LEGEND

Video 23: IOL explanation through corneal tunnel

CASE SCENARIO 8: IOL REFIXATION USING PIERCE TECHNIQUE

Case Summary

A 64-year-old female who had undergone cataract surgery 2 years ago reported a sudden drop in vision. There was no history of trauma.

On examination, the best-corrected distance visual acuity was 6/9. A single-piece IOL was displaced nasally, partly covering the pupillary area. The posterior capsule was damaged, and the anterior capsular rim appears incomplete **(Fig. 8A)**. The anterior vitreous phase appeared compromised. The retina was healthy, and the peripheral retinal examination was normal.

Treatment Plan

(Pierce technique: Piercing IOL at haptic-optic junction with sutures and anchoring to the sclera)

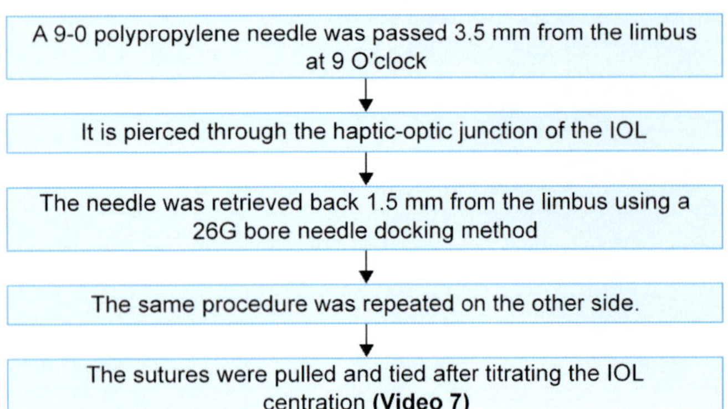

Thought Process

Decision	*Rationale*
Refix the existing IOL	Single piece without eyelets using the pierce technique
Use of 9-0 polypropylene	Piercing the IOL is easier than Gore-Tex
To place the IOL in the sulcus	Single piece with large haptics—not suitable for sulcus placement
IOL removal and SFIOL	Alternate and conventional option
Anterior vitrectomy	To clear the disturbed vitreous

(IOL: intraocular lens; SFIOL: scleral fixation of intraocular lens)

OUTCOME SUMMARY

The IOL was well centered in the postoperative period **(Fig. 8B)**. The pierced portion of the IOL was well covered under the dilated pupil. The vision improved to 6/6p with minimal astigmatism correction.

KEY POINTS

- Pierce technique is an alternative option to refix single-piece IOLs.
- 9-0/10-0 polypropylene sutures are preferable over Gore-Tex sutures.
- Closed-globe internal fixation offers a minimally invasive and cost-effective advantage.

VIDEO LEGEND

Video 24: IOL refixation using pierce technique

CASE SCENARIO 9: IOL REFIXATION USING GORE-TEX SUTURES (4 POINT FIXATION)

Case Summary

A 67-year-old lady presented with a recent onset of decreased vision in her right eye. She had undergone cataract surgery with the IOL placement done as a second procedure with vitrectomy and sutured scleral fixation of a PMMA IOL 25 years back.

The best-corrected distance visual acuity was 6/18. The pupil was dilated with anterior synechiae. An inferiorly subluxated rigid PMMA IOL was noted, with the suture snapped at one end and the other end suture exposed over the conjunctiva **(Fig. 9A—white arrow)**.

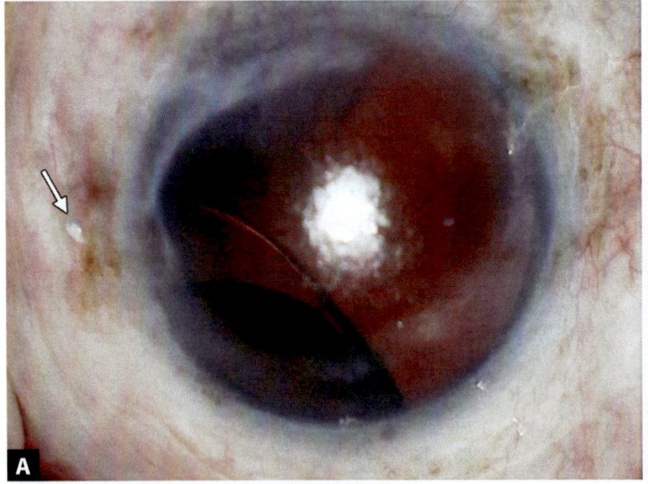

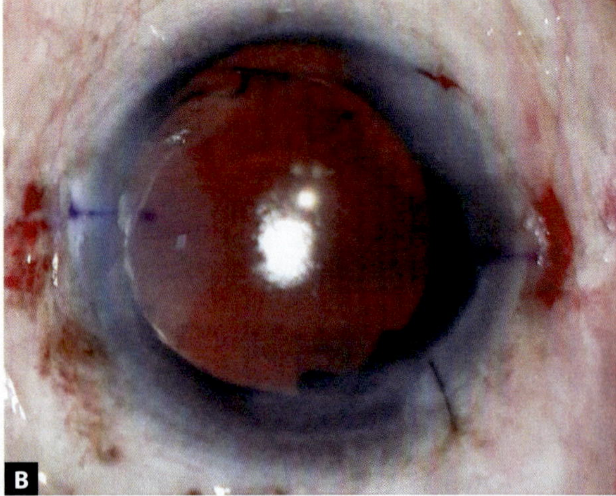

Figs. 9A and B: (A) An inferiorly subluxated rigid PMMA IOL with suture exposure (white arrow); (B) The postoperative image of the existing IOL refixated using a Gore-Tex suture. (IOL: intraocular lens; PMMA: polymethyl methacrylate)

Treatment Plan

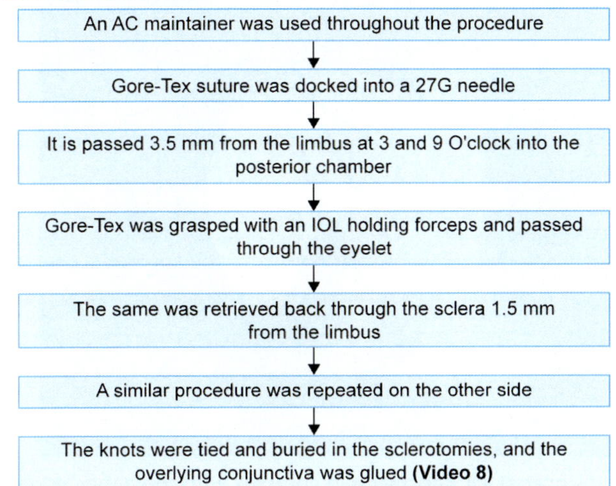

Thought Process

Decision	*Rationale*
To refix the same IOL	Being a PMMA IOL having haptics with eyelets, a refixation avoids the need for a newer IOL
To fix the same IOL in a closed globe manner	Removal and refixation of a rigid IOL needs larger scleral cutdowns. The iris being adherent to the peripheral cornea, tunnels can further compromise corneal health
Using Gore-Tex sutures instead of 9-0 polypropylene	10-0 polypropylene sutures have low strength with a tendency to break
AC maintainer or sclerotome infusion port	Since it was a vitrectomized eye, both options are feasible
4-point fixation	Gives more stability than the older 2-point fixation

(IOL: intraocular lens; PMMA: polymethyl methacrylate)

OUTCOME SUMMARY

The IOL was well centered **(Fig. 9B)**, and vision improved to 6/9 with a spherical equivalent of 1.5 D.

KEY POINTS

- Dislocation of scleral fixated sutured SFIOLs is not uncommon in the long term.
- They can often be refixed internally with sutures, avoiding large scleral cutdowns to remove the IOL.
- Internal refixation minimizes tissue damage and is also cost-effective.

VIDEO LEGEND

Video 25: IOL refixation using gore-tex sutures (4 point fixation)

CASE SCENARIO 10: IOL REFIXATION WITH CAPSULAR BAG USING GORE-TEX SUTURE (8-POINT FIXATION)

Case Summary

A 51-year-old gentleman had his right eye operated on 11 years ago and presented to us with diminished vision of 2 weeks' duration. He had undergone surgery for a traumatic cataract, and the surgery was apparently uneventful.

The best-corrected distance visual acuity was 6/60 in the right eye, and a grossly decentered IOL bag complex was floating in the anterior vitreous **(Fig. 10A)**, with a plate-haptic IOL design **(Fig. 10B)**. The vitreous was clear, and the retina was healthy, attached with normal periphery.

Treatment Plan

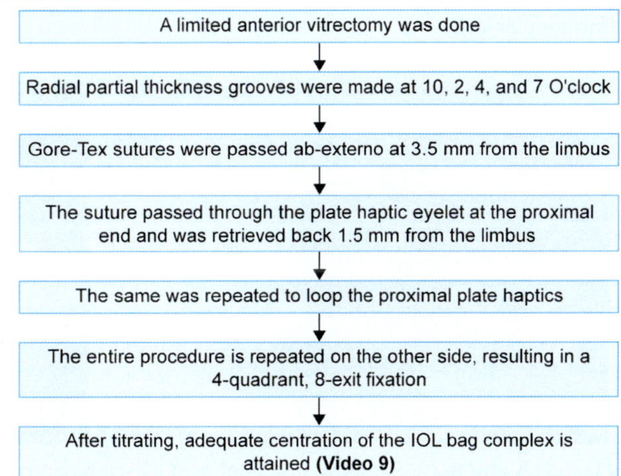

Thought Process

Decision	*Rationale*
To refix the existing IOL	The larger aperture in the plate haptics can serve as eyelets for the suture and can be fixed to the sclera
To fix the existing IOL along with the capsular bag	Fixing the entire IOL-bag complex prevents haptics from coming in contact with the posterior iris and thus reduces iris chaffing
Using Gore-Tex sutures instead of 9-0 polypropylene	10-0 polypropylene sutures have low strength with a tendency to break
25 G good anterior vitrectomy or complete vitrectomy	As suture is passed at 4 quadrants, the areas should be free of vitreous hence good anterior vitrectomy must but a complete vitrectomy with adequate base shaving is preferred
8-point fixation	Gives more stability than the conventional 4-point fixation

(IOL: intraocular lens)

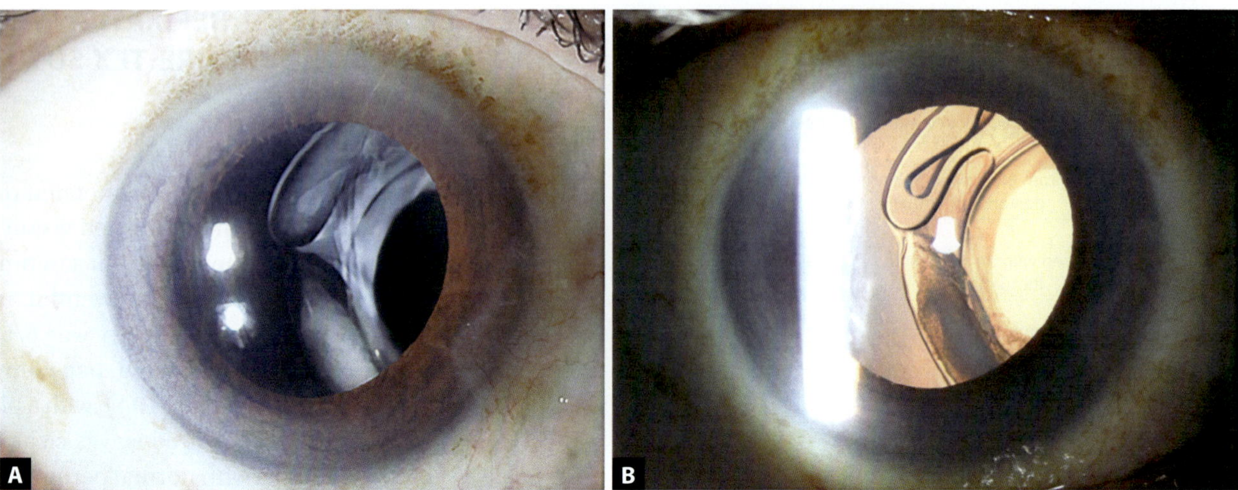

Figs. 10A and B: (A) Anterior segment of the right eye showing a nasally dislocated IOL capsular bag complex with the haptic edge at the pupillary center; (B) Retroilluminated image that revealed the plate haptic IOL design within the dislocated capsular bag. (IOL: intraocular lens)

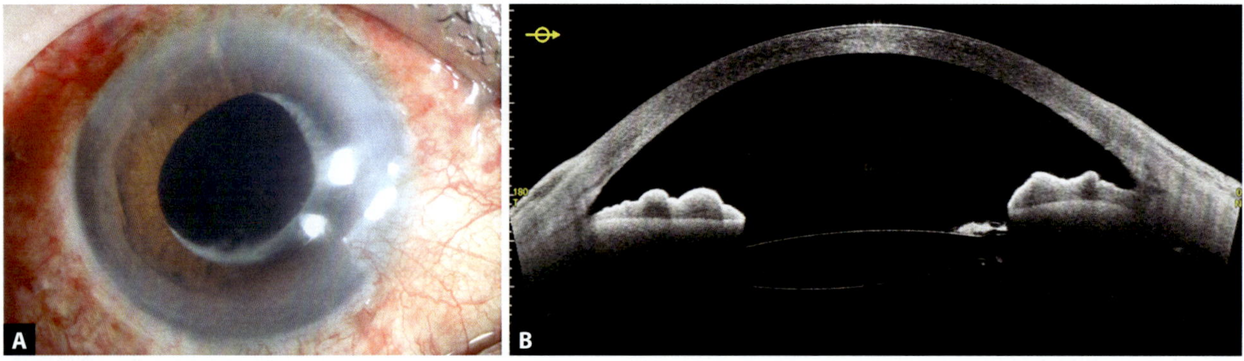

Figs. 11A and B: (A) Slit-lamp image of post IOL-bag complex fixation showing adequate centration; (B) Anterior segment OCT imaging, showing minimal tilt, adequate vaulting, and good centration. (IOL: intraocular lens)

OUTCOME SUMMARY

The bag complex was well centered postoperatively. Anterior segment OCT showed acceptable tilt and minimal decentration with an adequate IOL-iris gap **(Figs. 11A and B)**.

KEY POINTS

- Whole-bag complex refixation prevents the conventional management of its removal.
- The capsular bag prevents haptic touch to the cornea, thereby preventing iris chuffing.
- This capsular bag fixation is feasible irrespective of the type of IOL present in the bag.

VIDEO LEGEND

Video 26: IOL refixation with capsular bag using Gore-tex suture (8 point fixation)

CASE SCENARIO 11: PLACEMENT OF SECONDARY IOL USING FLANGED TECHNIQUE

Case Summary

A 64-year-old male had undergone lensectomy and anterior vitrectomy for traumatic anterior subluxation of the lens 6 weeks back. He was referred for a secondary IOL implantation.

The best-corrected distance vision was 6/8p in the right eye. The anterior segment showed a dilated and fixed pupil (traumatic mydriasis) and aphakia with no capsular remnants **(Fig. 12A)**. Fundus examination revealed a healthy-looking retina with a normal periphery. The intraocular pressure was 14 mm Hg without any medications.

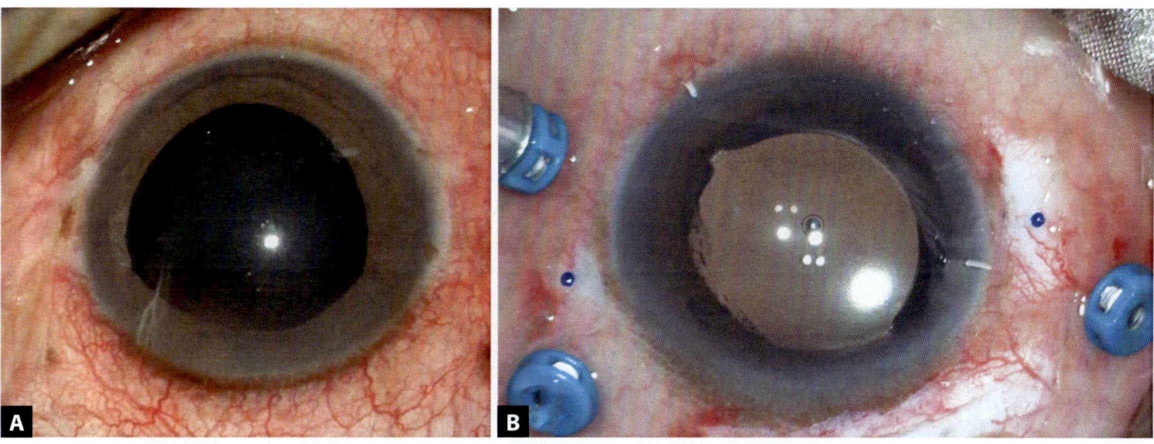

Figs. 12A and B: (A) Anterior segment image of the right eye with a clear cornea, traumatic mydriasis, and aphakia; (B) Intraoperative picture of a well-centered IOL and flanged sutures at 3 and 9 o'clock positions. (IOL: intraocular lens)

Treatment Plan

A superior sclerocorneal tunnel (6.5-mm wide) was created for the insertion of a rigid PMMA IOL with eyelets in the haptics

↓

A complete vitrectomy was done, including PVD induction and peripheral base shaving

↓

5-0 polypropylene suture is passed 2 mm from the limbus and brought through the sclerocorneal tunnel

↓

The thread is passed through the eyelet of the haptic and flanged

↓

The same procedure is repeated on the other end

↓

The IOL is positioned under the iris, and the sutures at 3 and 9 O'clock are cut and flanged adequately, ensuring good centration of the IOL **(Video 10)**

Thought Process

Decision	*Rationale*
Scleral fixation of IOL	As the capsular bag has been removed during the primary surgery. In dilated fixed pupils, iris claw IOL is not an ideal option
Large diameter PMMA IOL	The larger optics cover a larger pupillary area, thereby preventing lens-edge shadow/positive scotomas
5-0 polypropylene sutures for flanging	Thicker and stronger suture, less chance of suture erosion/breakage
Complete vitrectomy (optional)	Complete vitrectomy in post-traumatic cases is desirable to prevent postoperative retinal complications
2-point fixation	Flanging of suture ends at 2 points for ease of use

(IOL: intraocular lens; PMMA: polymethyl methacrylate)

OUTCOME SUMMARY

The IOL was well centered at the end of the surgery **(Fig. 12B)**. The flanges are well buried under the conjunctiva. At 6 weeks post-surgery, vision improved to 6/6.

KEY POINTS

- The flanging technique offers an alternative technique to the conventional ab-externo suture loop method.
- Adequate flange size and securing it under the conjunctiva is paramount.
- The thicker suture makes it longer lasting than 9-0/10-0 polypropylene sutures.

SUMMARIZED KEY POINTS: INTRAOCULAR LENS DISLOCATION MANAGEMENT AND SECONDARY INTRAOCULAR LENS IMPLANTATION

- The dislocated IOL should be removed as a planned procedure, provided there are no complications such as raised IOP, vitreocorneal touch, retinal detachment, vitreous hemorrhage, or endophthalmitis.
- The presence of an intact anterior capsular rim can be used for sulcus placement of 3-piece IOLs.
- Pre-existing 3-piece IOLs can be fixed to the sclera by tucking haptics into scleral pockets using different techniques.
- Other IOLs can be refixed using various sutured techniques, such as the lasso or pierce technique.

FURTHER READING

1. Canabrava S, Canêdo Domingos Lima AC, Ribeiro G. Four-Flanged Intrascleral Intraocular Lens Fixation Technique: No Flaps, No Knots, No Glue. Cornea. 2020;39(4):527-8.
2. Choudhary A, Sehgal G, Jayadev C, Krishnappa NC. Closed globe refixation of the IOL-bag complex with the ab-externo 8-exit-4-point fixation technique. Indian J Ophthalmol. 2025;73(3):442-5.
3. Choudhary A, Sehgal G, Jayadev C, Krishnappa NC. Modified ab-externo scleral fixation method for dislocated scleral fixated intraocular lenses. Indian J Ophthalmol. 2025;73(3):450-4.
4. Domingues M, Brito P, Falcão M, Monteiro T, Falcão-Reis F. Cupid fixation for repositioning subluxated intraocular lens. J Cataract Refract Surg. 2011;37(9):1571-5.
5. Gabor SG, Pavlidis MM. Sutureless intrascleral posterior chamber intraocular lens fixation. J Cataract Refract Surg. 2007;33(11):1851-4.
6. Rao SK, Gopal L, Fogla R, Lam DS, Padmanabhan P. Ab externo 4-point scleral fixation. J Cataract Refract Surg. 2000;26(1):9-10.

VIDEO LEGEND

Video 27: Placement of secondary IOL using flanged technique

CHAPTER 13

Decision Making in Surgical Management of Intraocular Tumors

Simakurthy Sriram, Meenakshi Mahesh, P Mahesh Shanmugam

ALGORITHMIC APPROACH TO SURGICAL MANAGEMENT OF INTRAOCULAR TUMORS

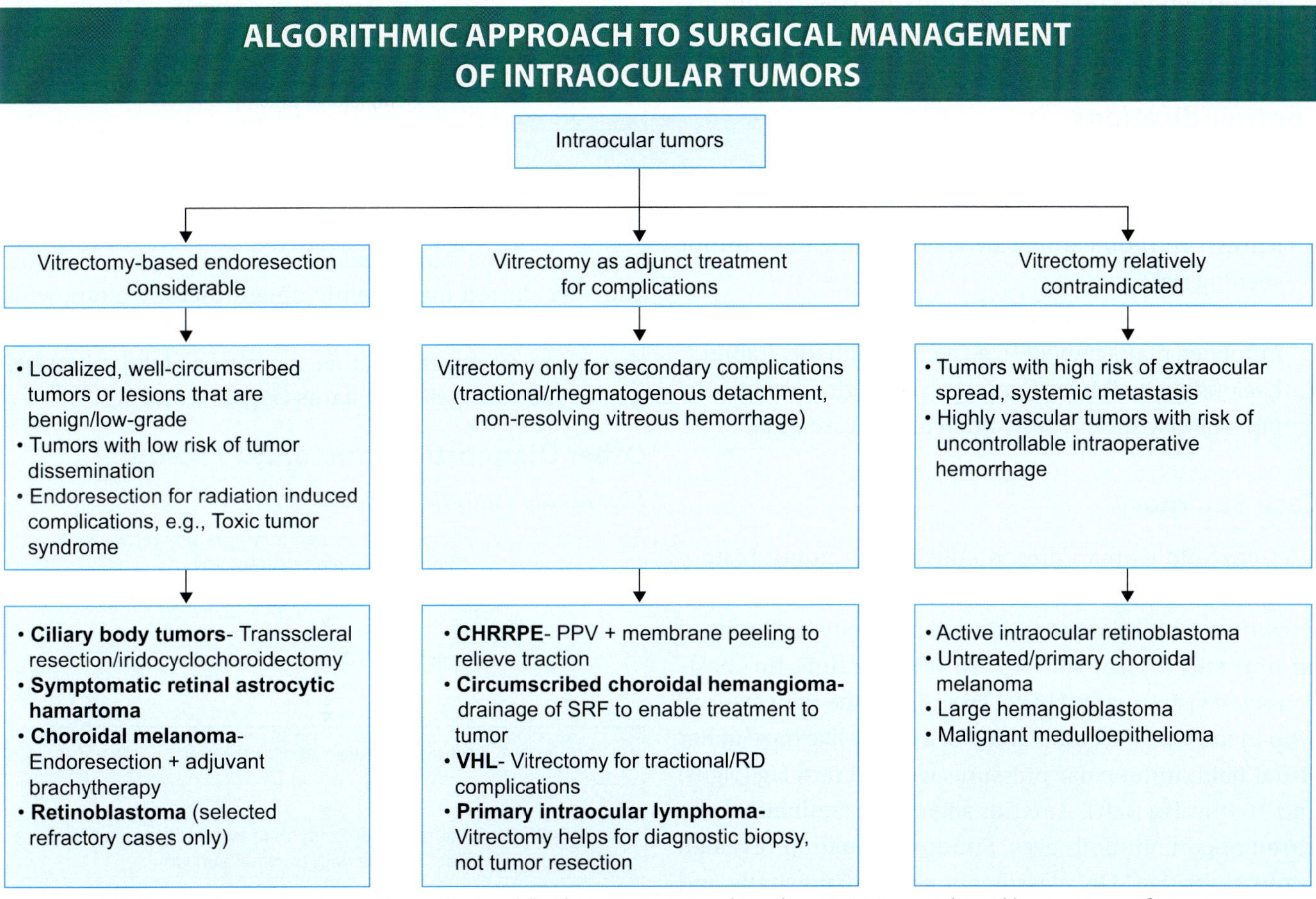

(PPV: pars plana vitrectomy; SRF: subretinal fluid; VHL: Von Hippel-Lindau; CHRRPE: combined hamartoma of retina and retinal pigment epithelium)

CASE SCENARIO 1: DIAGNOSTIC SURGICAL PROCEDURES

Diagnostic vitrectomy and adjunct procedures such as fine needle aspiration biopsy (FNAB) and intralesional biopsy play an important role in evaluation of intraocular mass lesions when clinical, and imaging techniques are nonconclusive. These techniques help in histopathological or cytological diagnosis with minimal risk of tumor spread when planned appropriately. Their use must be tailored to the suspected pathology, tumor location, and surgical feasibility.

Indications

- When diagnosis is uncertain—unexplained mass lesion, atypical uveitis, or masquerades which are unresponsive to corticosteroids or immunosuppressants

- Suspected intraocular lymphoma or metastasis to uveal tissue
- Amelanotic or atypical mass lesions: To differentiate between melanoma, hemangioma, or metastasis, pigmented or vascular lesions such as melanocytoma, CHRRPE (combined hamartoma of retina and retinal pigment epithelium)
- Molecular or genetic profiling—molecular confirmation of lymphoma (IgH rearrangement) or gene expression analysis (uveal melanoma).

Contraindications

- Extensive necrotic or hemorrhagic tumors with poor yield and high perforation risk
- Known retinoblastoma or lesions with high tumor seeding risk
- Eyes with no visual potential where diagnosis will not influence management (e.g., enucleation inevitable)
- Lesions accessible by noninvasive imaging or aqueous tap—biopsy should be avoided unless essential.

Case Summary

A 53-year-old woman presented with a 2-month history of blurred vision in both eyes. She had been diagnosed elsewhere with bilateral intermediate uveitis and started on oral and topical steroids. At presentation, her best-corrected visual acuity (BCVA) was 6/9 in the right eye and 6/6p in the left. She complained of a cloud-like haze in her visual field. Intraocular pressures were 15 mm Hg (right) and 16 mm Hg (left). Anterior segment examination was unremarkable in both eyes. Fundus evaluation revealed grade 1 vitritis (SUN classification) with snowballs and yellowish subretinal deposits. A uveitis workup was negative for infectious or autoimmune etiologies. 2 weeks later, her vision declined to 6/18 (right) and 6/9 (left) with worsening of intraocular inflammation. Given the progressive course and presence of subretinal deposits, primary intraocular lymphoma was suspected, and diagnostic vitrectomy was planned after discontinuation of steroids.

Treatment Plan

Vitreous biopsy:

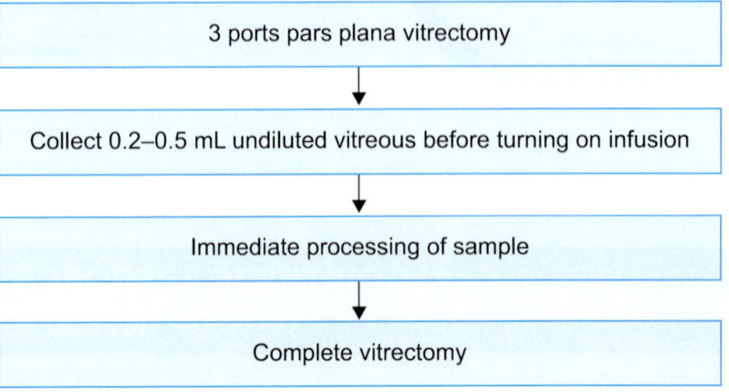

Outcome Summary

Cytological analysis confirmed primary intraocular lymphoma. The patient underwent oncologic evaluation and was started on systemic chemotherapy along with intravitreal methotrexate. At 6 months postoperatively, she showed a well-attached retina, regression of the subretinal lesion, and stable clinical status **(Figs. 1A and B)**.

Other Diagnostic Vitrectomy Procedures

Fine needle aspiration biopsy:

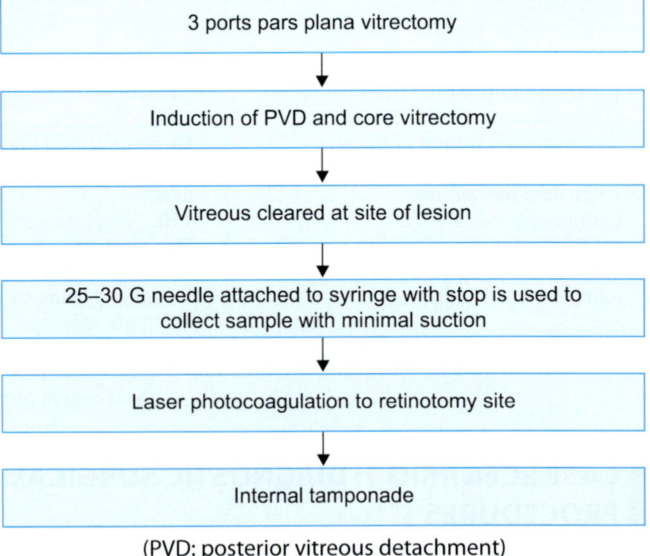

(PVD: posterior vitreous detachment)

Fine needle aspiration biopsy can also be performed via transscleral route under indirect ophthalmoscope

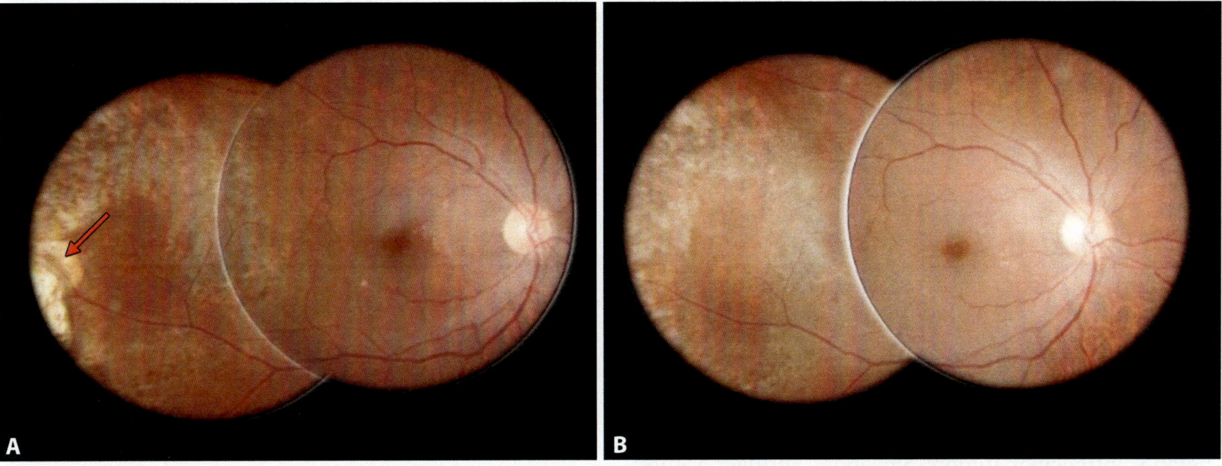

Figs. 1A and B: (A) Immediate postoperative fundus photo showing clear vitreous media with subretinal lesion (red arrow); (B) 6 months postoperative fundus photo showing resolution of subretinal lesions.

visualization. However, it has steep learning curve and is prone to complications such as massive intraocular hemorrhage, retinal break formation resulting from inappropriate movement of the needle within the eye. The laterally and vertically inverted image seen through the indirect ophthalmoscope and the need to operate with one hand (other hand holding the condensing lens) makes the technique challenging. In eyes where FNAB is done without vitrectomy, it is not imperative to laser the retinotomy site as it seldom results in a retinal detachment.

Incisional biopsy:

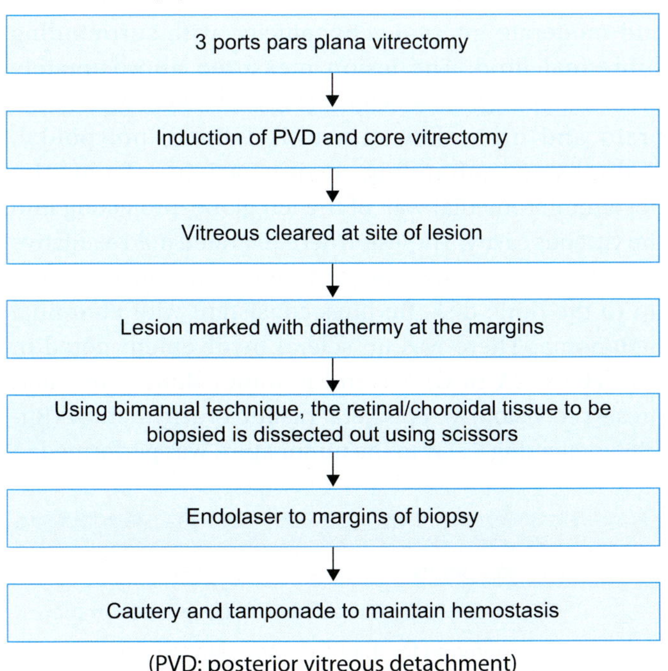

(PVD: posterior vitreous detachment)

Thought Process

Procedure	*Key points*
Vitreous biopsy	• Stop steroids prior to planned procedure to avoid false negative • Undiluted sample increases diagnostic yield • Can consider vitrectomy under air, but compression of the vitreous to the retina by air and visualization issues make it difficult • Using low cut rate and large gauge surgery prevents cell damage • Immediate and early fixing of the sample slide using HEPES increases diagnostic yield
FNAB	• Can be done transscleral or transvitreal • Transvitreal route helps in real time visualization and increases diagnostic yield
Incisional biopsy	• Localizing lesion with diathermy helps in maintaining hemostasis • Laser to margins prior to retinectomy helps in securing the edges of the retinectomy • PFCL-assisted incisional biopsy preferred • In cases where choroidal biopsy is planned, deep penetrating diathermy is used • Enlargement of sclerotomy may be needed depending on size of the tissue biopsied, if aphakic can be brought out through the limbus

(FNAB: fine needle aspiration biopsy; PFCL: perfluorocarbon liquid)

KEY POINTS

- Obtain undiluted vitreous before starting infusion.
- Maintain closed system and minimal manipulation to prevent tumor seeding.

- Coordinate with cytopathologist for immediate fixation.
- Use tamponade and local photocoagulation for hemostasis.
- Limit biopsy to eyes where results influence management.

FURTHER READING

1. Chhablani J. Diagnostic vitreous biopsy in suspected intraocular lymphoma. Indian J Ophthalmol. 2018;66(10): 1395-400.
2. Eide N, Walaas L. Fine-needle aspiration biopsy and other biopsies in intraocular tumors. Curr Opin Ophthalmol. 2009;20(6):488-92.
3. Khetan V. Intraocular Tumors. Singapore: Springer Nature; 2020.
4. Shields CL, Shields JA. Intraocular Tumors: An Atlas and Textbook, 3rd edition. Netherlands: Wolters Kluwer; 2016.

VIDEO LEGENDS

Video 28: 1a: Diagnostic vitrectomy.
Video 29: 1b: Fine needle aspiration biopsy.
Video 30: 1c: Incisional biopsy.

CASE SCENARIO 2: PLAQUE BRACHYTHERAPY IN MANAGEMENT OF CHOROIDAL MELANOMA

Background

Brachytherapy is a localized radiation therapy that delivers high doses of radiation directly to intraocular tumors via a radioactive plaque that is sutured over sclera. This technique preserves both globe architecture and visual function and provides survival outcomes comparable to enucleation for medium sized choroidal melanoma. The choice of radioactive isotopes—iodine 125 or ruthenium 106—depends on tumor thickness (*see* **Table 1**). Though, safe procedure, long-term complications include cataract and radiation retinopathy. This technique needs precision dosimetry and plaque placement.

Indications

- *Uveal melanomas*: Medium-sized choroidal melanomas with base diameter ≤16 mm and thickness ≤10 mm
- *Retinoblastoma:* Solitary, recurrent, or residual tumors with basal diameter ≤16 mm and thickness ≤8 mm
- *Choroidal hemangioma*: Circumscribed lesions causing exudative retinal detachment and not responsive to laser or photodynamic therapy
- *Vasoproliferative tumors*

Contraindications

- *Tumor size limits*: Tumors exceeding 18–20 mm in basal dimension or >10–12 mm in thickness.
- Tumors with extrascleral extension or optic nerve invasion beyond lamina cribrosa.
- Diffuse infiltrative retinoblastoma or vitreous seeding.
- Painful blind eyes where enucleation is more appropriate.

Case Summary

A 50-year-old male presented with a 2-year history of blurred vision in the left eye. Best-corrected visual acuity was 6/6 in the right eye and 6/6p in the left. Right eye examination was within normal limits. Left eye anterior segment was normal and fundus examination of the left eye revealed a peripapillary, dome-shaped brownish mass involving the inferior disk margin, associated with an inferior exudative retinal detachment and absence of drusen or orange pigment. B-scan ultrasonography demonstrated a choroidal mass located inferonasal to the optic disk, exhibiting moderate-to-high surface reflectivity and moderate internal echogenicity, with surrounding subretinal fluid. The lesion measured approximately 11.4 × 5.3 mm (base × height) **(Figs. 2A to C)**. MRI of the brain and orbit showed a well-defined, polypoidal, endophytic enhancing lesion arising from the posteroinferomedial wall of the left globe, projecting into the vitreous cavity. The lesion demonstrated mild exudative enhancement along the posterior wall and extended up to the optic disk, findings consistent with choroidal melanoma. There was no scleral involvement noted in MRI **(Figs. 2A to C)**. Given the tumor dimensions and preserved vision, an episcleral plaque brachytherapy (Ru-106), delivering 85 Gy to the tumor apex, was performed.

TABLE 1: Applicability of plaque types.

Plaque type	*Maximum tumor thickness*	*Maximum basal diameter*	*Key points*
Iodine (I-125)	≤10 mm	≤16–20 mm	Preferred for thicker tumors, deeper penetration
Ruthenium (Ru-106)	≤6–8 mm	≤16–20 mm	Preferred for thinner tumors, limited penetration

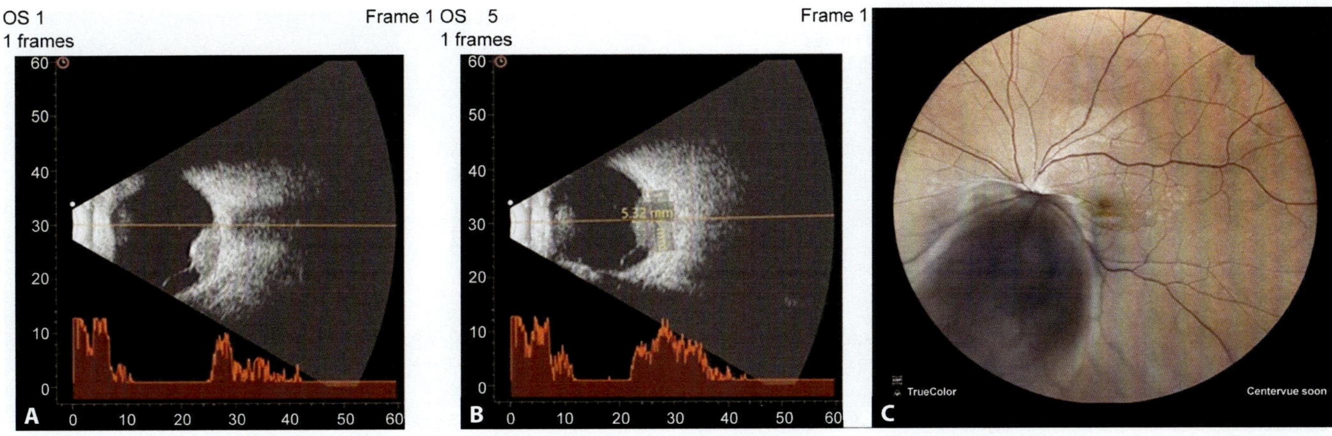

Figs. 2A to C: (A and B) Preoperative B-scan showing a dome-shaped choroidal mass lesion with moderate–high surface reflectivity and moderate internal echogenicity with adjacent subretinal fluid with tumor dimensions (W*H – 11.44 * 5.32 mm); (C) Fundus photograph showing a choroidal melanoma in inferonasal quadrant.

Planning Brachytherapy

Treatment planning is based on tumor size, location, and isotope activity. The objective is to deliver the prescribed dose to the tumor apex while sparing critical structures.

- *Dose to tumor apex*: 70–100 Gy for choroidal melanoma, 40–50 Gy for retinoblastoma, and 20–30 Gy for hemangioma
- *Isotopes used*: Iodine-125 (low-energy, deeper penetration), Ruthenium-106 (beta emitter, shallow penetration), Palladium-103 (shorter half-life)
- *Shielding*: The radioactive plaque material is designed to allow unidirectional radiation exposure toward the vitreous cavity.
- *Isolation room*: With radiation monitor affixed

Treatment Plan

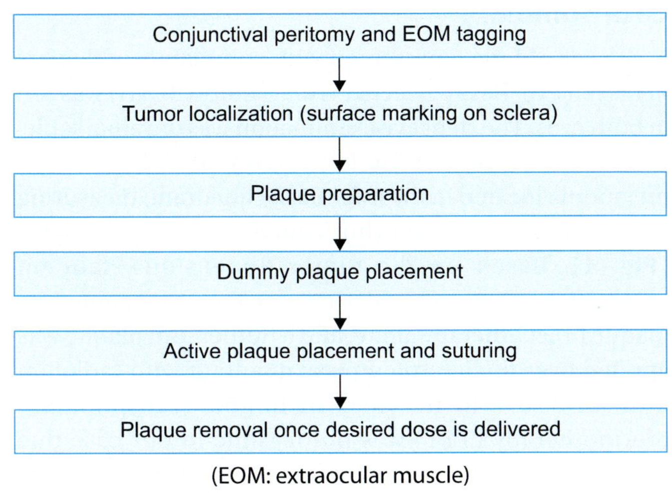

(EOM: extraocular muscle)

Thought Process

Step	*Rationale*
Episcleral localization	Allows accurate placement of the plaque over the tumor
Plaque placement	Tilt or displacement could lead to underdosing
Plaque preparation	Ensures appropriate penetration and dosing based on tumor thickness and location, while minimizing exposure to critical structures

OUTCOME SUMMARY

On follow-up, the lesion demonstrated progressive regression with development of macular hard exudates and edema, which were managed with a steroid implant. At 6 months post-treatment, the choroidal melanoma had regressed, visual acuity improved to 6/6, and mild optic disk pallor persisted **(Figs. 3A to C)**.

KEY POINTS

- Brachytherapy provides effective local control with globe preservation in selected intraocular tumors.
- Isotope selection and duration depend on tumor thickness and proximity to critical structures.
- Accurate plaque positioning and dosimetric planning are vital to success.
- Long-term follow-up is essential to detect recurrence and radiation-related complications.

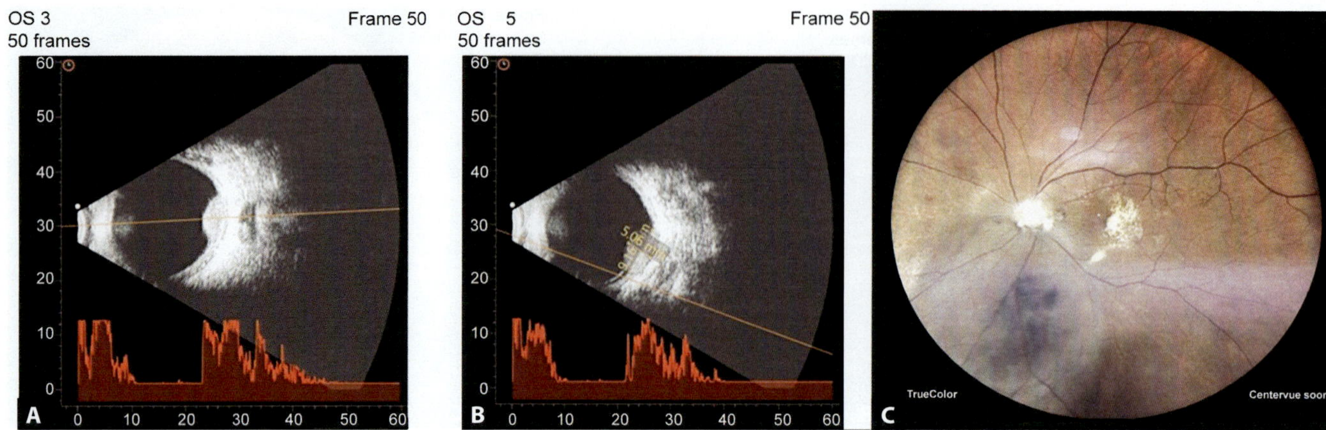

Figs. 3A to C: (A and B) Preoperative B-scan showing a dome-shaped choroidal mass lesion with moderate–high surface reflectivity and moderate internal echogenicity with adjacent subretinal fluid with tumor dimensions (W*H – 9.25 * 5.03 mm); (C) Fundus photograph showing a regressing choroidal melanoma in inferonasal quadrant.

- Adjuvant transpupillary thermotherapy (TTT) can be done for thicker melanomas when treating with Ru 106-sandwich therapy.

FURTHER READING

1. American Brachytherapy Society Ophthalmic Oncology Task Force. ABS consensus guidelines for plaque brachytherapy for ocular melanoma and retinoblastoma. Brachytherapy. 2014;13(1):1-14.
2. Fionda B, Pagliara MM, Chyrek AJ, Guix B, O'Day RFJ, Fog LS, et al. Ocular Brachytherapy (Interventional Radiotherapy): Preserving the Vision. Clin Oncol (R Coll Radiol). 2023;35(8):e445-52.
3. Khetan V. Intraocular Tumors. Singapore: Springer Nature; 2020.
4. Lim J, Teo AWJ, Siow TR, Chan KP, Tan GSW. Innovations in brachytherapy. Taiwan J Ophthalmol. 2025;15(1):62-72.
5. Tuncer S. Brachytherapy in the Management of Uveal Melanomas. Turk J Ophthalmol. 2014;44(1):43-8.

VIDEO LEGEND

Video 31: Brachytherapy for intraocular tumors.

CASE SCENARIO 3: ENDORESECTION AS PART OF MANAGEMENT OF CHOROIDAL MELANOMA

Background

Ab-interno resection of choroidal melanoma was first described by Peyman and Cohen. The term and refined technique of endoresection was popularized by Damato. Though technically challenging, it is a viable eye-preserving option for selected patients, as an alternative to enucleation or radiotherapy. There is no extra risk of metastasis post choroidal endoresection as compared to brachytherapy.

Indications

Endoresection is suitable for:

- Tumors unsuitable for brachytherapy or radiotherapy
- Medium-sized posterior melanomas (height 8–10 mm, diameter <16 mm)
- Cases where globe preservation is desired and the tumor does not involve the ciliary body or optic nerve

Contraindications

- Basal diameter >16 mm
- Ciliary body involvement
- Optic nerve involvement

Case Summary

A 38-year-old male presented with complaints of floaters in his left eye. Best-corrected visual acuity (BCVA) was 6/6 in both eyes. The right eye examination was unremarkable. Fundus evaluation of the left eye revealed a choroidal melanoma located in the inferonasal quadrant, measuring 10.22 × 9.75 × 7.91 mm (horizontal × vertical × height) **(Fig. 4)**. Based on the tumor dimensions, tandem brachytherapy was advised. However, the patient opted for plaque brachytherapy alone, and a Ruthenium plaque was applied over the inferotemporal quadrant with radiation dose of 85 Gy to the apex of tumor. Transpupillary thermotherapy (TTT) was not feasible in our case due to the pedunculated nature of the tumor. The tumor was

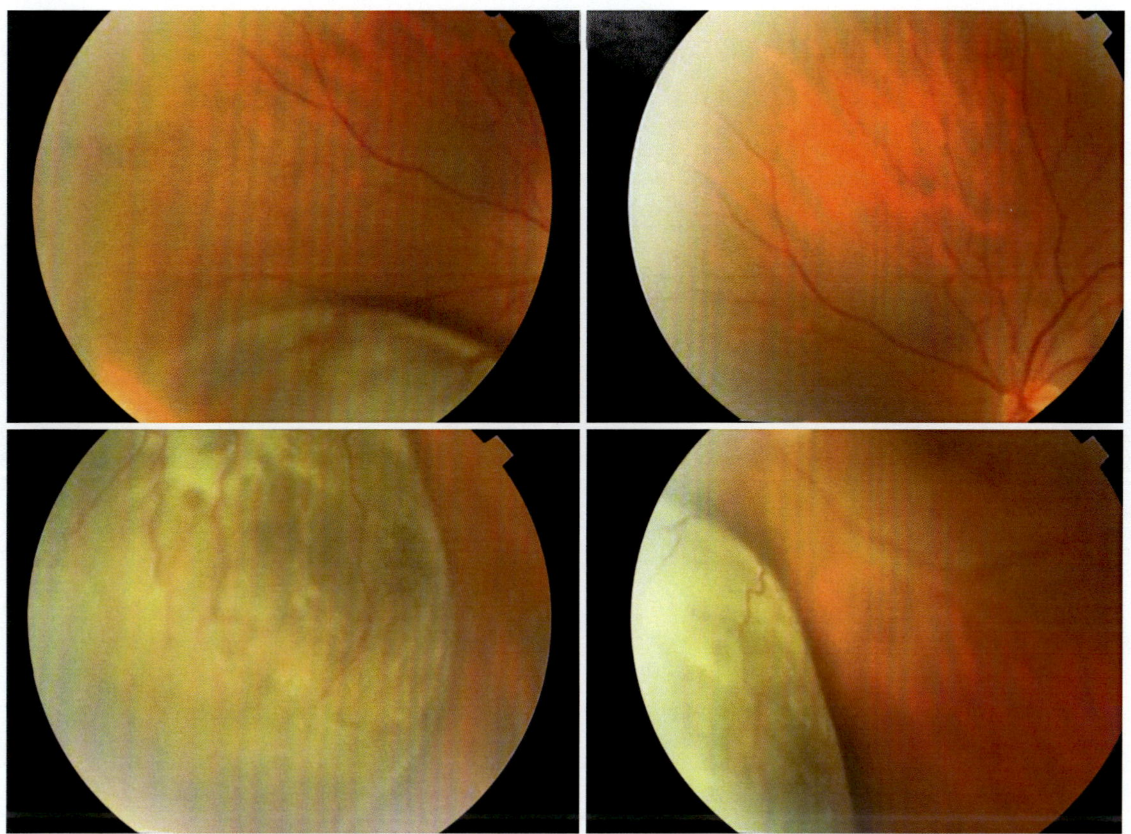

Fig. 4: Fundus photo showing dome-shaped pigmented elevated mass lesion in inferonasal quadrant suggestive of choroidal melanoma.

stable without further growth in the follow-up period. However, 6 months after brachytherapy, endoresection of the tumor was performed as patient developed toxic tumor syndrome.

Treatment Plan

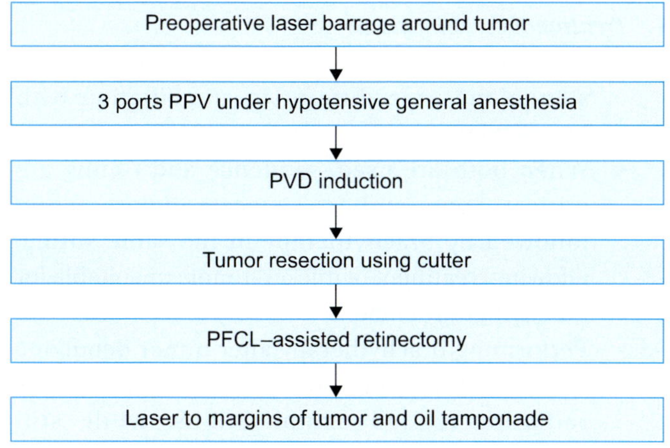

(PFCL: perfluorocarbon liquid; PPV: pars plana vitrectomy; PVD: posterior vitreous detachment)

Thought Process

Step	*Rationale*
Preoperative laser photo-coagulation	• Decreases vascularity to tumor • Acts as barrage to minimize risk of subsequent retinal detachment due to retinectomy
Anesthesia	General anesthesia is usually preferred to maintain controlled hypotension and minimize the risk of intraoperative choroidal hemorrhage
Tumor resection	The tumor is removed piecemeal using vitrectomy cutter
Hemostasis	• Elevate the bottle height (gravity-assisted fluidics) or set active fluidics at high IOP • Cautery done to bleeders
Endo laser	• Done to tumor margins—helps identify margins of resection and follow-ups • Done to tumor bed—to destroy tumor cells adherent to sclera, which cannot be removed satisfactorily
Tamponade	PFCL—silicone oil exchange is preferred to reduce risk of air embolism

(IOP: intraocular pressure; PFCL: perfluorocarbon liquid)

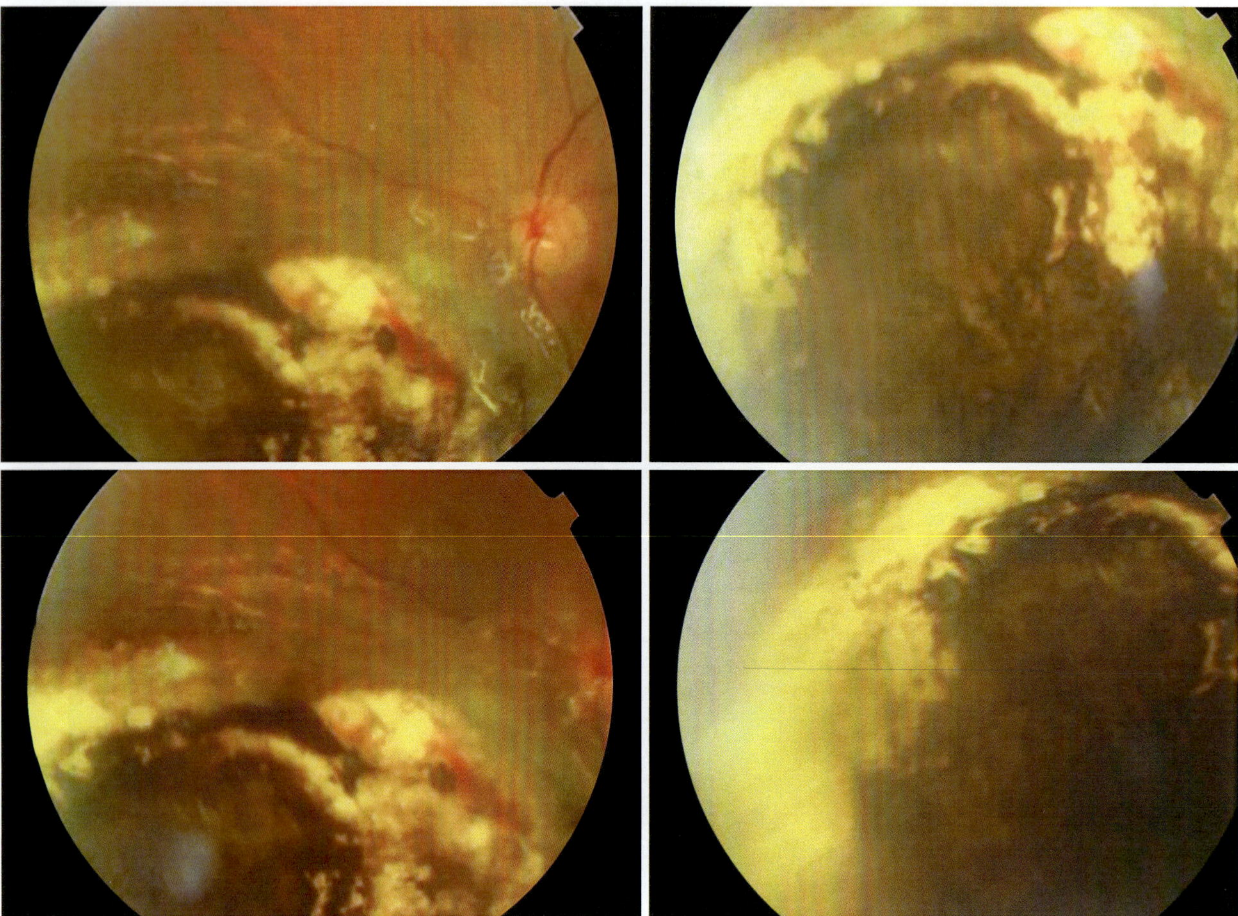

Fig. 5: Postoperative image of left eye fundus showing areas of tumor endoresection surrounded by laser scars and well-attached retina with silicone oil tamponade.

OUTCOME SUMMARY

Postoperatively, the patient is stable without growth of melanoma. Patient underwent silicone oil removal with epiretinal membrane (ERM) peeling at 4 months follow-up period **(Fig. 5)**.

KEY POINTS

- Endoresection is a globe-salvaging surgical option for selected cases of choroidal melanoma, especially when conventional radiotherapy or brachytherapy is unsuitable or as an adjunct to brachytherapy.
- Proper patient selection and meticulous surgical technique are essential to minimize intraoperative and postoperative complications.
- *Possible complications* include vitreous hemorrhage, retinal detachment, proliferative vitreoretinopathy, residual or recurrent tumor, radiation retinopathy (in combined cases), and endophthalmitis.
- Preoperative laser and careful intraoperative hemostasis help reduce tumor dissemination risk.
- Long-term follow-up is mandatory to monitor for local recurrence or secondary complications.
- *Treatment combinations*:
    - Endoresection can be performed as a standalone procedure or in combination with brachytherapy.
    - When both are used, sequence and timing are critical. Some authors advocate endoresection followed by brachytherapy in the same sitting, allowing treatment of thicker tumors unsuitable for brachytherapy alone.
    - Performing brachytherapy after tumor debulking reduces total radiation dose and minimizes radiation-related complications, while still ensuring tumor control.

FURTHER READING

1. Anguita R, Kiilgaard JF. Endoresection of choroidal melanoma: practical and safety considerations. Eye. 2025;39:1875-7.
2. Damato B, Groenewald C, McGalliard J, Wong D. Endoresection of choroidal melanoma. Br J Ophthalmol. 1998;82(3):213-18.
3. Garcia-Arumi J, Distefano LN, Quijano C. Endoresection of a high equatorial choroidal melanoma. Retin Cases Brief Rep. 2015;9(1):30-2.
4. Peyman GA, Cohen SB. Ab interno resection of uveal melanoma. Int Ophthalmol. 1986;9(1):29-36.

VIDEO LEGEND

Video 32: Endoresection in choroidal melanoma.

CASE SCENARIO 4: VITRECTOMY FOR MANAGEMENT OF RRD, IN EYE WITH RETINOBLASTOMA

Background

Vitrectomy, although seldom practiced in eyes with retinoblastoma, can be considered in cases with retinal detachment, vitreous hemorrhage, tractional detachments, or to salvage the only seeing eye. In a study by Li et al., on 28 retinoblastoma patients who underwent vitrectomy as a treatment for intraocular retinoblastoma, and followed up for almost 6 years, 35.7% patients underwent enucleation ultimately, but the 5-year survival rate was almost 96%. Factors carrying worse prognosis were eyes with higher stage and posterior location of the tumor. Shields et al. published a study of 11 patients who were unsuspected prior to surgery to have RB. They did not recommend vitrectomy in eyes with RB. If performed in unsuspected cases, they recommended enucleation with combined adjuvant chemotherapy, radiotherapy, or both.

Indications

- *Rhegmatogenous retinal detachments (RRD)*: In eyes with active or regressed tumors
- Sequelae of radiation retinopathy such as vitreous hemorrhage, anterior hyaloid proliferation
- Macular holes
- Tractional retinal detachment
- Recalcitrant tumors, especially in one eyed patient

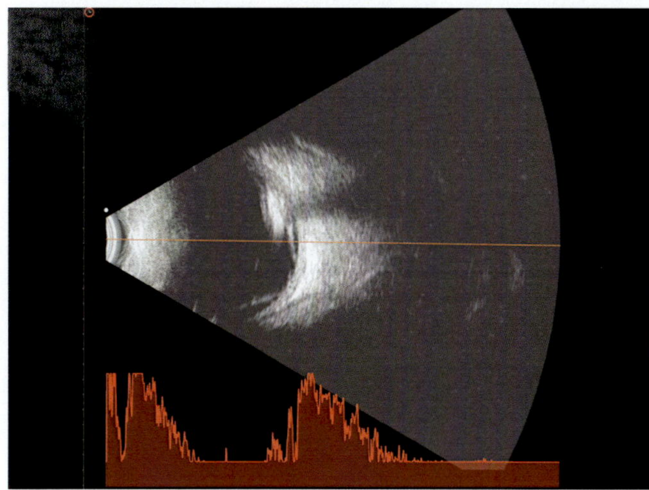

Fig. 6: B-scan image depicting mass lesion abutting the optic disk with hyperechoic regions within it, and a hyperechoic membranous structure inferior to the optic disk suggestive of retinoblastoma with inferior retinal detachment.

Contraindications

- Active, viable tumor—relative contraindication
- Diffuse vitreous seeding
- Cases with suspicion of extraocular extension

Case Summary

A 2-year-old boy, who was a known case of bilateral retinoblastoma, was referred to us. He had been treated with transpupillary thermotherapy (TTT) and cryotherapy previously, along with 8 cycles of intravenous chemotherapy. Following the last TTT in the right eye, he was noted to have an RRD involving the macula, with an active tumor. On examination, the right eye showed a partly active tumor inferonasal to the disk, just abutting the disk margin. Multiple breaks were seen within the tumor, and along the nasal edge of the tumor, with an inferior retinal detachment (RD). The B-scan was done, which was consistent with retinoblastoma with an inferior RD **(Fig. 6)**. The left eye had poor prognosis, due to macular scarring secondary to regressed tumor and calcific residue, with partly active subretinal seeds. Considering the one-eyed status, difficult configuration of RD, and presence of multiple breaks, including those within the tumor, vitrectomy with silicone oil tamponade was planned **(Figs. 7 and 8)**.

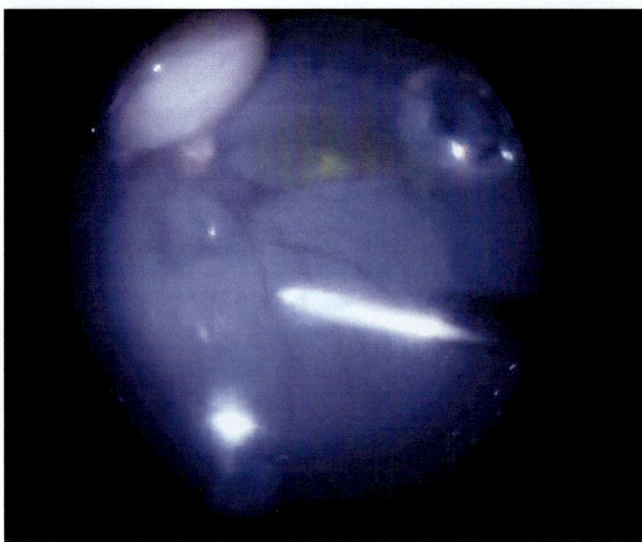

Fig. 7: Preoperative image showing a partly active tumor inferonasal to the disk, just abutting the disk margin. Multiple breaks were seen within the tumor, and along the nasal edge of the tumor, with an inferior retinal detachment (RD).

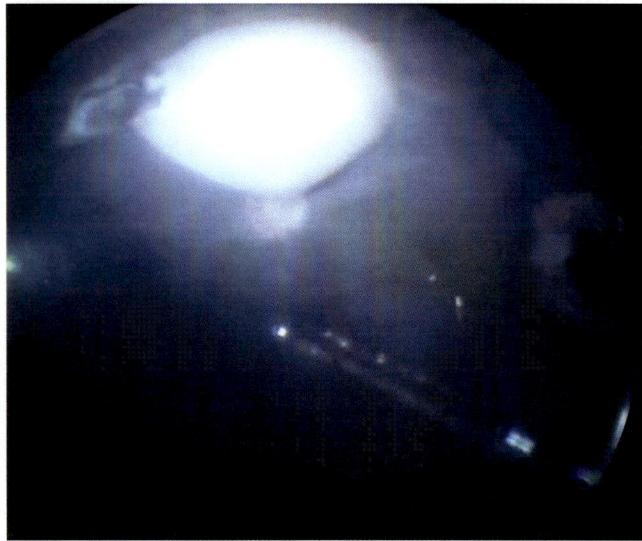

Fig. 8: Intraoperative image at end of procedure showing attached retina following thorough vitrectomy, dissection of bridging tissue, and partial tumorectomy. Silicone oil injection seen.

Treatment Plan

Dilution and mixture of chemotherapeutic agent in the infusion
↓
Insertion of valved sclerotomy cannulae
↓
Posterior vitreous detachment induction
↓
Dissection of any bridging tissue/Endo-resection or partial tumorectomy in rare cases
↓
Identification of breaks
↓
Fluid air exchange
↓
Endo-laser over and around the tumor, and the break sites. In anterior tumors, cryotherapy can be considered
↓
Injection of distilled water in the vitreous cavity-for 3 minutes, along with the chemotherapeutic agent
↓
Drainage retinotomy
↓
Silicone oil tamponade
↓
Suturing of ports, along with triple freeze thaw cryotherapy followed by injection of subconjunctival distilled water

Thought Process

Step	*Rationale*
Chemotherapeutic agent	Due to the local toxic effects of melphalan, topotecan is preferred
Valved cannulae	Avoids extraocular spillage of the retinoblastoma cells/vitreous seeds Limit instrument exchanges and turn off the infusion while doing so
PVD induction and vitrectomy	• Vitreous over the tumor and areas of cryotherapy/TTT scar is densely adherent and may not be easily removed with cutter • Overlying vitreous is truncated and freed from the rest of the posterior hyaloid and trimmed close to the tumor • Areas of peripheral CRA with densely adherent vitreous, may need a localized retinectomy • Triamcinolone is used to stain the vitreous, and for PVD induction

Contd...

Contd...

Step	Rationale
Identification of breaks	If the break is not identifiable, or beneath the tumor, a cautery is done around the calcific residue, with limited retinectomy
Fluid air exchange	• Using active suction • Usage of active suction from the machine (rather than a passive aspiration with a flute needle where the egressed fluid may spill on to the surgical field) to avoid spillage of contents. In case passive aspiration is used, the flute can be connected to a syringe without the plunger to collect the aspirate in the syringe
Distilled water injection	Francis et al. validated the in vitro usage of sterile distilled water immersion for 3 minutes to kill almost 99% of the viable retinoblastoma cells
Suture and cryo to the port sites	Neutralize any cells that may have egressed out

(PVD: posterior vitreous detachment; TTT: transpupillary thermotherapy)

OUTCOME SUMMARY

The child remained stable for 6 months post-surgery, with regressed tumors and an attached retina. He developed a posterior capsular cataract, 4 months postoperative. A lens aspiration with intraocular lens implantation was performed, and he remains on periodic follow-up thereafter. He is disease free and has ambulant vision.

KEY POINTS

Unique features of RRD in retinoblastoma:

- May not follow Lincoff's rules due to the tumor and areas of chorioretinal scarring
- Difficult localization of the break (may be within the CRA or obscured by the tumor/calcific residue/vitreous seeding/hemorrhage)
- The breaks are usually posteriorly located and the presence of RRD appears to aid in tumor propagation within the eye.

Additional steps in special scenarios:

- Sutureless band buckle with/without segmental buckle to help in cases of dense vitreous adhesions or scarring. In rare cases, a macular buckle is also used.
- Endoresection of the tumor/tumor fracture.
    - When the tumor mass tents up the retina, precluding reattachment of the break
    - Inaccessible breaks beneath the tumor

FURTHER READING

1. Francis JH, Xu XL, Gobin YP, Marr BP, Brodie SE, Abramson DH. Death by water: precautionary water submersion for intravitreal injection of retinoblastoma eyes. Open Ophthalmol J. 2014;8:7-11.
2. Li L, He T, Su Y, Wu L, Chen C. The Results of Pars Plana Vitrectomy in the Treatment of Intraocular Retinoblastoma: A Retrospective Study and Literature Review. Technol Cancer Res Treat. 2021;20:15330338211048634.
3. Shields CL, Honavar S, Shields JA, Demirci H, Meadows AT. Vitrectomy in eyes with unsuspected retinoblastoma. Ophthalmology. 2000;107(12):2250-5.

VIDEO LEGEND

Video 33: Vitrectomy in retinoblastoma.

CASE SCENARIO 5: IRIDOCYCLECTOMY IN MANAGEMENT OF CILIARY BODY MELANOMA

Background

Iridocyclectomy is indicated in some localized tumors involving the iris and ciliary body. The technique has been described first in 1911 by Zinn, following which it has evolved over the years. Although most performed together, isolated iridectomy or cyclectomy is also done in tumors localized to the iris or ciliary body alone.

In a study that investigated the long-term outcomes of the procedure in 52 patients, with varying lesion types, almost 43% maintained good visual acuity, with about 29% needing enucleation, and 10% undergoing melanoma metastasis over the follow-up period. In a similar study on long-term survival rates and functional results of 39 patients following iridocyclectomy, the outcomes were noted to be encouraging, with low rates of recurrence and complications.

With regards to the procedure for ciliary body melanomas on 107 cases, the cell type emerged to be the most significant prognostic feature 6% needed enucleation, and local complications such as recurrence and metastasis, although rare were noted to occur early.

Indications

- Iris melanomas
- Malignant lesions of ciliary body—adenocarcinoma and melanoma
- Ciliary body cysts, causing complications such as obscuring the angle
- Foreign body granuloma

- Ciliary body medulloepithelioma, leiomyoma, and schwannoma
- Iridociliary melanocytoma
- Resection of lesion along with segmental iridocyclectomy can be performed for lesions involving less than 3 clock hours.
- Larger lesions may require localized iridocyclectomy, followed by brachytherapy. A thorough histopathological analysis of the margins should be done.

Contraindications

- Diffuse spread of the lesion
- Extraocular extension is a relative contraindication.
- Large tumor size involving more than 4–5 clock hours—resection of this extent of ciliary body may result in irretractable hypotony.

Case Summary

A 24-year-old man was presented with complaints of diminution of vision in the left eye. He was evaluated elsewhere for a cystic lesion involving the iris root and ciliary body. The MRI findings showed a T1 hyperintense, T2 hypointense lesion along the inferior iris/ciliary body involvement. The presenting vision was 6/9 N10 in that eye, with normal intraocular pressure. A cystic lesion was noted inferiorly, between the iris and lens with a prominent vessel over the iris, prominent episcleral vessel inferiorly, and pigment dispersion in the anterior chamber **(Figs. 9 to 11)**. With a strong suspicion of ciliary body melanoma, an iridocyclectomy was planned. The histopathology was suggestive of low-grade adenocarcinoma from the nonpigmented epithelium of the ciliary body, with epithelioid cells.

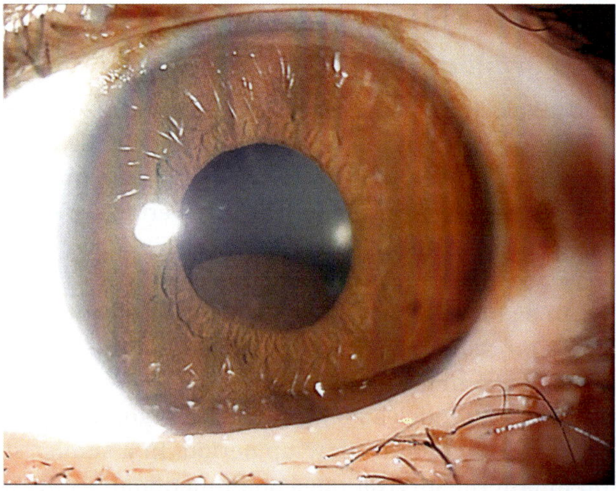
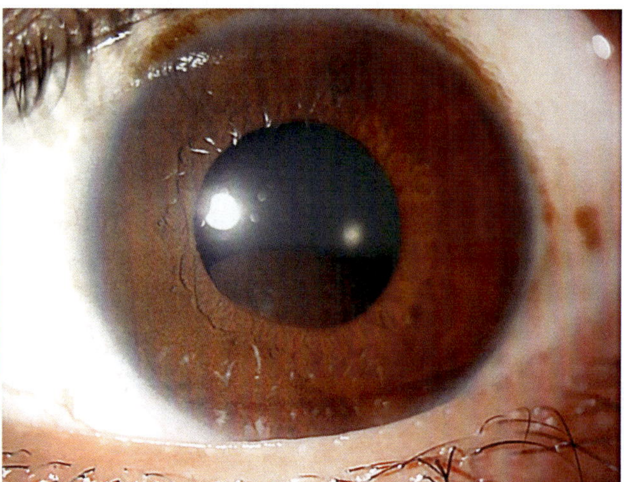

Fig. 9: Depicting a cystic lesion inferiorly between the iris and lens and pigment dispersion in the anterior chamber.

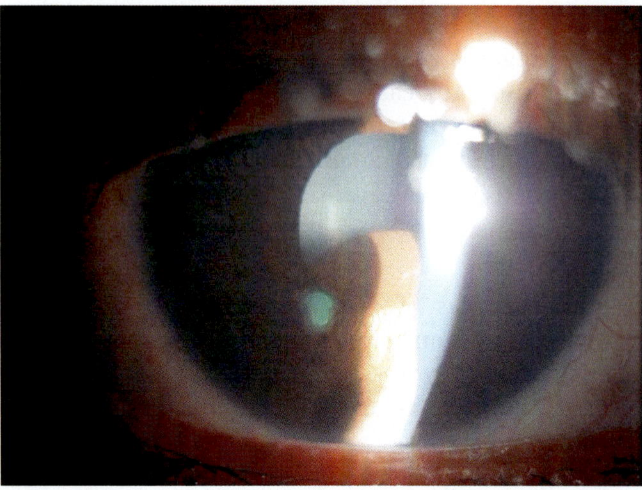

Fig. 10: Slit beam image showing retro-iridal bulge, with irregular anterior chamber.

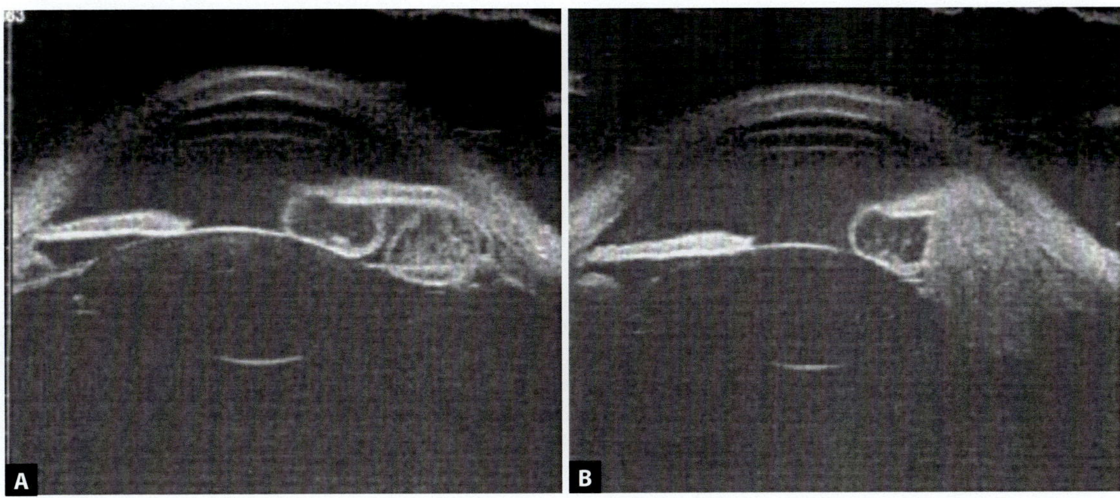

Figs. 11A and B: UBM showing moderately echogenic cysts at 7 o'clock and 6 o'clock, respectively. (UBM: ultrasound biomicroscopy)

Treatment Plan

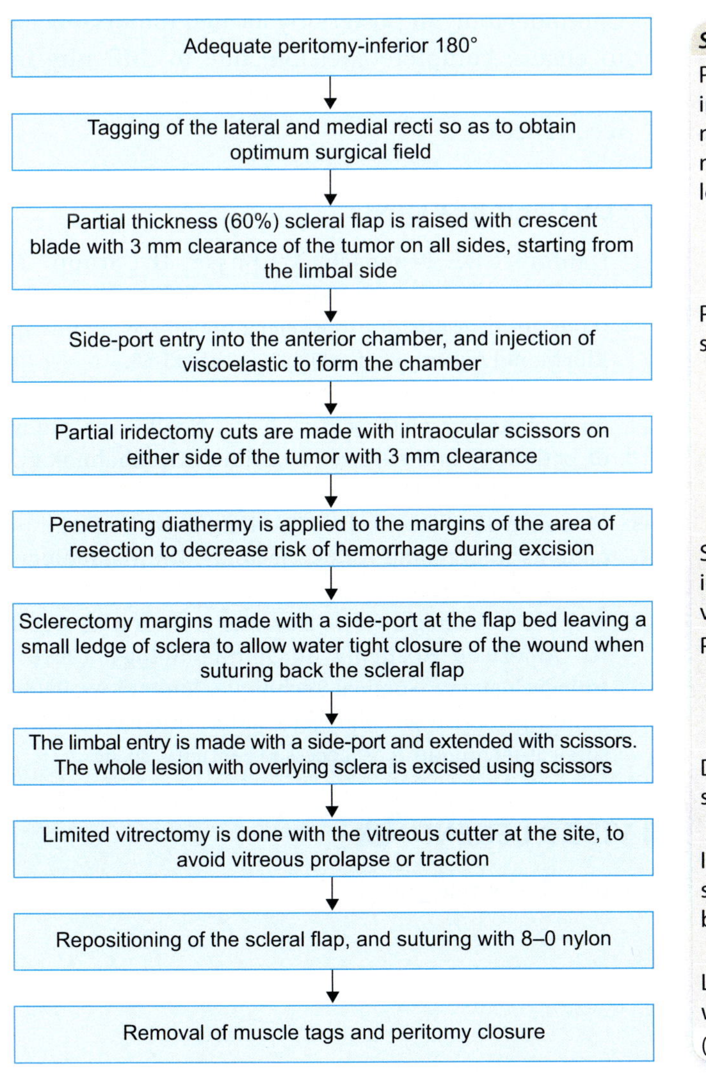

Thought Process

Step	*Rationale*
Preoperative imaging and precise measurement and mapping of the lesion on the sclera	Multiple imaging modalities such as B-scan, UBM, and MRI are to be used so as to correctly locate the location, extent, measurement, and to rule out involvement of other ocular structures. Intraoperative transillumination is also performed to precisely map the tumor on the scleral surface
Partial thickness scleral flap	• Meticulous dissection with a crescent blade is done, to ensure correct thickness of the flap, and to avoid untoward entry into the globe • The size of the flap is determined by the extent of lesion, with a 3-mm clear margins • Allows water-tight closure
Side port entry into the AC and viscoelastic injection	Done to form the chamber well. Inadvertent lens touch or endothelial touch can be avoided by performing this step
Partial iridectomy	Careful iridectomy should be performed to involve the entire extent of the lesion with 2–3 mm of surrounding normal iris, and should be complete till the root of iris
Diathermy to the scleral bed edges	Adequate diathermy avoids extensive bleed, and makes the dissection with scissors easier
Initial entry with side port followed by scissor dissection	Helps to gauge thickness of the dissection and is more precise. A ledge of sclera left along the margins allows water-tight closure of the wound after excision
Limited vitrectomy with vitreous cutter	Avoids hypotony, further vitreous prolapse and traction

(UBM: ultrasound biomicroscopy)

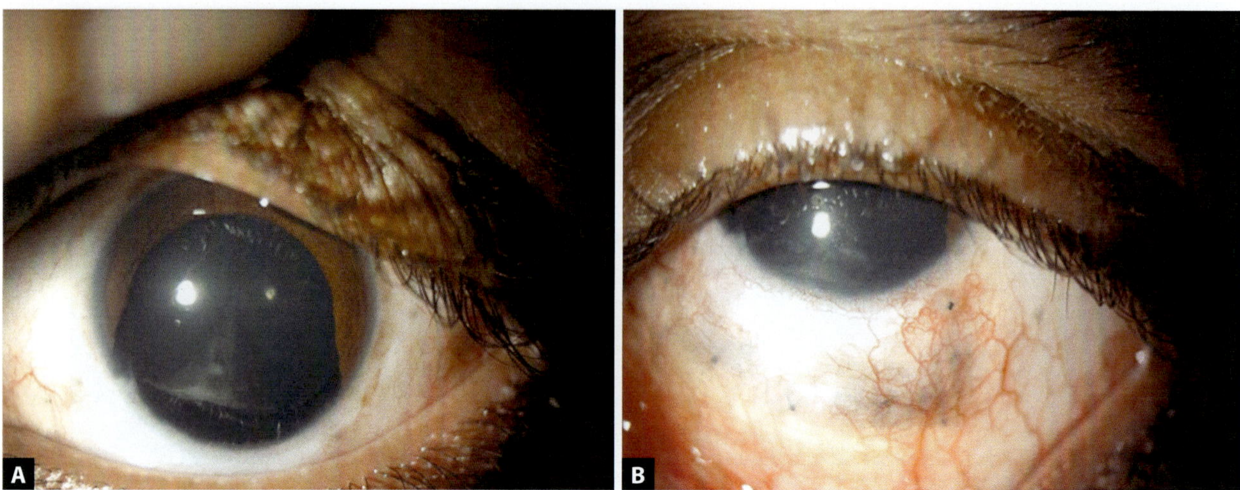

Figs. 12A and B: (A) Postinferior segmental iridocyclectomy. Slit lamp image shows localized lens changes; (B) Prominent episcleral vessel persists, with no recurrence of the tumor.

OUTCOME SUMMARY

Considering the presence of epithelioid cells on HPE, and the young age of presentation, the patient was advised adjuvant brachytherapy, which he denied. Hence, he remains on close follow-up and is stable for 1 year now, with a BCVA of 6/6, minimal cataractous changes and no recurrence of the tumor **(Figs. 12A and B)**.

KEY POINTS

- Careful dissection of the scleral flap—slow and precise dissection (but of sufficient thickness) to avoid entry into the globe
- Use of pre-placed sutures to suture the sclera back in place immediately to minimize chances of hypotony-related expulsive hemorrhage
- Precise preoperative measurement of the lesion and careful resection to excise in toto, with 3-mm clear zone on all sides
- Vitrectomy at the site should be done carefully, to just remove the prolapsed vitreous and extensive vitrectomy is avoided, in view of impending hypotony.

Additional steps in special scenarios:

- Full-thickness eye wall resection with scleral patch graft—in cases of iridociliary melanoma with subconjunctival/extrascleral extension.
- Choroidectomy in posteriorly located tumors—need to ensure complete excision, due to difficulty in assessment of margins, and higher chances of delayed recurrences

FURTHER READING

1. Daubner D, Prokosch V, Busse H, Stupp T. Langzeitergebnisse nach Iridozyklektomie bei Iristumoren [Long-term results of iridocyclectomy for iris tumours]. Klin Monbl Augenheilkd. 2008;225(12):1045-50.
2. Forrest AW, Keyser RB, Spencer WH. Iridocyclectomy for melanomas of the ciliary body: a follow-up study of pathology and surgical morbidity. Ophthalmology. 1978;85(12):1237-49.
3. Memmen JE, McLean IW. The long-term outcome of patients undergoing iridocyclectomy. Ophthalmology. 1990;97(4):429-32.
4. Singh AD, Echegaray JJ, Davanzo J, Fekrat S, Scott IU; American Academy of Ophthalmology. (2018). Iridocyclectomy: Surgical Technique. [online] Available from https://www.aao.org/eyenet/article/iridocyclectomy-surgical-technique. [Last accessed February, 2026]

VIDEO LEGEND

Video 34: Iridocyclectomy.

CHAPTER 14

Decision Making in Surgical Management of Uveitic Pathologies

Atul Arora, Vishali Gupta, Amer F Alsouldi, Lisa J Faia

INFECTIOUS UVEITIC CONDITIONS

Atul Arora, Vishali Gupta

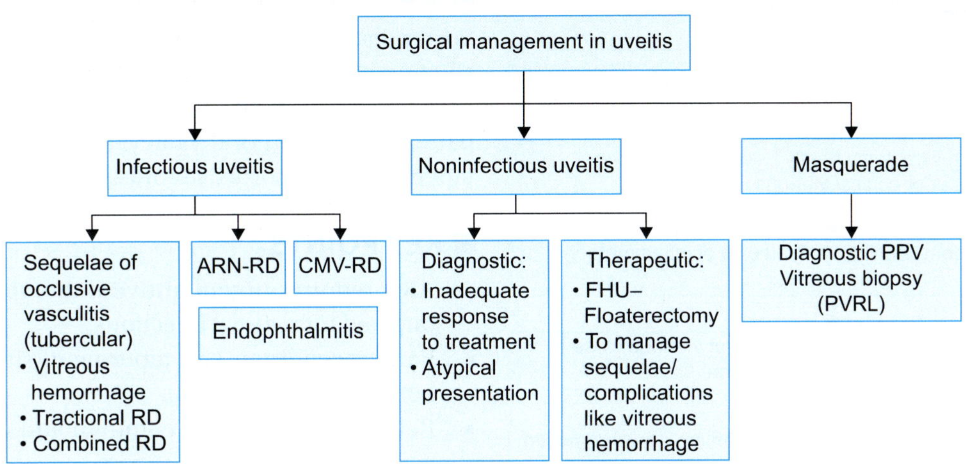

ALGORITHMIC APPROACH TO SURGICAL MANAGEMENT IN UVEITIS

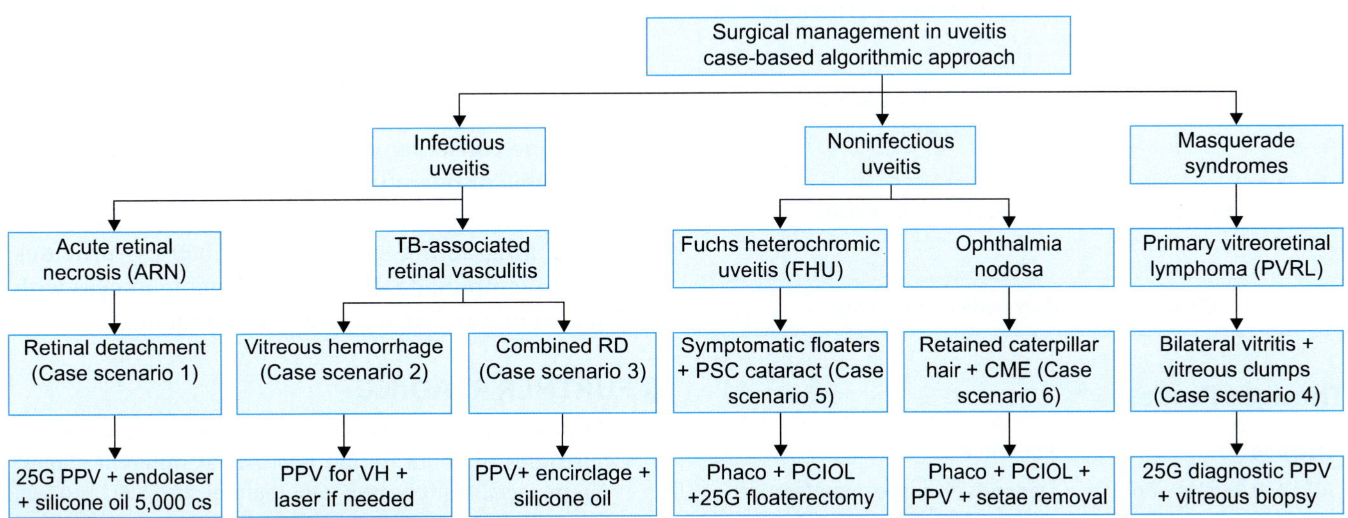

CASE SCENARIO 1: RETINAL DETACHMENT IN ACUTE RETINAL NECROSIS

Case Summary

A 48-year-old woman presented with diminution of vision in her left eye since past 10 days. On examination, her visual acuity was light perception, with granulomatous keratic precipitates, 2+ anterior chamber (AC) cells, vitritis, disc edema, and peripheral patches of necrotizing retinitis. AC tap polymerase chain reaction (PCR) was positive for herpes simplex virus (HSV), confirming viral etiology.

She was treated with intravenous acyclovir (10 mg/kg/dose) for 21 days. Systemic corticosteroids (prednisolone 1 mg/kg/day) were added 48 hours after initiating antiviral cover. Additionally she also receive aspirin 75 mg OD. The retinitis lesions gradually healed with well-demarcated edges and reduction in inflammation.

At 8 weeks, she developed a retinal detachment, a known complication of acute retinal necrosis (ARN), for which she underwent 25 G pars plana vitrectomy (PPV) + Endolaser + silicone oil tamponade (5,000 cs).

Treatment Plan

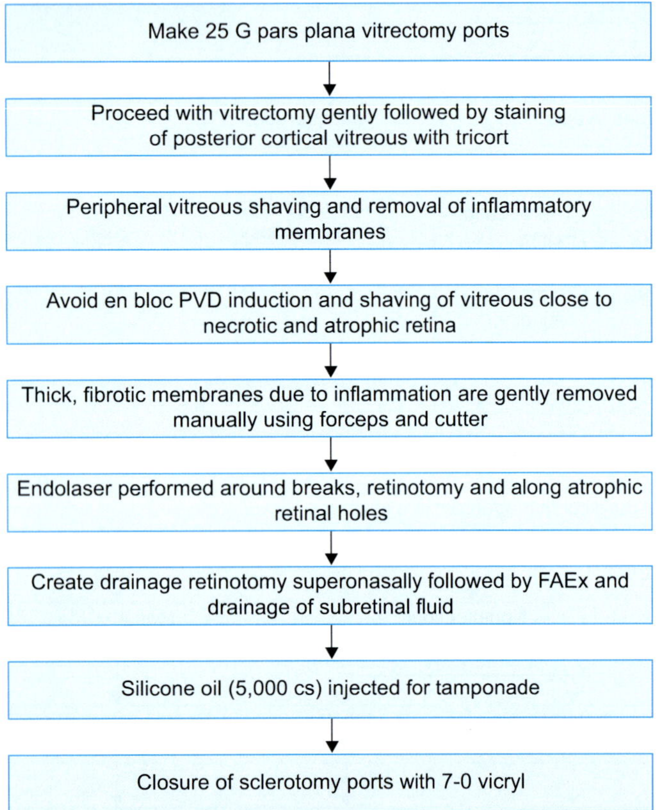

Thought Process

Decision	*Rationale*
Add belt/buckle or not	Depends on surgeon preference; preferred in young patients with adherent vitreous
Avoid en bloc PVD induction	Vitreous is adherent to thinned, atrophic retina; PVD induction with suction can result in formation of large iatrogenic breaks
Peripheral vitreous shaving and removal of inflammatory membranes	Adherent peripheral vitreous is removed via shaving close to retina at a high cut rate and low vacuum
Silicone oil (5,000 cs) is used for tamponade	Allows longer tamponade with late emulsification
Suturing of sclerotomy ports	To avoid postoperative hypotony and rebleed

OUTCOME SUMMARY

Postoperatively, the retina remained well attached under silicone oil, media clarity improved, and inflammation remained controlled on systemic antiviral therapy. The patient continued oral valacyclovir for 3 months with a tapering dose of corticosteroids.

KEY POINTS

- ARN requires urgent antiviral therapy, supported by targeted intravitreal injections.
- Early recognition and tapering of steroids only after antiviral cover is critical.
- Retinal detachment is common and mandates timely vitrectomy.
- Peripheral vitreous is often densely adherent in inflammatory retinopathies, making careful vitreous base shaving essential to prevent tractional recurrence and iatrogenic breaks.
- Induction of posterior vitreous detachment (PVD) should be conservative, as forceful en bloc elevation in atrophic or necrotic retina can lead to large retinal tears.
- Use of long-acting silicone oil (5,000 cs) provides durable tamponade, especially valuable in eyes with fragile retina and high risk of redetachment.

FURTHER READING

1. Fu H, Tao Q, Yang F, Zhang X. Clinical characteristics and outcomes of acute retinal necrosis at different stages: A retrospective study. BMC Ophthalmol. 2025;25(1):107.
2. Gore J, Kelgaonkar A, Patel A, Basu S, Pathengay A. Clinical features and management of eyes with acute retinal necrosis presenting with rhegmatogenous retinal detachment. Indian J Ophthalmol. 2025;73(Suppl 1):S95-S99.
3. Mooss VS, Murthy KR, Babu K, Tirumalai AA. Clinical profile and treatment outcomes in acute retinal necrosis in a South Indian patient population. Indian J Ophthalmol. 2025;73(6):858-63.

VIDEO LEGEND

Video 35: Retinal detachment in acute retinal necrosis

CASE SCENARIO 2: VITREOUS HEMORRHAGE AS A SEQUELAE OF OCCLUSIVE RETINAL VASCULITIS

Case Summary

A 23-year-old Asian Indian male presented with decreased vision in his right eye (OD) since past week. He gave history seeing floaters in both his eyes since past 3 months and was given a short course of oral steroids elsewhere with no improvement in symptoms. At presentation, his visual acuity was hand motions close to face (HMCF) in his right eye and 6/12 in his left eye. Anterior segment examination did not show any sign of inflammation. Fundus examination showed media grade 4 due to vitreous hemorrhage in OD, while vitreous cells were present in OS. Ultrasonography of OD showed vitreous cavity filled with pinpoint echoes suggestive of vitreous attachment and attached retina.

Laboratory investigations revealed a positive Mantoux and interferon gamma release assay (IGRA) test. Contrast-enhanced computed tomography (CECT) chest showed healed lesions suggestive of infective/tubercular etiology. Serology for syphilis and human immunodeficiency virus were negative.

The patient was taken up for PPV in OD (surgical steps are given in flowchart below).

Treatment Plan

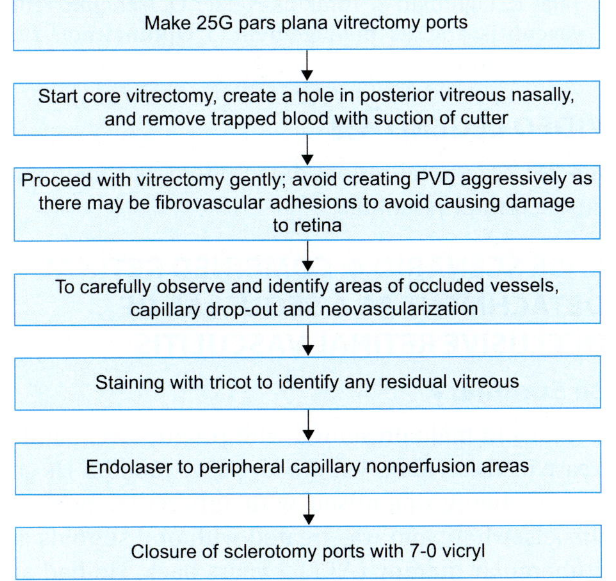

Thought Process

Decision	*Rationale*
Preoperative ultrasonography	To look for status of retina, posterior vitreous detachment, fibrovascular adhesions and tractional retinal detachment
Create a hole in posterior vitreous to remove trapped blood	To avoid inadvertent injury to retina in cases of traction/pulled up retina; removing trapped blood clears media, allowing better visualization of underlying retina
To carefully observe and identify areas of occluded vessels, capillary drop-out and neovascularization	• To assess need for intraoperative laser photocoagulation • In cases with florid neovascularization, anti-VEGF can be added at the end of surgery
Suturing of sclerotomy ports	To avoid postoperative hypotony and rebleed

OUTCOME SUMMARY

Post-PPV, media cleared and visual acuity improved to 6/24 in OD. Fundus fluorescein angiography done post PPV showed active retinal vasculitis in both the eyes. The patient was started on oral steroids (1 mg/kg/day) alongwith 4 drug antitubercular therapy (isoniazid 5 mg/kg/day, rifampicin 10 mg/kg/day, pyrazinamide 25 mg/kg/day, and ethambutol 15 mg/kg/day).

KEY POINTS

- Dense vitreous hemorrhage in retinal vasculitis warrants early vitrectomy, especially when fundus visualization is inadequate or tractional changes cannot be ruled out clinically.
- Preoperative ultrasonography is essential to assess retinal status, identify PVD, and detect early traction, guiding safe surgical planning.
- Intraoperative identification of ischemic and occluded vessels is critical, as targeted laser and adjunctive anti-VEGF (vascular endothelial growth factor) may be required depending on neovascular activity.
- Postoperative management must address the underlying systemic etiology, with prompt initiation of corticosteroids and appropriate anti-tubercular therapy to prevent recurrence and bilateral progression.

FURTHER READING

1. Motlagh MN, Javid CG. Rapid and progressive decline despite early intervention in a case of bilateral hemorrhagic

occlusive retinal vasculitis. Am J Ophthalmol Case Rep. 2020;17:100595.
2. Tien MC, Kaplan AJ. Severe Occlusive Retinal Vasculitis in an Immunocompetent Patient with Chronic CMV Anterior Uveitis. Ocul Immunol Inflamm. 2025;33(2):308-9.

CASE SCENARIO 3: TRACTIONAL RETINAL DETACHMENT AS A SEQUELA OF OCCLUSIVE RETINAL VASCULITIS

Case Summary

A 28-year-old Asian Indian female presented with progressive vision loss in her left eye (OS) over 2 weeks. She reported floaters and photopsia in OD for 4 months, previously treated with topical steroids elsewhere without relief. At presentation, visual acuity was 6/60 in OD and 6/9 in OS. Anterior segment was quiet. Fundus examination showed grade 3 media haze in OD. Ultrasonography of OD revealed vitreous hemorrhage, and fibrovascular proliferation with tractional retinal detachment (TRD) at the macula. The patient was taken up for PPV in OD.

Treatment Plan

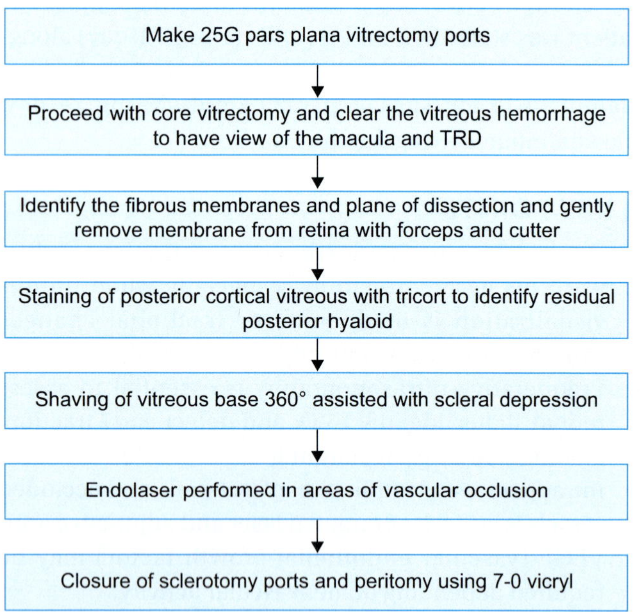

Thought Process

Decision	Rationale
Preoperative ultrasonography	Define TRD geometry, vitreoretinal traction, and macula threat to plan peeling approach
Peel fibrovascular membranes and TA-assisted posterior hyaloid removal	Relieve traction, prevent progression to rhegmatogenous RD; exposes underlying retina
Avoid en bloc PVD induction	Underlying fibrovascular adhesions may result in iatrogenic retinal breaks if a forceful PVD is induced
Identify occluded vessels and capillary nonperfusion	Guide targeted endolaser to hypoxic retina, reducing neovascular drive

OUTCOME SUMMARY

Post-PPV, TRD flattened, macula attached, and visual acuity improved to 6/18 in OD at 1 month. Fundus fluorescein angiography (FFA) confirmed peripheral nonperfusion but no new vessels.

KEY POINTS

- TRD in occlusive vasculitis demands prompt PPV to relieve traction before macula involvement.
- Preoperative ultrasonography (USG) is vital for delineating traction planes and surgical risks.
- Intraoperative membrane peeling with laser/anti-VEGF addresses ischemia and prevents recurrence.

FURTHER READING

1. Menia NK, Alcibahy Y, Pichi F, Neri P, Agarwal A. An Update on Noninfectious Retinal Vasculitis. Ophthalmologica. 2024;1-4.
2. Talat L, Lightman S, Tomkins-Netzer O. Ischemic retinal vasculitis and its management. J Ophthalmol. 2014; 2014:197675.

VIDEO LEGEND

Video 36: Tractional retinal detachment as a sequela of occlusive retinal vasculitis

CASE SCENARIO 4: COMBINED RETINAL DETACHMENT AS A SEQUELAE OF OCCLUSIVE RETINAL VASCULITIS

Case Summary

A 25-year-old male presented with progressive, painless decrease in vision in his left eye for past 3 months. He gave history of being diagnosed with tubercular posterior uveitis elsewhere and was treated with oral steroids and antitubercular therapy (ATT) 2 years back. He had also underwent scatter laser photocoagulation at that time for occlusive retinal vasculitis. At presentation to our center, his visual acuity was counting-fingers. Fundus examination showed vitreous hemorrhage. USG showed inferior TRD. The patient was taken up for PPV with encirclage in OD (surgical steps are given in flowchart).

Treatment Plan

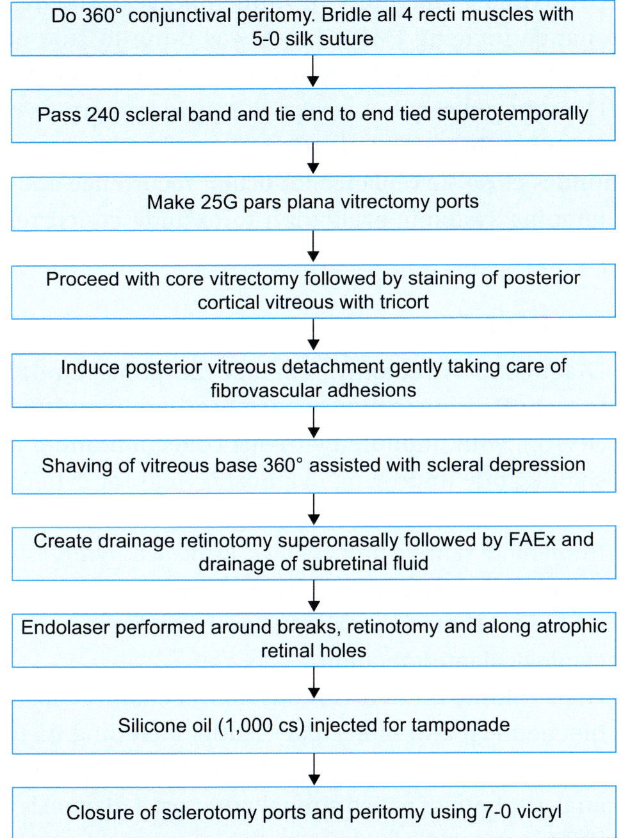

Thought Process

Decision	*Rationale*
Add belt/buckle or not	Adding belt/buckle is preferred as traction is usually peripheral in vasculitis combined retinal detachments
Avoid en bloc PVD induction	Underlying fibrovascular adhesions may result in iatrogenic retinal breaks if a forceful PVD is induced
Peripheral vitreous shaving	Adherent peripheral vitreous is removed via shaving close to retina at a high cut rate and low vacuum
Silicone oil (1,000 cs) is used for tamponade	Due to inferior breaks, it allows for longer tamponade as compared to gas

OUTCOME SUMMARY

Postoperatively, the retina remained well-attached under silicone oil and media clarity improved. The visual acuity improved to 3/60. Silicon oil removal (SOR) was done at 3 months. The patient maintained visual acuity of 3/60 post SOR.

KEY POINTS

- Tractional/combined retinal detachment in occlusive vasculitis often arises from peripheral fibrovascular adhesions, making combined scleral buckle and vitrectomy a rational strategy to relieve traction and support peripheral retina.
- USG plays an important role in preoperative assessment, allowing confirmation of combined retinal detachment, identification of site and extent of traction, and presence/absence of PVD.
- Induction of PVD should be conservative, as long-standing inflammatory adhesions predispose to large iatrogenic retinal breaks if en bloc elevation is attempted.
- Meticulous vitreous base shaving with scleral depression is essential to eliminate residual traction and prevent postoperative recurrence, especially when inferior pathology is present.

FURTHER READING

1. Talat L, Lightman S, Tomkins-Netzer O. Ischemic retinal vasculitis and its management. J Ophthalmol. 2014; 2014:197675.

VIDEO LEGEND

Video 37: Combined retinal detachment as a sequelae of occlusive retinal vasculitis

CASE SCENARIO 5: DIAGNOSTIC VITRECTOMY ESTABLISHES THE DIAGNOSIS OF PRIMARY VITREORETINAL LYMPHOMA

Case Summary

A 42-year-old Asian Indian female presented with complains of floaters and diminution of vision her left eye (OS) for past 2 months. Upon examination, her visual acuity was 6/9 and 6/18 in the right eye (OD) and OS, respectively. Anterior segment did not show any sign of inflammation. Fundus examination showed 1+ vitreous cells in OD while vitreous haze and 3+ vitreous cells were present in OS. Laboratory investigations revealed a negative tuberculin skin test, and IGRA. Serology for syphilis and human immunodeficiency virus were negative. Given the bilateral involvement and the presence of vitreous clumps, a masquerade etiology was suspected. The left eye underwent 25 G PPV with vitreous biopsy for diagnostic evaluation.

Treatment Plan

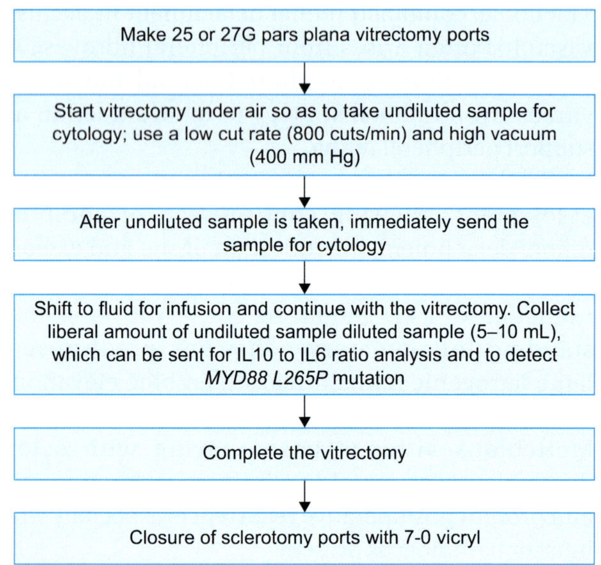

Thought Process

Decision	*Rationale*
Start vitrectomy under air	To collect undiluted sample so as to increase yield to obtain malignant cells
Use a low cut rate (800 cuts/min) and high vacuum (400 mm Hg)	To avoid distortion of cell morphology in the collected sample
To transport the sample for cytology immediately	Lymphoma cells degenerate rapidly once removed from the eye; prompt fixation and processing minimizes cellular degradation and increases positivity for cytology, which is often low-sensitivity in PVRL
Shift to fluid to complete vitrectomy	Diluted vitreous can be used for biochemical assays. The IL-10 to IL-6 ratio is a key biomarker—an elevated ratio strongly supports PVRL. Collecting a larger diluted sample increases the reliability of cytokine and molecular testing (PCR for *MYD88 L265P* mutation, immunoglobulin gene rearrangement, etc.)
Suturing of sclerotomy ports	To avoid postoperative hypotony and rebleed

OUTCOME SUMMARY

Following diagnostic vitrectomy, adequate undiluted and diluted vitreous samples were obtained for cytology, flow cytometry interleukin 10 (IL-10)/IL-6 ratio analysis, and PCR for *MYD88 L265P* mutation. The investigations supported a diagnosis of primary vitreoretinal lymphoma, prompting initiation of weekly intravitreal methotrexate and rituximab injections in both the eyes. Magnetic resonance imaging (MRI) brain was done to rule out central nervous system (CNS) lymphoma and was normal.

Over the subsequent weeks, the vitritis progressively regressed with marked clearing of media. The patient continues close surveillance for ocular recurrence and is undergoing systemic evaluation to exclude concurrent CNS lymphoma.

KEY POINTS

- Diagnostic vitrectomy remains the gold standard for confirming primary vitreoretinal lymphoma (PVRL), with undiluted vitreous collection under air significantly improving diagnostic yield for cytology and flow cytometry.
- Immediate sample processing is critical, as lymphoma cells are fragile and rapidly undergo degeneration, making prompt transport essential for accurate cytological interpretation.
- High-volume diluted vitreous allows comprehensive biochemical and molecular testing, including IL-10/IL-6 cytokine ratio and *MYD88 L265P* mutation analysis, both of which strongly support a diagnosis of PVRL.
- Early initiation of intravitreal methotrexate and rituximab after diagnosis leads to rapid reduction in vitreous infiltrates, but long-term surveillance is mandatory due to the high risk of ocular recurrence and possible CNS involvement.

FURTHER READING

1. Dalal M, Casady M, Moriarty E, Faia L, Nussenblatt R, Chan CC, Sen HN. Diagnostic procedures in vitreoretinal lymphoma. Ocul Immunol Inflamm. 2014;22(4):270-6.
2. Iuliano L, Marchese A, Miserocchi E, Corbelli E, Bongiovanni L, Ponzoni M, et al. Subretinal lavage during diagnostic vitrectomy: an adjunctive technique for cell sampling in suspected vitreoretinal lymphoma. Retin Cases Brief Rep. 2025.

VIDEO LEGEND

Video 38: Diagnostic vitrectomy in primary vitreoretinal lymphoma

CASE SCENARIO 6: SYMPTOMATIC FLOATERS IN FUCHS' HETEROCHROMIC UVEITIS MANAGED WITH FLOATERECTOMY

Case Summary

A 40-year-old male presented with gradually increasing floaters and intermittent blurring of vision in his right eye (OD) for the past 6 months. He denied any complaints of pain, redness, or photophobia. Upon clinical examination his visual acuity was 6/12 in OD and 26/6 in the left eye (OS) Anterior segment examination showed stellate keratic precipitates, minimal AC inflammation, and diffuse iris stromal atrophy. Additionally, a posterior subcapsular cataract was present. Posterior segment evaluation revealed dense vitreous opacities but no active retinitis, vasculitis, or cystoid macular edema. Optical coherence tomography (OCT) confirmed absence of cystoid macular edema. Anterior and posterior segment examination of OS was normal. Based on clinical findings, a diagnosis of Fuchs' heterochromic uveitis (FHU) was made. The patient underwent phacoemulsification with posterior chamber intraocular lens (PCIOL) implantation and 25 G PPV (floaterectomy) in OD.

Treatment Plan

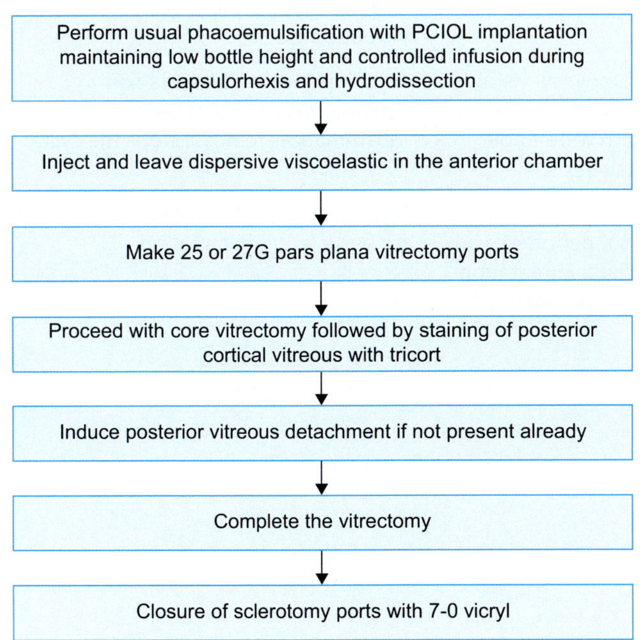

Thought Process

Decision	*Rationale*
Opt for surgery rather than medical therapy	Floaters in FHU result from vitreous degeneration, not active inflammation; steroids do not improve symptoms
Phacoemulsification: Maintain low bottle height and controlled infusion during capsulorhexis and hydrodissection	Reduces turbulence and prevents sudden pressure fluctuations that may trigger hyphema from fragile angle vessels typical of FHU (Amsler's sign)
Inject dispersive viscoelastic and leave viscoelastic in the anterior chamber before starting posterior segment surgery	Tamponades the angle vessels to reduce the risk of bleeding, stabilizes the AC, and dilates the pupil required for adequate view while performing vitrectomy

OUTCOME SUMMARY

The patient underwent uneventful 25 G floaterectomy. The vitreous opacities were effectively removed, and the retina remained stable intraoperatively. Postoperatively, the media became clear. Visual acuity improved to 6/6, and the patient reported significant subjective improvement in contrast sensitivity and disappearance of floaters.

KEY POINTS

- FHU is characterized by low-grade, chronic inflammation, with prominent vitreous opacities and posterior subcapsular cataract (PSC) often contributing more to visual symptoms than active uveitis.
- Symptomatic floaters in FHU do not respond to corticosteroids, as the underlying pathology is degenerative vitreopathy rather than active intraocular inflammation; hence, surgery is the only effective treatment.
- Phacoemulsification in FHU requires special precautions due to fragile angle vessels—maintaining low infusion pressure minimizes the risk of Amsler's sign (intraoperative hyphema).
- Leaving dispersive viscoelastic in the AC before vitrectomy stabilizes the chamber, protects the endothelium, and tamponades friable vessels, reducing bleeding risk during combined surgery.
- 25 G floaterectomy provides significant visual and symptomatic improvement, with rapid recovery and minimal postoperative inflammation in eyes with stable FHU.

FURTHER READING

1. Keles S, Ondas O, Ates O, Ekinci M, Kartal B, Arpali E et al. Phacoemulsification and Core Vitrectomy in Fuchs' Heterochromic Uveitis. Eurasian J Med. 2017;49(2): 97-101.
2. Scott RA, Sullivan PM, Aylward GW, Pavésio CE, Charteris DG. The effect of pars plana vitrectomy in the management of Fuchs heterochromic cyclitis. Retina. 2001;21(4):312-6.

CASE SCENARIO 7: INTERMEDIATE UVEITIS WITH CYSTOID MACULAR EDEMA SECONDARY TO RETAINED CATERPILLAR HAIR (OPHTHALMIA NODOSA)

Case Summary

A 40-year-old male was referred with a 3-year history of recurrent episodes of redness, ocular irritation, and painless decrease of vision in his left eye (OS). He had previously been diagnosed elsewhere as a case of intermediate uveitis and treated with multiple courses of topical and systemic corticosteroids. Symptoms recurred each time therapy was tapered, and the patient was advised initiation of immunosuppressive therapy before referral.

At presentation, his best-corrected visual acuity was 6/6 in OD and 6/60 in OS. Slit-lamp examination of OS revealed 2+ AC cells, 2+ flare, and PSC. Fundus evaluation showed 2+ vitreous cells, vascular sheathing, and cystoid macular edema (CME). OCT confirmed large cystoid spaces with subfoveal serous detachment. On FFA diffuse vascular leakage was present in OS. Anterior and posterior segment examination of OD was normal. A detailed history revealed that a caterpillar had fallen into his eye three years earlier, causing acute irritation. While the superficial hair had been removed at that time, the recurrent inflammation raised suspicion of retained intraocular setae. Given the recurrent inflammation and visually significant CME, the patient underwent combined cataract extraction with PCIOL implantation and PPV, with removal of all visible setae.

Treatment Plan

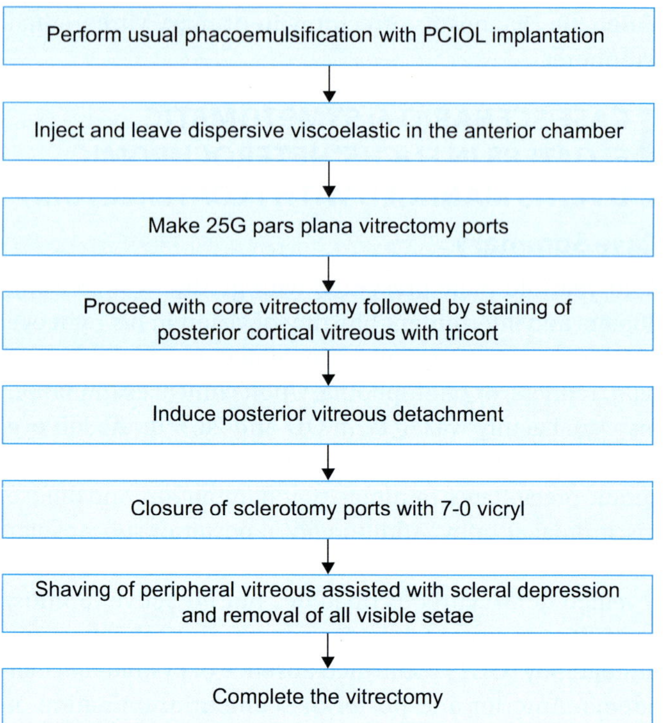

Thought Process

Decision	*Rationale*
Opt for combined phacoemulsification + PPV	Phacoemulsification with PCIOL gives room for anterior vitrectomy and removal of embedded hair from vitreous base
Remove all visible setae during PPV with wide-angle viewing	Mechanical irritation and toxin (thaumetopoein) from setae perpetuate inflammation; removal stops the cycle
Carefully inspect 360° periphery with scleral indentation intraoperatively	Additional missed hair may act as nidus for persistent inflammation

OUTCOME SUMMARY

The patient had an uncomplicated surgery with successful removal of all detectable caterpillar hair. At 2 months postoperatively, the eye was quiet, vitreous inflammation had resolved, and OCT demonstrated complete resolution of CME with restoration of foveal contour. His visual acuity improved to 6/12, eventually reaching 6/9 at 1 year. No recurrence of inflammation was noted, and long-term systemic immunosuppression was avoided.

KEY POINTS

- Retained caterpillar hair (ophthalmia nodosa type V) can mimic chronic intermediate uveitis, and repeated relapses despite corticosteroids should prompt reevaluation of history for prior insect exposure.
- Peripheral scleral-indented examination is critical, as setae are often located in the far periphery or pars plana and can be easily overlooked without meticulous inspection.
- Persistent vitreous inflammation and CME result from mechanical irritation and toxin release (thaumetopoein) from embedded setae, making medical therapy alone insufficient.
- Combined phacoemulsification and PPV allows both visual rehabilitation and complete removal of intraocular setae, effectively eliminating the nidus responsible for chronic inflammation.
- Comprehensive 360° peripheral inspection and removal of all visible setae are essential to prevent recurrence, and complete extraction leads to rapid resolution of inflammation and CME without the need for long-term immunosuppression.

FURTHER READING

1. Ashkenazy N, Rosenfeld PJ, Davis JL. Multimodal imaging in the diagnosis and management of ophthalmia nodosa. Am J Ophthalmol Case Rep. 2022;28: 101692.
2. González-Martín-Moro J, Altares-Mateos V, Padeira Iranzo V, Mittendrein V, Miralles Pechuan V, Picasso-Simón L, et al. The Multiple Faces of Setae Induced Ocular Inflammation (Ophthalmia Nodosa): A Review. Semin Ophthalmol. 2026;41(1):79-98.
3. Hom-Choudhury A, Koukkoulli A, Norris JH, Mokete B, Backhouse OC. A hairy affair: tarantula setae-induced panuveitis requiring pars plana vitrectomy. Int Ophthalmol. 2012;32(2):161-3.

NONINFECTIOUS UVEITIC CONDITIONS

Amer F Alsouldi, Lisa J Faia

SURGICAL APPROACH FOR NONINFECTIOUS UVEITIS

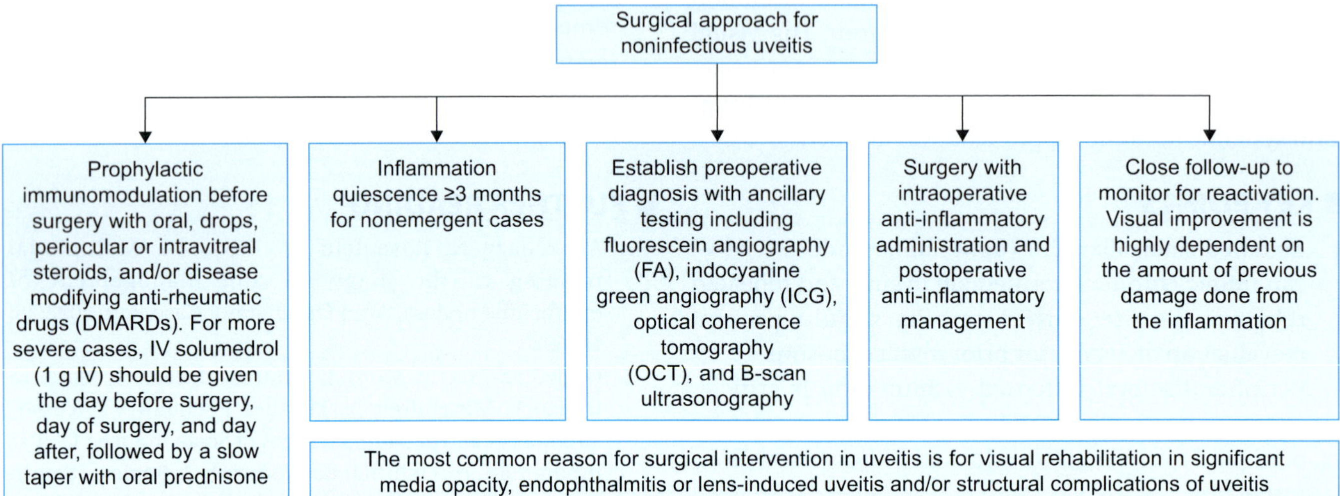

CASE SCENARIO 1: MANAGEMENT OF MACULAR HOLE IN BIRDSHOT RETINOCHOROIDOPATHY

Case Summary

A 62-year-old female with a known diagnosis of birdshot retinochoroidopathy on infliximab [Remicade (Janssen Biotech Inc., Raritan, New Jersey)] 5 mg/kg infusion every 6 weeks presents with a chronic full-thickness macular hole in the left eye. The patient had previously received several subtenon kenalog injections in the left eye, though the inflammation in the left eye had remained quiescent for greater than 3 months. Her vision was 20/40 and 20/HM (hand motion) in the right and left eye, respectively **(Figs. 1A and B)**.

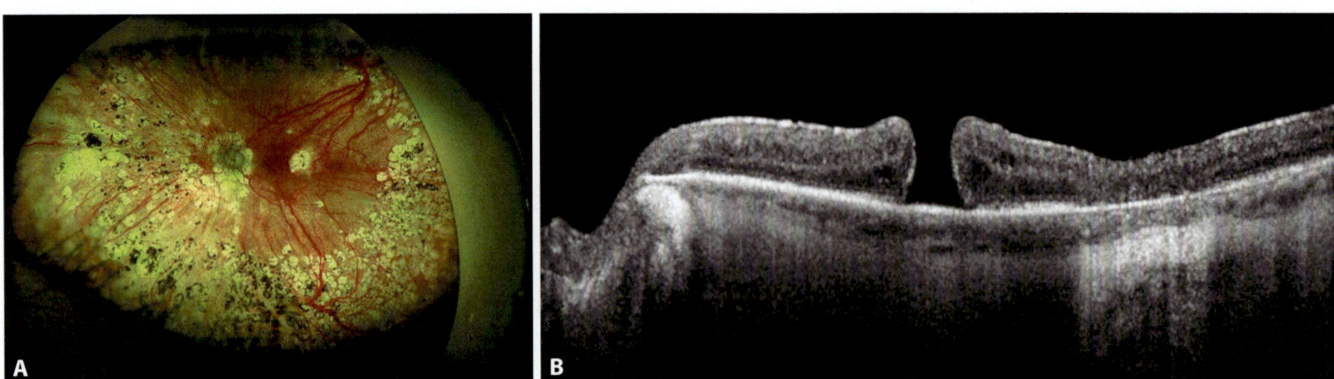

Figs. 1A and B: (A) Color fundus photograph depicts numerous small, oval, cream-colored hypopigmented lesions scattered across the posterior pole and midperiphery, radiating from the optic disc; (B) Optical coherence tomography (OCT) demonstrating a full-thickness macular hole.

Treatment Plan

Surgical intervention was planned for the left eye and 1 month prior to the surgery the patient was started on predfort eyedrop four times a day in the left eye

↓

Surgical steps included 23G pars plana vitrectomy, internal limiting membrane peel, and sulfur hexafluoride (SF6) gas placement

↓

Intraoperative subtenon kenalog injection

↓

Facedown positioning was maintained for 3 days after the surgery

Thought Process

Decision	*Rationale*
Inflammation quiescence ≥3 months for nonemergent cases	A longer quiescent period reduces the chance of postoperative inflammatory reactivation and complications
Operate on a "hot eye" only when necessary (e.g., endophthalmitis, retinal detachment, diagnostic vitrectomy) and minimize inflammation perioperatively	Some indications cannot wait, but surgeons should proceed cautiously and make every effort pre-, intra-, and postoperatively to eliminate inflammation
After 3 months quiet without escalation, consider prophylactic immunomodulation (often a one-step increase)	Even when quiet, surgical manipulation can trigger reactivation; modest prophylaxis may prevent future recurrence

OUTCOME SUMMARY

Postoperative vision improved to 20/200 after 1 month of follow-up. The patient's uveitis has been controlled with Infliximab infusion three years after the surgery **(Fig. 2)**.

KEY POINT

For retinal surgery in patients with preexisting uveitis and on immunosuppressions, additional steps apart from routine surgical care including good preoperative control of the inflammation and a plan for escalation of inflammatory control before surgery are essential to ensure success.

FURTHER READING

1. Callaway NF, Gonzalez MA, Yonekawa Y, Faia LJ, Mandelcorn ED, Khurana RN, et al. Outcomes of Pars Plana Vitrectomy for Macular Hole in Uveitis Patients. Retina. 2018;38(Suppl 1):S41-S48.

VIDEO LEGEND

Video 39: Management of macular hole in birdshot retinochoroidopathy

CASE SCENARIO 2: MANAGEMENT OF FOCAL TRACTIONAL RETINAL DETACHMENT WITH INTERMEDIATE UVEITIS

Case Summary

A 15-year-old male with idiopathic and recurrent intermediate uveitis refractory to mycophenolate mofetil [CellCept (Roche, Basel, Switzerland)] monotherapy presented with a focal tractional retinal detachment and intermediate uveitis precluding adequate fundus examination in the left eye. On subsequent visits, the examination revealed persistent inflammation and therefore the patient was continued on CellCept 1,500 mg orally twice a day and adalimumab [Humira (AbbVie, North Chicago, Illinois)] 40 mg/0.4 mL every other week was initiated. His vision was 20/15 and 20/40 in the right

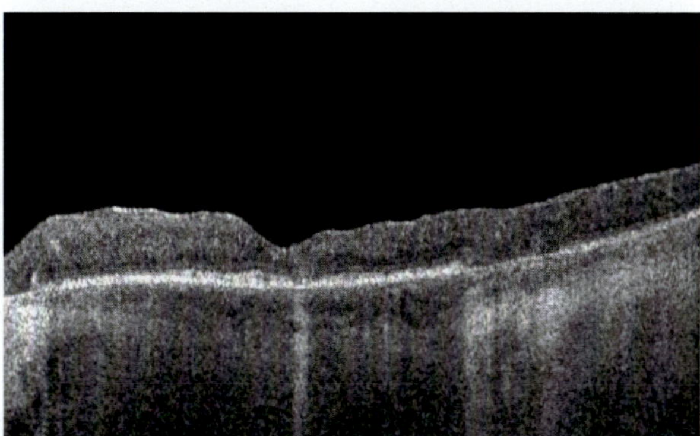

Fig. 2: Follow-up optical coherence tomography (OCT) demonstrates successful closure of a full-thickness macular hole. Partial reconstitution of the ellipsoid (IS/OS) zone is also evident.

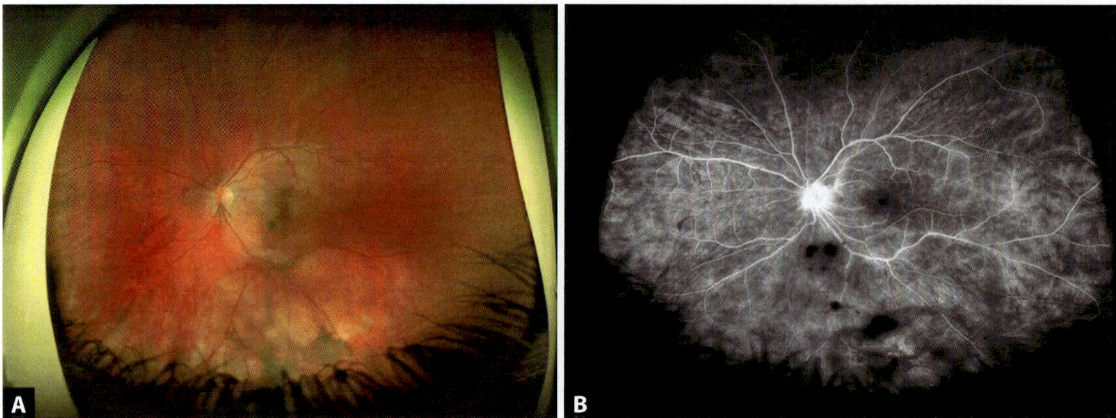

Figs. 3A and B: (A) Color fundus photograph depicts a localized area of tractional retinal elevation associated with peripheral snowbanking along the inferior ora serrata, noted on physical examination; (B) Late-phase fluorescein angiography of the left eye demonstrates widespread vascular leakage involving both arterial and venous arcades. Areas of capillary dropout are present.

and left eye, respectively. The focal tractional detachment threatened the macula and the patient was symptomatic, so surgical intervention was planned **(Figs. 3A and B)**.

Treatment Plan

Two weeks prior to the surgery the patient was started on predfort eyedrop four times a day in the left eye

↓

The patient underwent a primary encircling scleral buckle procedure using a type 41 band and cryotherapy

↓

With intraoperative adjuvant subtenon Kenalog injection

Thought Process

Decision	*Rationale*
Avoid pars plana vitrectomy when you can	In the second case, the young patient is phakic with a clear lens; scleral buckle preserves accommodation and reduces cataract risk
If starting/changing systemic immunomodulation (other than oral prednisone), allow 4–6 weeks before operating	Many systemic agents need 4–6 weeks to take effect—operating sooner can be premature

OUTCOME SUMMARY

Postoperative vision improved to 20/20 after 1 month of follow-up. The patient was continued on CellCept 1,500 mg orally twice a day and Humira 40 mg/0.4 mL every other week for 1 year postoperatively. Since then, the patient's uveitis has been controlled with adalimumab-adaz (Hyrimoz, Sandoz, Bracknell, United Kingdom) 40 mg/0.4 mL infusion every other week, 7 years after his initial surgery date **(Fig. 4)**.

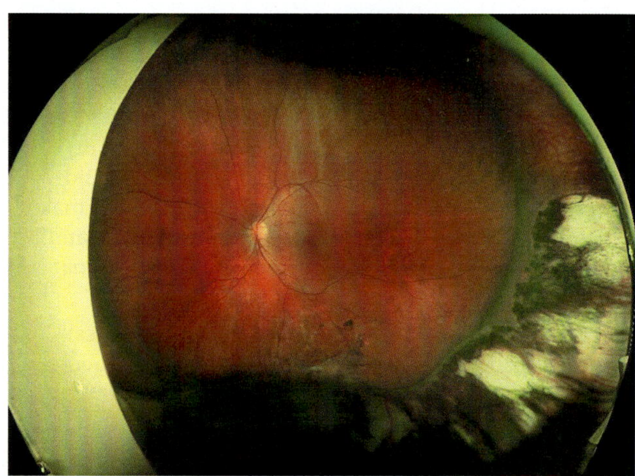

Fig. 4: Postoperative color fundus photograph of the left eye demonstrates resolution of prior vitreoretinal traction and successful retinal reattachment. An encircling scleral buckle is visible well-demarcated cryotherapy scars are present.

KEY POINTS

- Care for a patient with ongoing uveitis can be challenging, and when a surgical intervention is necessary the disease can be even more difficult to handle.
- Close follow-up and long term follow up is essential to monitor for inflammation recurrence after the surgery.

FURTHER READING

1. Faia LJ. Surgical Management of Uveitis Patients. Curr Surg Rep. 2015;3(12):38.

CHAPTER 15

Recent Advances in Retinal Surgeries

Saloni Kapoor, Jay Chhablani

ADVANCES IN RETINAL SURGERY: GENE THERAPY

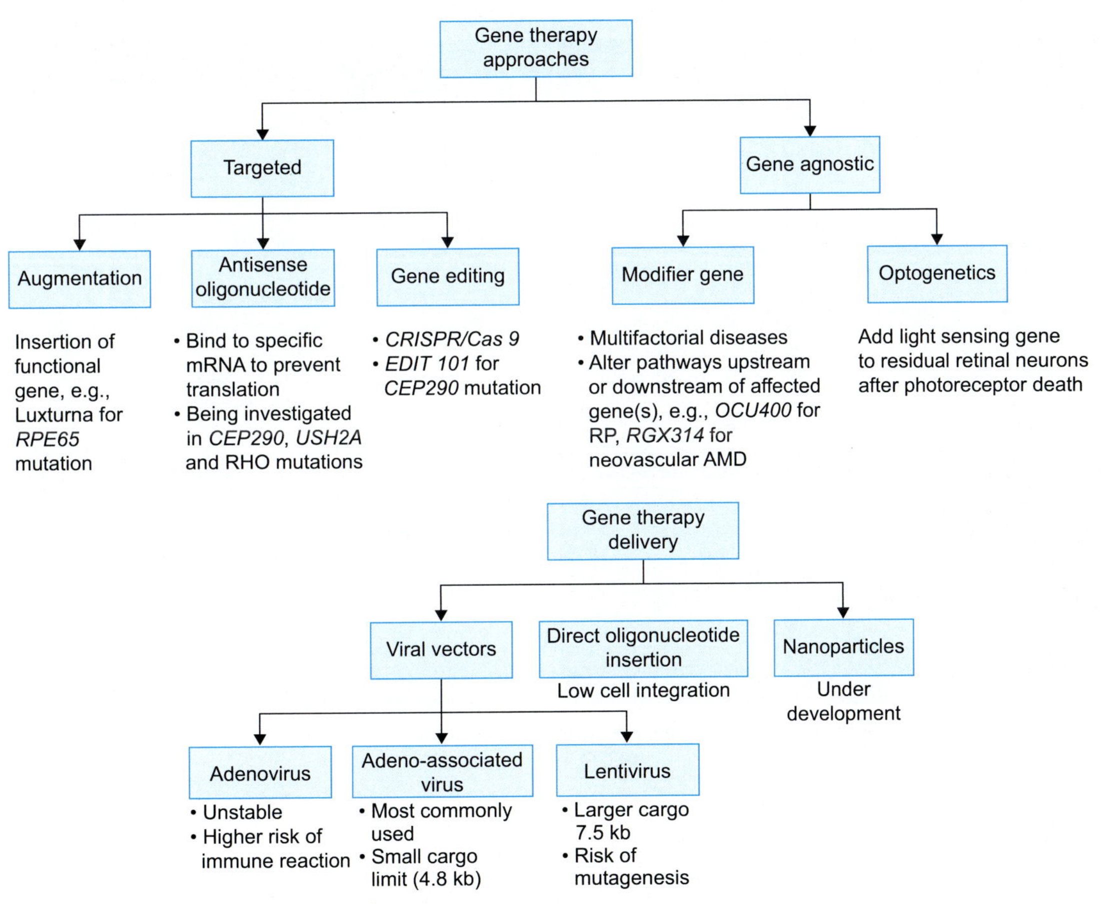

(AMD: age-related macular degeneration)

CASE SCENARIO 1: GENE THERAPY IN MANAGEMENT OF AMD

Case Summary

A 73-year-old female with a history of nonexudative age-related macular degeneration (AMD) in both eyes presented for a routine follow-up. Optical coherence tomography (OCT) demonstrated new subretinal fluid over previously seen pigment epithelial detachments. She received intravitreal anti-vascular endothelial growth factor (VEGF) therapy with improvement in subretinal fluid. Over the next 3 years, she needed 21 anti-VEGF injections. Her visual acuity declined from 20/25 to 20/40 during this period despite consistent treatment.

Given the anatomic volatility observed on OCT and the burden of ongoing anti-VEGF injections, the patient was selected for gene therapy **(Figs. 1 and 2)**.

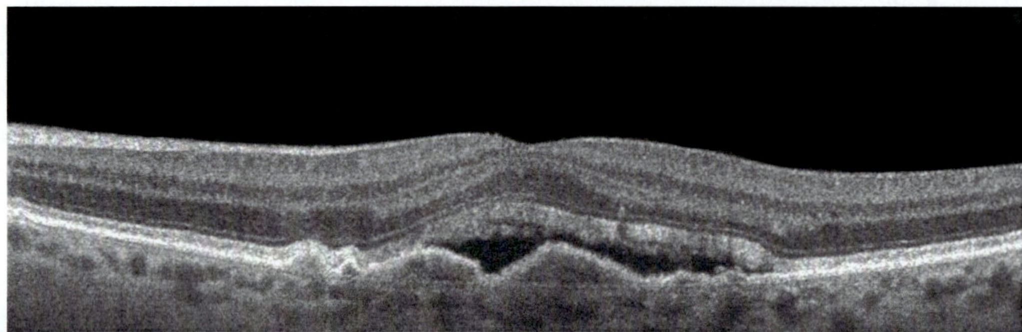

Fig. 1: Spectralis optical coherence tomography demonstrating subretinal fluid over pigment epithelial detachments.

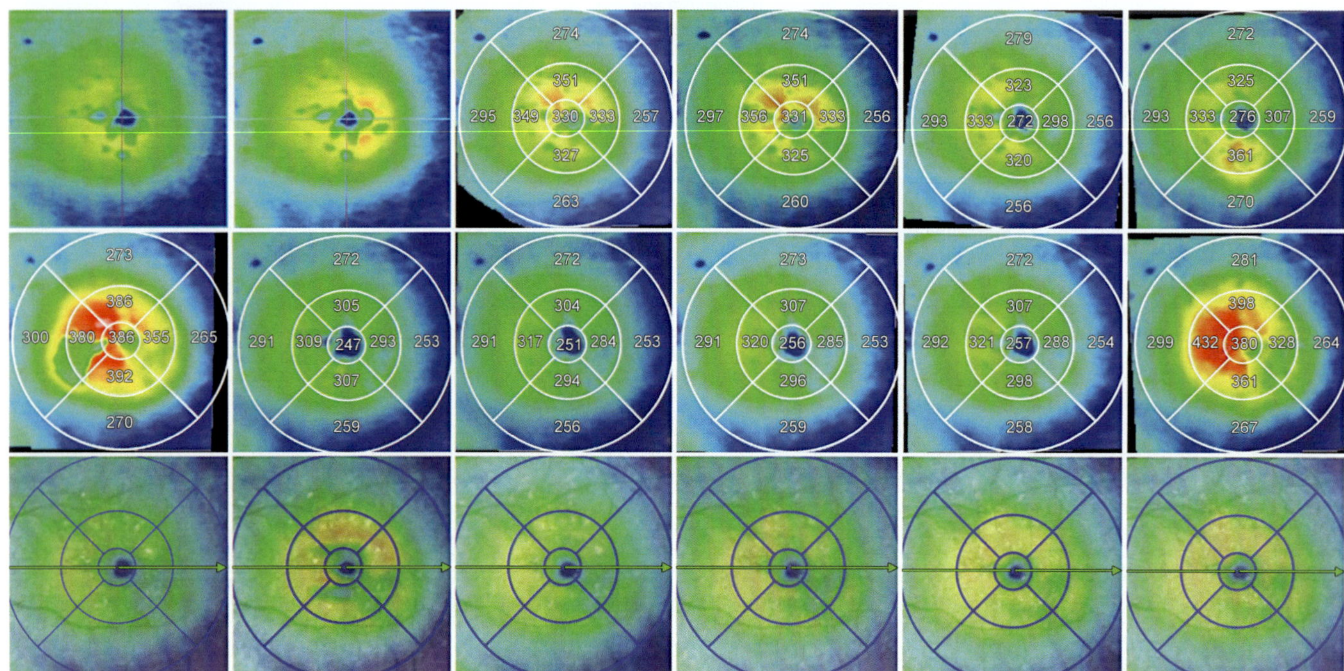

Fig. 2: Variation in subretinal fluid volume over 3 years despite consistent intravitreal anti-vascular endothelial growth factor (VEGF) injections.

Treatment Plan

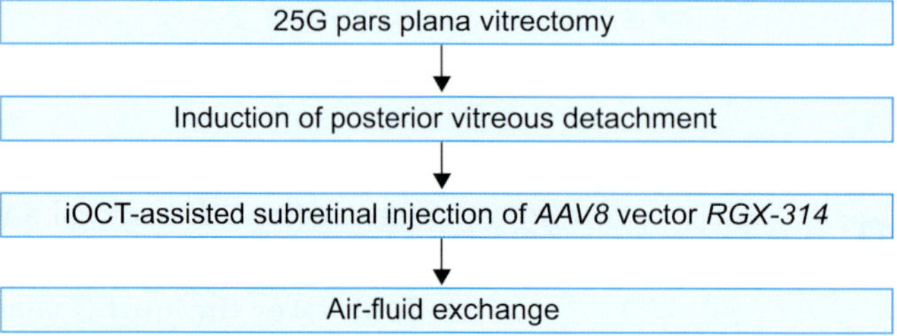

Thought Process

Decision	*Rationale*
Consider gene therapy	Good response to anti-VEGF, high treatment burden with multiple anti-VEGF injections per year
RGX-314	Favorable safety profile in phases 1 and 2 trials. Availability and patient willing to enroll in clinical trial
Subretinal versus suprachoroidal route	Subretinal route offers high transduction efficiency with localized expression
Close follow-up	Postsurgical inflammation can occur

(VEGF: vascular endothelial growth factor)

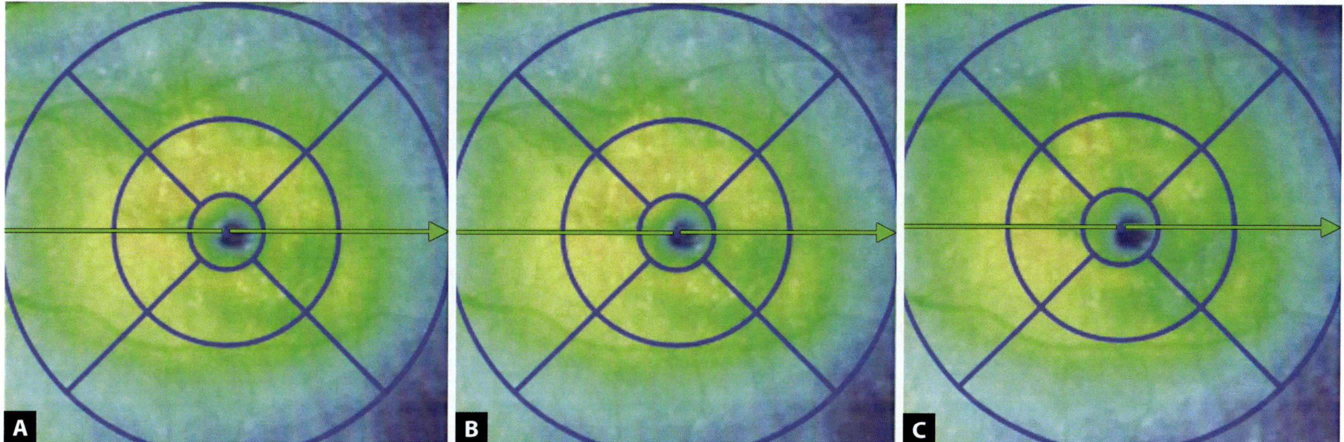

Figs. 3A to C: Variation in macular thickness minimized over 1 year after *RGX-314* subretinal gene therapy.

OUTCOME SUMMARY

Visual acuity stabilized between 20/25 and 20/30. Only one injection of anti-VEGF was required in the 2 weeks following surgery. No further anti-VEGF injection required in 16 months of follow-up **(Figs. 3A to C)**.

KEY POINTS

- Gene therapy in neovascular AMD offers the potential to reduce treatment burden and maintain anatomical stability.
- Ideal candidates include patients with demonstrated sustained response to anti-VEGF therapy and frequent anti-VEGF requirements.
- With the exception of voretigene neparvovec-rzyl (Luxturna), gene therapies are still undergoing clinical trials. While promising, safety and efficacy concerns remain.

FURTHER READING

1. Campochiaro PA, Avery R, Brown DM, Heier JS, HO AC, Huddleston SM, et al. Gene therapy for neovascular age-related macular degeneration by subretinal delivery of RGX-314: a phase 1/2a dose-escalation study. Lancet. 2024;403(10436):1563-73.
2. Drag S, Dotiwala F, Upadhyay AK. Gene Therapy for Retinal Degenerative Diseases: Progress, Challenges, and Future Directions. Invest Ophthalmol Vis Sci. 2023;64(7):39.
3. Sahel JA, Boulanger-Scemama E, Pagot C, Arleo A, Galluppi F, Martel JN, et al. Partial recovery of visual function in a blind patient after optogenetic therapy. Nat Med. 2021;27(7):1223-9.

ALGORITHMIC APPROACH TO IMPROVED VISUALIZATION FOR VITREORETINAL SURGERY

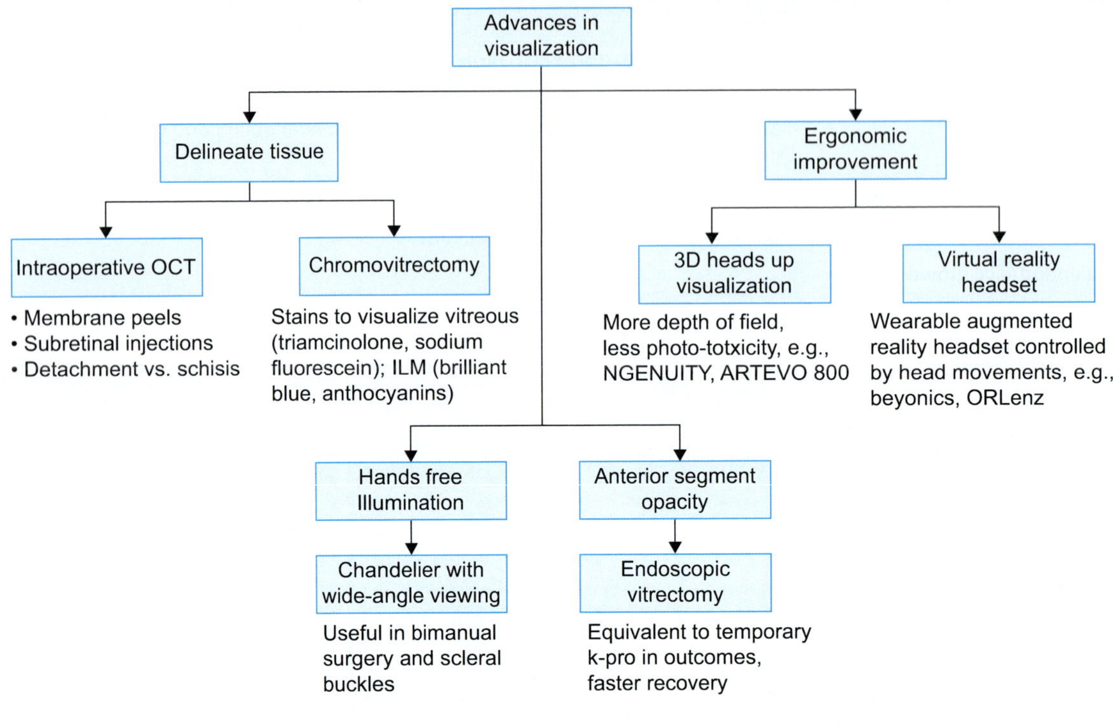

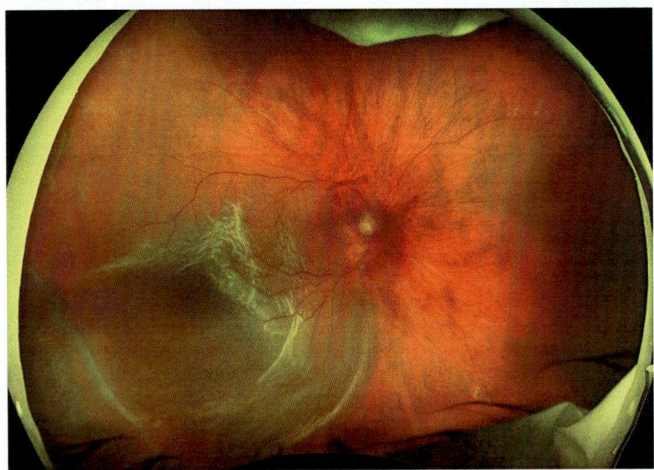

Fig. 4: Ultra-widefield fundus image demonstrating macula-off rhegmatogenous retinal detachment extending from 5:30 to 11 o'clock.

CASE SCENARIO 2: CHANDELIER ASSISTED SCLERAL BUCKLE IN MANAGEMENT OF RRD

Case Summary

A 52-year-old phakic male presented with sudden onset of floaters and flashes in his right eye for 3 days, followed by a progressive shadow in the superior visual field. Best-corrected visual acuity was HM. Fundus examination revealed a macula-off rhegmatogenous retinal detachment extending from 5:30 to 11 o'clock, with a horseshoe tear at 10 o'clock, an operculated hole at 8 o'clock, and lattice degeneration at 12 and 4 o'clock. The patient had no prior ocular surgeries or systemic illnesses **(Figs. 4 and 5)**.

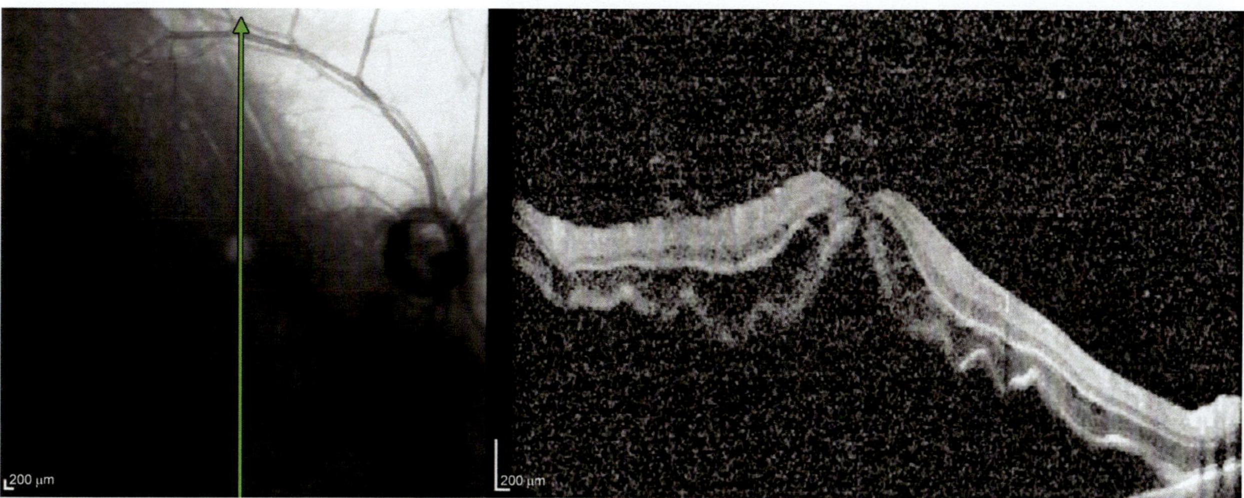

Fig. 5: Optical coherence tomography showing macula off with inner retinal corrugations.

Treatment Plan

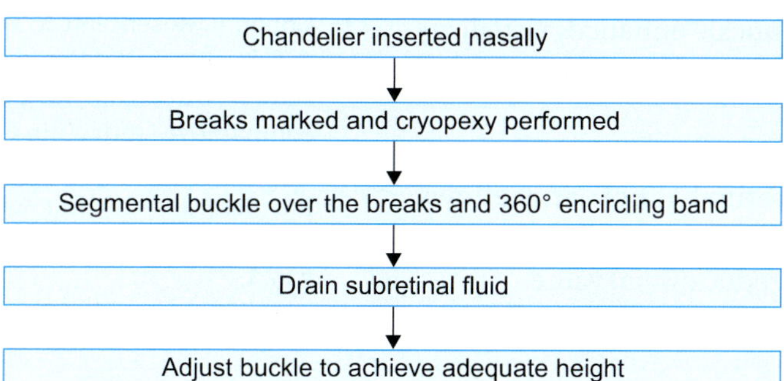

Thought Process

Decision	*Rationale*
Avoid pars plana vitrectomy	Patient is phakic with a clear lens; scleral buckle preserves accommodation and reduces cataract risk
Use chandelier-assisted scleral buckle	Provides wide-angle illumination using the microscope and eliminated need for multiple checks with indirect ophthalmoscopy
Position chandelier nasally	Prevents inadvertent contact with the detached retina or retinal breaks during manipulation
Apply cryopexy around all breaks and lattice areas	Strengthens chorioretinal adhesion and reduces recurrence risk
Place segmental buckle (10–8 o'clock) with 360° encircling band	Provides focal support for identified breaks and prophylactic support for lattice areas

OUTCOME SUMMARY

The chandelier-assisted scleral buckle procedure was performed successfully with clear intraoperative visualization. The retina reattached with appropriate buckle indentation supporting both the horseshoe tear and operculated hole. Subretinal fluid resolved within 1 week. At 1-month follow-up, the retina remained attached and visual acuity improved to 20/25. At 6 months, the retina was stable with no proliferative vitreoretinopathy or new breaks **(Fig. 6)**.

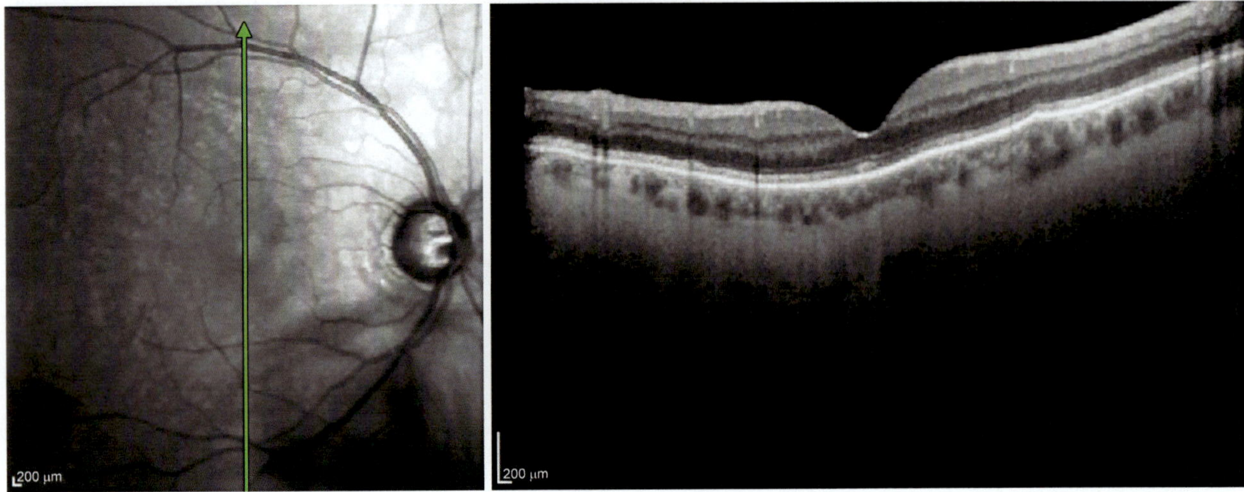

Fig. 6: Optical coherence tomography showing reattachment of the macula with reconstitution of the EZ band.

KEY POINTS

- Chandelier-assisted scleral buckle enhances visualization and eliminates the need for intraoperative indirect ophthalmoscopy.
- Chandelier placement away from the retinal detachment minimizes risk of retinal touch and allows comfortable manipulation.
- Can enhance efficiency and educational value.

FURTHER READING

1. Cohen E, Rosenblatt A, Bornstein S, Loewenstein A, Barak A, Schwartz S. Wide-angled endoillumination vs. traditional scleral buckling surgery for retinal detachment—a comparative study. Clin Ophthalmol. 2019;13:287-93.
2. Narayanan R, Tyagi M, Hussein A, Chhablani J, Apte RS. Scleral buckling with wide-angled endoillumination as a surgical educational tool. Retina. 2016;36(4):830-3.

CHAPTER 16

Decision Making in Surgical Management of Endophthalmitis

Manoj Shettigar, Taraprasad Das, Vivek Dave

ALGORITHMIC APPROACH TO ENDOPHTHALMITIS MANAGEMENT

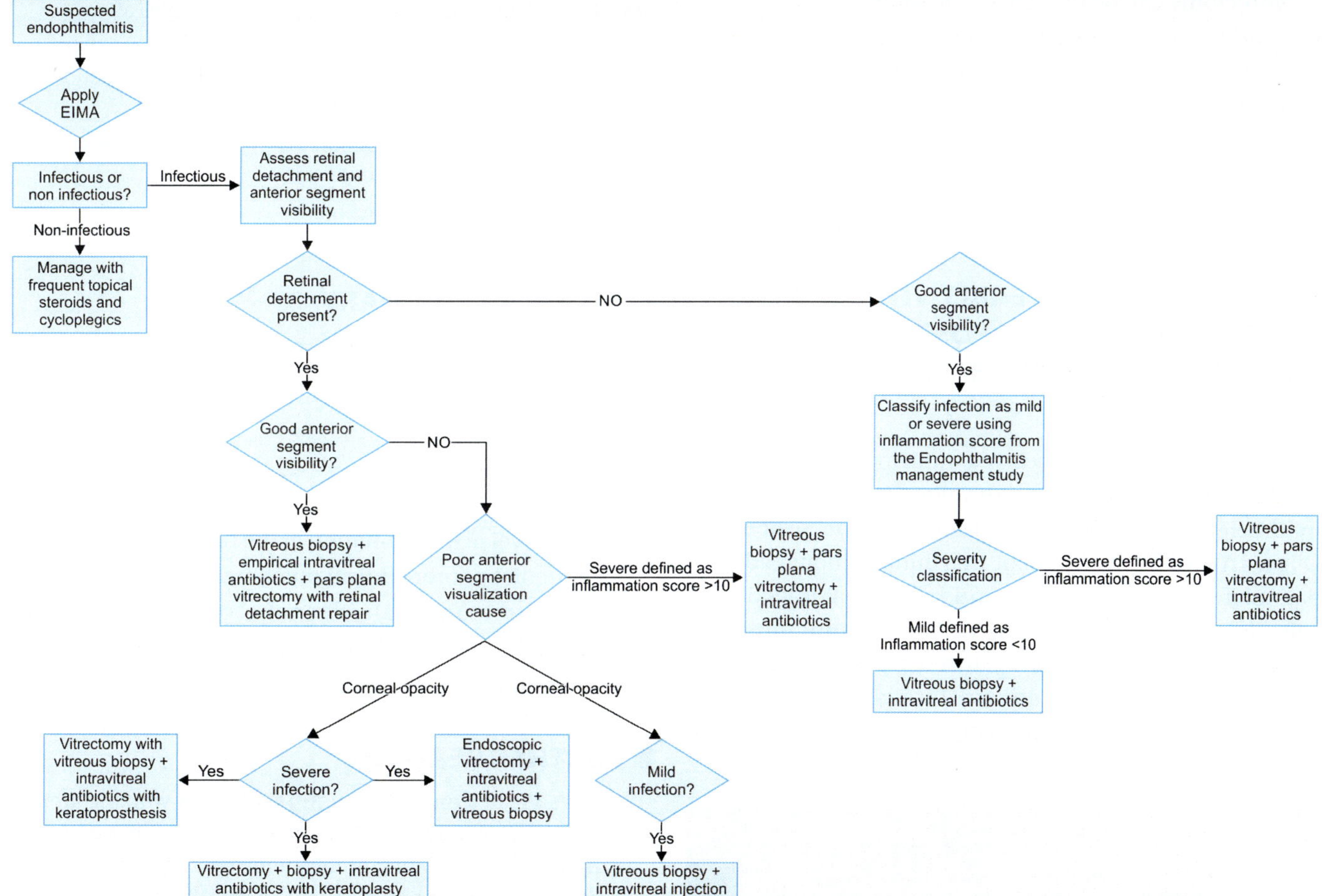

INTRODUCTION

Endophthalmitis is a rare but severely vision-threatening ocular condition. It is considered an ophthalmic emergency due to its potential for rapid progression and devastating impact on vision. While most cases are infectious, noninfectious (sterile) endophthalmitis can also occur due to retained lens material after surgery, toxic agents, or low-virulence organisms.

Management includes early recognition and appropriate surgical intervention, collection of a vitreous sample for diagnosis, and injection of intravitreal antibiotics.

Attached is a flowchart outlining a simple approach to the surgical management of endophthalmitis.

Common Riders Applicable to all Cases

- Preoperative B-scan is a surrogate marker of endophthalmitis, not diagnostic of it. Echoes on the B scan need to be taken in the context of baseline echoes in the other eye vitreous cavity, the associated increase in choroidal thickness, and other clinical signs and symptoms.

- If, in a phakic eye, a lens abscess is seen concurrently, it needs to be removed entirely during the vitrectomy.
- In cases with retinal breaks during vitrectomy, concurrent retinal detachment or a drug-resistant endophthalmitis, silicone oil endotamponade is preferred.
- After a couple of intravitreal injections with a sensitive drug, the vitreous cavity is mainly sterile, and the residual vitreous echoes can be observed with anti-inflammatory therapy, or over time, an optical vitrectomy can be offered for the same.
- While systemic therapy in terms of intravenous (IV) antibiotics and oral antibiotics is proposed and used in many protocols, intravitreal antibiotics are the mainstay, and the rest if at all are supplementary.
- Topical antibiotics, while proposed and used in most protocols, show no significant additional benefit unless there is a concurrent corneal infection.

CASE SCENARIO 1: EARLY VITRECTOMY IN MANAGEMENT OF POST ANTI VEGF INJECTION ENDOPHTHALMITIS

Case Summary

A 57-year-old male who received intravitreal bevacizumab for diabetic macular edema developed endophthalmitis in the left eye after 4 days following the procedure **(Figs. 1A and B)**. The patient was initially managed with pars plana vitrectomy (PPV) and intravitreal injection of ceftazidime and vancomycin. Vitreous culture indicated that endophthalmitis was caused by *Staphylococcus Warneri sensitive to vancomycin.* Intravitreal injection of 1 mg/0.1 mL vancomycin and 4 mg/0.1 mL dexamethasone was repeated.

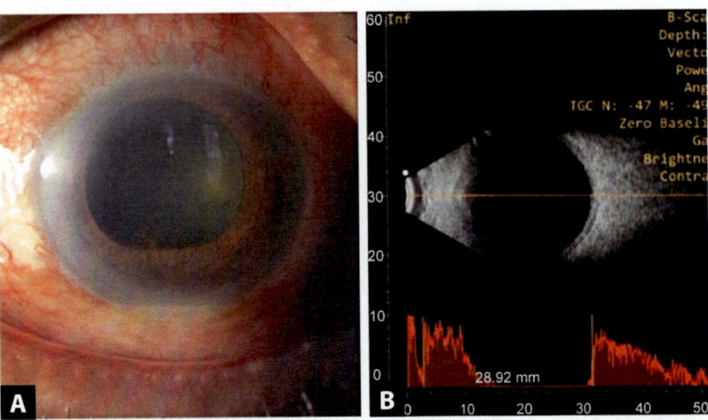

Figs. 1A and B: (A) Slit-lamp examination showed 4+ cells and hypopyon and (B) minimal dot echoes in the vitreous cavity were noted in the B scan.

Treatment Plan

Early vitrectomy

↓

Regular follow-up is necessary to identify recurrence or complications such as retinal detachment

Thought Process

Decision	*Rationale*
Povidine iodine eyedrops	Can lower endophthalmitis rates after intravitreal injections
Vitreous biopsy	Helps to differentiate sterile inflammation from infectious endophthalmitis
Early vitrectomy	PVD induction to remove all exudates from the vitreous cavity

(PVD: posterior vitreous detachment)

OUTCOME SUMMARY

The patient's visual acuity improved to 20/160, and ranibizumab therapy for diabetic macular edema was resumed.

KEY POINTS

- A high level of inflammation at the time of presentation can predict poorer clinical outcomes.
- Early vitrectomy can clear the ocular media and reduce the toxic load, thereby minimizing the risk of irreversible retinal damage.

FURTHER READING

1. Dave VP, Belenje A, Dogra A, Das T; EMS working group. Application and validation of a novel inflammatory score in the clinical grading of infectious endophthalmitis: The endophthalmitis management study - Report 2. Indian J Ophthalmol. 2023;71(2):396-400.
2. Das T, Sahoo J, Belenje A, Joseph J, Pandey S, Kapoor A, et al. Design and Validation of Endophthalmitis Infectivity Measurement Algorithm in Post Cataract Acute Endophthalmitis: EMS Report No. 6. Transl Vis Sci Technol. 2024;13(8):10.

VIDEO LEGEND

Video 40: Early vitrectomy in postintravitreal injection endophthalmitis

CASE SCENARIO 2: IOL EXPLANTATION IN POST CATARACT SURGERY ENDOPHTHALMITIS

Case Summary

A 64-year-old man developed endophthalmitis along with keratitis 1 month after cataract surgery **(Figs. 2A and B)**. The patient underwent AC wash with intraocular lens (IOL) explantation, pars plana vitrectomy (PPV), and intravitreal injection of ceftazidime and vancomycin. Vitreous culture indicated that the *Nocardia* species was *sensitive to vancomycin.* The smear showed no organisms, but the culture grew *Nocardia*. The infection resolved with tablet ciprofloxacin 750 mg BD, repeat intravitreal vancomycin and topical 5% fortified vancomycin eye drops.

Treatment Plan

Vitreous biopsy and culture is essential

↓

Empirical topical fortified therapy

Thought Process

Decision	Rationale
Intravitreal dexamethasone	Protects the retina from collateral damage.
Fortified topical antibiotics	Medications can undergo passive diffusion into the deep stroma and, at higher concentrations, reach the aqueous humor
IOL explantation	Prevents the formation of biofilm and prevents the recurrence of infection

(IOL: intraocular lens)

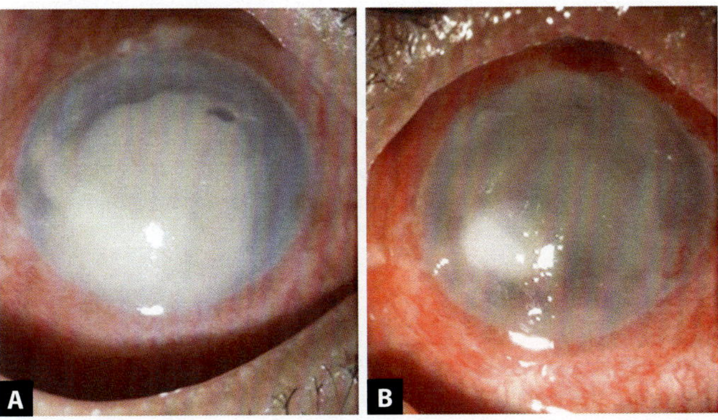

Figs. 2A and B: (A) Slit-lamp examination showed stromal infiltration along with exudation in AC; (B) The stromal infiltrate at the nasal margins began to consolidate and resolve, and the AC exudates gradually resolved over time with topical 5% fortified vancomycin eye drops.

OUTCOME SUMMARY

The infection resolved with tablet ciprofloxacin 750 mg BD, repeat intravitreal vancomycin and topical 5% fortified vancomycin eye drops.

KEY POINTS

- The presence of deep stromal infiltrates and hypopyon suggests a fulminant infection, for which fortified topical antibiotics are indicated.
- IOL explantation can be crucial in preventing the recurrence of infection.

FURTHER READING

1. Dave VP, Pathengay A, Nishant K, Reddy VS, Pappuru RR, Das T. Management of Endophthalmitis with and without Topical Antibiotics: A Case-Control Study. Ophthalmologica. 2021;244(3):208-12.
2. Jalali S, Das T, Gupta S. Presumed noninfectious endophthalmitis after cataract surgery. J Cataract Refract Surg. 1996;22(10):1492-7.
3. Panahi P, Mirzakouchaki-Borujeni N, Pourdakan O, Arévalo JF. Early Vitrectomy for Endophthalmitis: Are EVS Guidelines Still Valid? Ophthalmic Res. 2023;66(1):1318-26.

CASE SCENARIO 3: ENDOSCOPIC VITRECTOMY IN MANAGEMENT OF POST TRAUMATIC ENDOPHTHALMITIS WITH OPAQUE MEDIA

Case Summary

A 6-year-old male presented with a decrease in vision in the right eye following with a wire. A corneal tear was noted with posterior stromal infiltrates, diffuse cellularity at the site of the tear, and hypopyon **(Fig. 3)**. Provisional

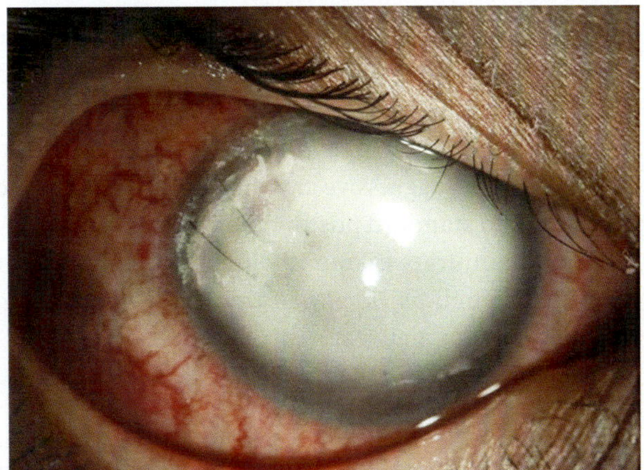

Fig. 3: Slit-lamp examination showing sutured corneal tear with posterior stromal infiltrates and diffuse cellularity at the site of corneal tear, with hypopyon.

diagnosis of right eye post-traumatic bacterial keratitis with endophthalmitis was made. Corneal scraping, corneal tear repair, and vitreous biopsy was performed with empirical intravitreal antibiotics of ceftazidime and vancomycin were injected under general anesthesia. Corneal scraping and vitreous biopsy revealed gram-positive cocci. Postoperatively, systemic cefazoline 50 mg/kg in three divided doses, topical 5% fortified vancomycin eye drops, and chloramphenicol 0.5% and cycloplegics. Culture showed the growth of *Clostridium tertium*.

Treatment Plan

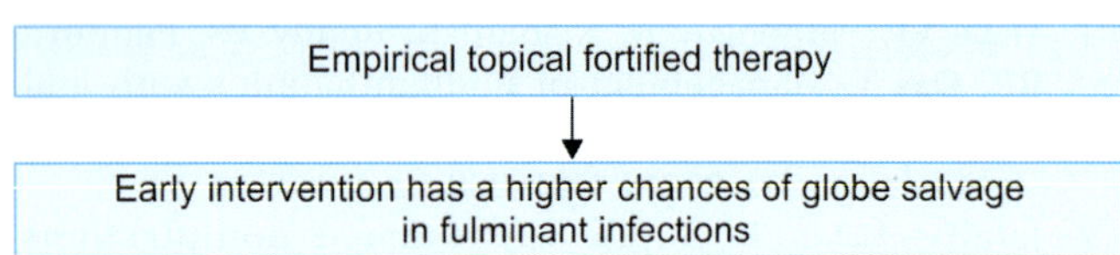

Thought Process

Decision	*Rationale*
Early wound closure	Decreases the chances of infection following globe injury
Fortified topical antibiotics	Deep stromal infiltrates and hypopyon suggest fulminant infection

OUTCOME SUMMARY

The child underwent pars plana lensectomy as there was lens abscess and vitrectomy and intravitreal antibiotics but ended up with phthisis.

KEY POINTS

- Pars plana lensectomy removes the infected lens, thereby eliminating a potential source of infection and associated toxins.
- The management of traumatic endophthalmitis requires a more aggressive and time-sensitive approach compared to standard postoperative cases.
- Traumatic injuries frequently involve highly virulent organisms such as *Bacillus cereus and may include* retained foreign material.

FURTHER READING

1. Dave VP, Pathengay A, Budhiraja I, Sharma S, Pappuru RR, Tyagi M, et al. Clinical presentation, microbiologic profile and factors predicting outcomes in bacillus endophthalmitis. Retina. 2018;38(5):1019-23.
2. Dave VP, Pappuru RR, Khader MA, Basu S, Tyagi M, Pathengay A. Endophthalmitis with opaque cornea managed with primary endoscopic vitrectomy and secondary keratoplasty: Presentations and outcomes. Indian J Ophthalmol. 2020;68(8):1587-92.

VIDEO LEGEND

Video 41: Endoscopic vitrectomy in management of endophthalmitis with opaque media.

CASE SCENARIO 4: MANAGEMENT OF CHRONIC ENDOPHTHALMITIS POSTCATARACT SURGERY

Case Summary

A 61-year-old female presented with complaints of diminution of vision in the left eye with redness and pain for 5 months, worsening over the past 20 days. There was history of cataract surgery several months prior. The patient initially had good vision following cataract surgery, but it worsened later. There were episodes of recurrent inflammation **(Figs. 4A and B)**. Presenting visual acuity in the left eye was hand motion. Provisional diagnosis of left eye chronic postsurgical endophthalmitis was made. Patient underwent LE AC wash, AC tap, vitreous biopsy, and PPV. Intraoperatively, posterior capsule membranotomy was done with a cutter, and preretinal exudates were noted in the vitreous cavity **(Fig. 4C)**. Intracameral moxifloxacin and empirical intravitreal vancomycin and ceftazidime were injected. Blood and urine culture results were negative. Smear and culture from the AC tap and vitreous biopsy did not reveal any organisms. PCR was negative for Eubacterial DNA, negative for *Priopionibacterium acnes*.

Treatment Plan

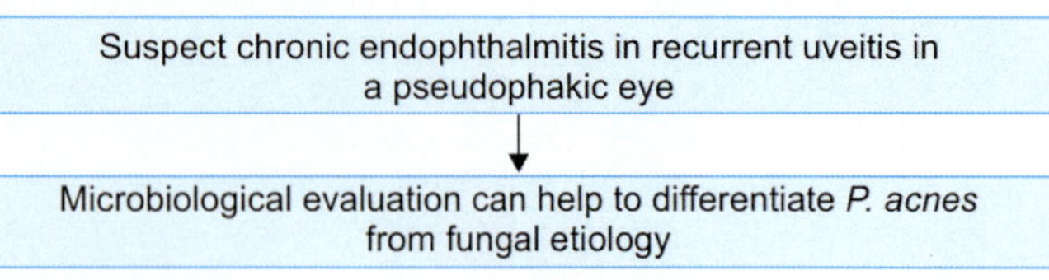

Thought Process

Decision	*Rationale*
Eradicate the persistent infection source	Biofilms on IOL and posterior capsule
Early IOL removal	The infection frequently resolves with antibiotic therapy; however, recurrence occurs when treatment is discontinued

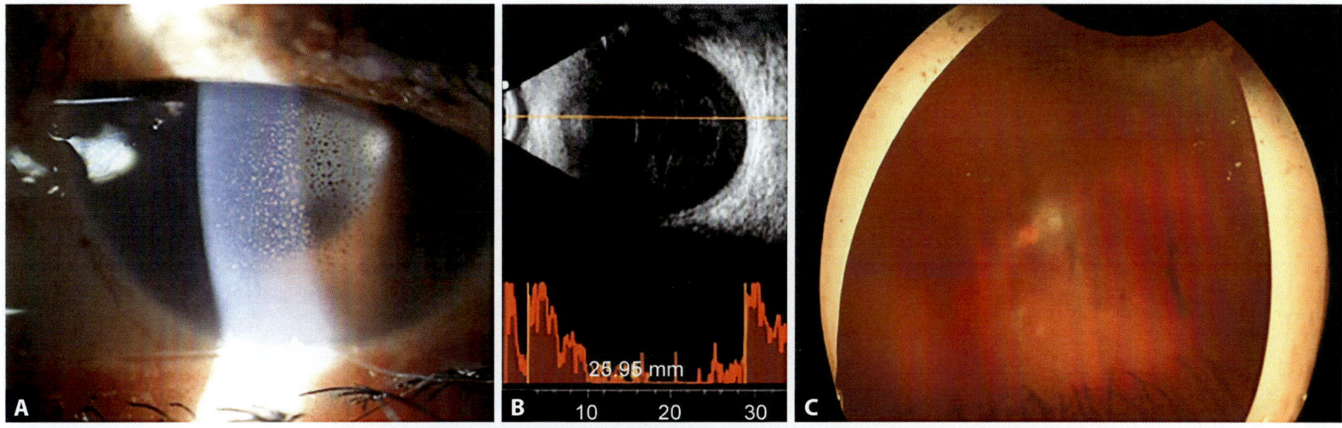

Figs. 4A to C: (A) Anterior segment examination showing large keratic precipitates, cells 3+, flare with intraocular pressure (IOP) 20 mm Hg. B-scan of the left eye showed low-to-moderate-intensity echoes in the mid- and posterior vitreous (B), and the retina was attached. (C) Ultra-widefield fundus photograph of left eye showing resolving vitritis and attached retina. Visual acuity in the left eye gradually improved over a period of 2 months and the retina was attached.

OUTCOME SUMMARY

Topical steroid medications and cycloplegics were continued till inflammation was resolved. At the 2-month follow-up, visual acuity in the left eye improved to 20/25; the eye was quiet, and the retina was attached.

KEY POINTS

- In cases of recurrent uveitis in a pseudophakic eye, chronic endophthalmitis remains a primary consideration in the differential diagnosis. Such cases often respond to initial steroid therapy, but symptoms typically recur once the corticosteroids are tapered.
- Total capsulectomy, along with IOL explantation, decreases the chances of recurrence by removing possible sequestered infectious material.

FURTHER READING

1. Dave VP, Pathengay A, Sharma S, Govindhari V, Karolia R, Pappuru RR, et al. Clinical presentations and comparative outcomes of primary versus deferred intraocular lens explantation in delayed-onset endophthalmitis. Indian J Ophthalmol. 2019;67(7):1101-4.

CASE SCENARIO 5: MANAGEMENT OF ENDOGENOUS ENDOPHTHALMITIS

Case Summary

A 35-year-old female presented with diminution of vision in the right eye with redness and pain for 3 days, and had a history of fever 1 week back. Fundus examination of right eye had hazy media due to vitritis, and a yellowish lesion 1.5 DD in size was seen on the macula with fuzzy borders **(Figs. 5A and B)**. A provisional diagnosis of right-eye endogenous endophthalmitis was made. *Candida* was suspected based on "rain cloud sign" morphology. Left eye fundus examination was within normal limits. The patient was initially managed with a right-eye PPV and intravitreal injections of ceftazidime and vancomycin, imipenem, and amphotericin B. Smear and culture results from the deep-vitreous biopsy did not reveal any organisms. Blood and urine cultures were negative. Intravitreal amphotericin was repeated after 5 days. Visual acuity improved after 2 months of oral tablet voriconazole 100 mg BD.

Treatment Plan

Rule out systemic source of infection such as: Infected IV line, endocarditis, and liver abscess

↓

Systemic antibiotics (antifungal) is essential along with intravitreal therapy

Thought Process

Decision	*Rationale*
Deep vitreous biopsy	Has higher diagnostic yield as load of infection is more concentrated in the posterior vitreous
Systemic antibiotics	Source of infection often travels via blood steam

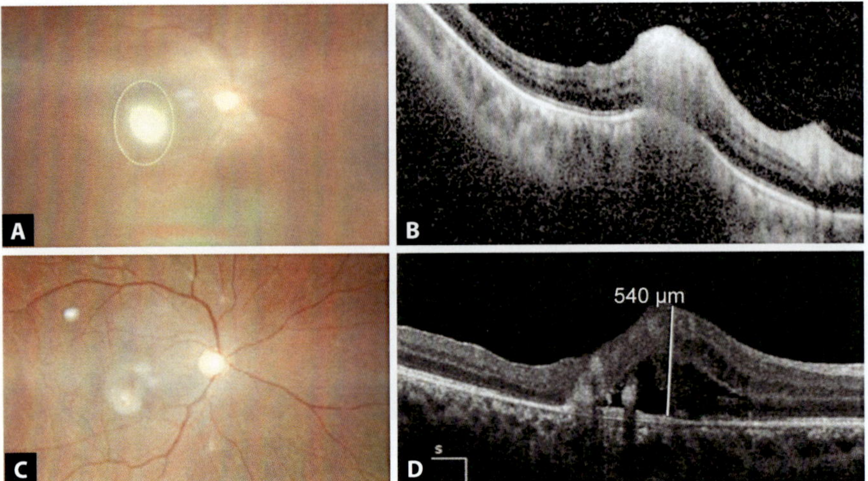

Figs. 5A to D: (A) On fundus examination, (A) the media was hazy due to vitritis, and a yellowish lesion 1.5 DD in size was seen on the macula with fuzzy borders. (B) OCT through the lesion showed hyperreflective dots in the posterior vitreous, hyperreflectivity involving all retinal layers in the lesion, with backshadowing and an elevated choroid underlying it, suggestive of retinochoroiditis. At 2 months of follow-up (C) vitritis gradually resolved with consolidation of lesion. (D) Follow-up OCT through the lesion showed reduced resolved dots in the posterior vitreous and reduced hyperreflectivity in the retinal layers in the lesion.

OUTCOME SUMMARY

At 2-months follow-up, the patient's best-corrected visual acuity improved to 20/125 **(Fig. 5C)**. The media was clearer. The lesion was noted to be regressing with scarring which is already evident **(Fig. 5D)**. OCT through the lesion showed reduced hyperreflectivity of the retinal layers with intraretinal cystic spaces and SRF with disorganization of outer retinal layers and loss of photoreceptor, some hyperreflectivity in the outer retinal layers suggestive of scarring, scans passing through the center of the lesion showed loss of all the retinal layers with scarring.

KEY POINTS

- In cases of suspected fungal endogenous endophthalmitis, characterized by vitreous opacities, immunocompromised status, or intravenous drug use, systemic azoles or amphotericin combined with intravitreal antifungals should be prioritized.
- Delayed treatment significantly increases the risk of bilateral blindness and mortality.

FURTHER READING

1. Dave VP, Pappuru RR, Tyagi M, Pathengay A, Das T. Endoscopic vitrectomy in endophthalmitis: initial experience of 33 cases at a tertiary eye care center. Clin Ophthalmol. 2019;13:243-51.

VIDEO LEGEND

Video 42: AC biopsy with PPV in chronic endophthalmitis.

Index

Page numbers followed by *f* refer to figure.

R

S

T